D0189174

EMQs and SBAs for Medical Finals

EMQs and SBAs for Medical Finals

Jonathan Bath MBBS BSc (Hons)
Fellow in Vascular Surgery
University of Pittsburgh Medical Center
Pittsburgh, USA

Rebecca Morgan MBBS BSc (Hons) DRCOG
GP ST3
Aberfeldy Practice
London, UK

Mehool Patel MBBS MD MRCP
Consultant Physician in Stroke and Elderly Medicine
University Hospital
Lewisham, UK

WILEY-BLACKWELL

A John Wiley & Sons, Ltd., Publication

This edition first published 2011 © 2011 by John Wiley & Sons, Ltd.
Previous edition © 2007 Jonathan Bath, Rebecca Morgan & Mehool Patel. Published by Blackwell Publishing.

Wiley-Blackwell is an imprint of John Wiley & Sons, formed by the merger of Wiley's global Scientific, Technical and Medical business with Blackwell Publishing.

Registered office: John Wiley & Sons, Ltd, The Atrium, Southern Gate, Chichester,
West Sussex, PO19 8SQ, UK

Editorial offices: 9600 Garsington Road, Oxford, OX4 2DQ, UK
The Atrium, Southern Gate, Chichester, West Sussex, PO19 8SQ, UK
111 River Street, Hoboken, NJ 07030-5774, USA

For details of our global editorial offices, for customer services and for information about how to apply for permission to reuse the copyright material in this book please see our website at www.wiley.com/wiley-blackwell.

The right of the author to be identified as the author of this work has been asserted in accordance with the UK Copyright, Designs and Patents Act 1988.

Library of Congress Cataloging-in-Publication Data
Bath, Jonathan.
EMQs and SBAs for medical finals / Jonathan Bath, Rebecca Morgan, Patel, Mehool.
p. ; cm.
Rev. ed. of: EMQs and MCQs for medical finals / Jonathan Bath, Rebecca Morgan, Mehool Patel. 2007.
Includes bibliographical references and index.
ISBN 978-0-4706-5444-6 (pbk. : alk. paper)
1. Medicine–Examinations, questions, etc.   I. Morgan, Rebecca.   II. Patel, Mehool.   III. Bath, Jonathan. EMQs and MCQs for medical finals.   IV. Title.
[DNLM: 1. Medicine–Great Britain–Examination Questions. W 18.2]
R834.5.B37 2011
610.76–dc22

2011007201

A catalogue record for this book is available from the British Library.

Set in 9.25/12pt Meridien by Aptara® Inc., New Delhi, India
Printed and bound in Malaysia by Vivar Printing Sdn Bhd

1   2011

Contents

Preface

The idea for the first edition of *EMQs and MCQs for Medical Finals* was to provide a solid question book that provided detailed explanations with the answers to enable the reader to learn not only why the answer was correct, but also why the other options were incorrect. At the time of publication in 2007, the number of question and answer books with this detailed answer format was limited, allowing *EMQs and MCQs for Medical Finals* to establish a niche, which has been quickly recognized by subsequent question and answer books to be the preferred format for examination preparation resources.

The second edition reflects feedback from many students, doctors and other readers and has led to many improvements. The title of the book has evolved to better describe the question format used in current examinations, question stems have been shortened to allow quick and precise reading of questions, and factual information has been updated where needed to reflect changes in clinical practice. Finally, the five practice examination papers have been indexed to allow for rapid review of specific areas, for example Cardiology or Vascular Surgery, as required.

We hope that these improvements will ensure that *EMQs and SBAs for Medical Finals* will continue to provide an excellent resource for identifying key examination topics and, more importantly, help to focus preparation on less familiar areas of knowledge for Finals.

Jonathan Bath
Pittsburgh

Rebecca Morgan
London

Abbreviations

AAA	abdominal aortic aneurysm
ABC	airway–breathing–circulation
ABG	arterial blood gas
ACE	angiotensin-converting enzyme
ACTH	adrenocorticotropic hormone
ADH	antidiuretic hormone
A&E	Accident and Emergency
AFP	alpha-fetoprotein
ALL	acute lymphocytic leukaemia
ALT	alanine transaminase
AML	acute myeloid leukaemia
AMT	abbreviated mental test
ANCA	antineutrophil cytoplasmic antibody
A/P	antero-posterior
APTT	activated partial thromboplastin time
ARMD	age-related macular degeneration
AST	aspartate transaminase
AV	atrioventricular
BCG	Bacille Calmette Guerin
BMI	body mass index
BPH	benign prostatic hyperplasia
bpm	beats per minute
CA 15-3	cancer antigen 15-3
CEA	carcino-embryonic antigen
CK	creatine kinase
CLL	chronic lymphocytic leukaemia
CML	chronic myeloid leukaemia
CMV	cytomegalovirus
CoA	coenzyme A
COPD	chronic obstructive pulmonary disease
CPP	cerebral perfusion pressure
CREST	calcinosis, Raynaud's phenomenon, oesophageal dysmotility, sclerodactyly and telangiectasia)
CSF	cerebrospinal fluid
CT	computed tomography
CT-PA	computed tomography with pulmonary angiography
DC	direct current

DCIS	ductal carcinoma *in situ*
ds-DNA	double-stranded DNA
ECG	electrocardiogram/electrocardiography
ECT	electroconvulsive therapy
EMDR	eye movement desensitization and reprocessing
ENT	ear, nose and throat
ERCP	endoscopic retrograde cholangiopancreatogram
ESR	erythrocyte sedimentation rate
ETT	exercise tolerance test
FAST	focused assessment with sonography for trauma
FENa	fractional excretion of sodium
GBM	glomerular basement membrane
GCS	Glasgow coma scale
γ-GGT	gamma glutamyl transpeptidase
GORD	gastro-oesophageal reflux disease
GP	general practitioner
G6PD	glucose-6-phosphatase
GTN	glyceryl trinitrate
hCG	human chorionic gonadotropin
5-HIAA	5-hydroxyindoleacetic acid
HIDA	hepatobiliary iminodiacetic acid
HIV	human immunodeficiency virus
HMG CoA	3-hydroxymethylglutaryl coenzyme A
HMMA	4-hydroxy methyl mandelate
HPV	human papilloma virus
HSV	herpes simplex virus
HTLV	human T-cell lymphotropic virus
ICP	intracerebral pressure
ICU	Intensive Care Unit
IgA	immunoglobulin A
IgE	immunoglobulin E
IgG	immunoglobulin G
IL	interleukin
IM	intramuscular
INR	international normalized ratio
IUCD	intrauterine contraceptive device
IV	intravenous
IVU	intravenous urogram
JVP	jugular venous pressure
LDH	lactate dehydrogenase
LFT	liver function test
LKM1	liver/kidney microsomal type I antibodies
LSD	lysergic acid diethylamide
MAOI	monoamine oxidase inhibitor
MAP	mean arterial pressure

MCV	mean corpuscular volume
MI	myocardial infarction
MMR	measles, mumps and rubella
MRI	magnetic resonance imaging
NMDA	N-methyl-D-aspartic acid
NSAID	non-steroid anti-inflammatory drug
NSE	neurone specific enolase
OGD	oesophagogastroduodenoscopy
$PaCO_2$	partial pressure of carbon dioxide in arterial blood
PaO_2	partial pressure of oxygen in arterial blood
PAS	Periodic acid Schiff
pCO_2	partial pressure of carbon dioxide in blood
PCP	phencyclidine
PDA	patent ductus arteriosus
PEFR	peak expiratory flow rate
PEG	percutaneous endoscopic gastrostomy
PFT	pulmonary function test
pO_2	partial pressure of oxygen in blood
PSA	prostate-specific antibody
PSC	primary sclerosing cholangitis
PTCA	percutaneous transluminal coronary angioplasty
PUVA	psoralen plus ultraviolet A
SA	sinoatrial
SIADH	syndrome of inappropriate ADH secretion
SLE	systemic lupus erythematosus
SSRI	selective serotonin reuptake inhibitor
TCA	tricyclic antidepressant
TFT	thyroid function test
THC	δ-1-tetrahydrocannabinol
TIBC	total iron binding capacity
TNF-α	tumour necrosis factor α
TPN	total parenteral nutrition
TRH	thyroid-releasing hormone
TSH	thyroid-stimulating hormone
TURP	transurethral resection of the prostate
vWF	von Willebrand factor
V/Q	ventilation–perfusion
VZV	varicella zoster virus

PART 1

Practice Papers

Questions

Single Best Answer Questions

1 Which area of the breast is most commonly affected by breast cancer?
   - ☐ **a.** Upper outer quadrant
   - ☐ **b.** Upper inner quadrant
   - ☐ **c.** Lower outer quadrant
   - ☐ **d.** Lower inner quadrant
   - ☐ **e.** Retro-areolar

2 A 75-year-old man is referred to cardiology for management of his newly diagnosed atrial fibrillation. His heart rate is 70–90 beats/minute (bpm) and he suffers from palpitations and occasional shortness of breath. He has no past history of cardiovascular disease. Which one of the following is the most appropriate next stage in his management?
   - ☐ **a.** Start digoxin for rate control
   - ☐ **b.** Warfarinization to reduce the risk of thromboembolism formation
   - ☐ **c.** Start a beta-blocker for associated hypertension
   - ☐ **d.** Organize an echocardiogram
   - ☐ **e.** Refer back to his general practitioner (GP) as his case can easily be managed in the community

3 Which one of the following is NOT a risk factor for breast cancer?
   - ☐ **a.** Nulliparity
   - ☐ **b.** Late pregnancy (>30 years)
   - ☐ **c.** Early menarche
   - ☐ **d.** Late menopause
   - ☐ **e.** High dietary dairy intake

EMQs and SBAs for Medical Finals, Second Edition. Jonathan Bath, Rebecca Morgan and Mehool Patel.
© 2011 John Wiley & Sons, Ltd. Published 2011 by John Wiley & Sons, Ltd.

4 A 38-year-old man attends Accident and Emergency (A&E) complaining of 12 hours of intermittent chest pain. His pain is central in location with no radiation but some associated nausea. He has a family history of cardiovascular disease. His troponin I is 0.05 (significant >0.1) and his electrocardiogram (ECG) shows no ischaemic changes. He asks you what will happen next. What should you tell him?

- ☐ **a.** He needs to be admitted for further bloods tests
- ☐ **b.** He requires an exercise tolerance test (ETT) before he is discharged
- ☐ **c.** An echocardiogram will be useful in his further management
- ☐ **d.** He can be safely discharged without further follow-up
- ☐ **e.** He should be started on aspirin

5 A 31-year-old man presents to his GP complaining of an itchy rash on his hands. On questioning, he reveals that he works as a dishwasher for a Chinese restaurant. On examination of his hands, there are multiple excoriated sites on the dorsum and over the fingers of both hands with cracking of the skin over an erythematous base. The most likely diagnosis is:

- ☐ **a.** Dermatitis
- ☐ **b.** Lichen planus
- ☐ **c.** Chemical burn
- ☐ **d.** Porphyria cutanea tarda
- ☐ **e.** Psoriasis

6 Optimal assessment of a breast lump in a 55-year-old woman is best described by which one of the following?

- ☐ **a.** Clinical examination, ultrasound, biopsy
- ☐ **b.** Clinical examination and mammogram
- ☐ **c.** Ultrasound, mammogram and biopsy
- ☐ **d.** Clinical examination, mammogram and biopsy
- ☐ **e.** Clinical examination, chest X-ray and biopsy

7 A 16-year-old boy with type I diabetes mellitus presents to hospital complaining of abdominal pain, nausea and vomiting. He has been feeling unwell for the last 3 days since he 'caught a cold' from his younger sister. Urine dipstick was taken that showed protein +, ketones ++, glucose +++. Which one of the following insulin regimens should this man be started on?

- [ ] **a.** Normal subcutaneous insulin with hourly blood glucose monitoring
- [ ] **b.** Sliding scale of insulin with hourly blood glucose monitoring
- [ ] **c.** Constant insulin infusion with hourly blood glucose monitoring
- [ ] **d.** Change of normal insulin regimen to once-daily long-acting insulin
- [ ] **e.** Increase of normal insulin regimen to double requirements

8 A 35-year-old man is admitted to the intensive care unit (ICU) with respiratory failure secondary to a fungal chest infection. His past medical history reveals acute myelogenous leukaemia, splenomegaly and a recent bone marrow transplant. His blood results reveal neutropenia and anaemia. Which one of the following should be avoided, unless absolutely necessary?

- [ ] **a.** Incision and drainage of a 4-cm subcutaneous abscess
- [ ] **b.** Digital rectal examination
- [ ] **c.** Regular suction of nasopharyngeal secretions
- [ ] **d.** Daily bloods taken via a central venous catheter
- [ ] **e.** Regular turning to avoid pressure sores

9 An 84-year-old woman re-presents to A&E 2 weeks after admission for control of an 'irregular heart beat' when she was started on digoxin. She now complains of dizziness and intermittent shortness of breath. Her drug history includes atenolol 100 mg od. Her ECG today shows a rate of approximately 40 bpm with no association between P waves and QRS complexes. What is the next step in her management?

- [ ] **a.** Insert a temporary pacing wire
- [ ] **b.** Give regular atropine
- [ ] **c.** Start amiodarone 200 mg tds
- [ ] **d.** Stop digoxin
- [ ] **e.** Take bloods, including drug levels

10 A 78-year-old woman is found by the warden in her apartment, sitting on the floor and very confused. Past medical history is remarkable for pernicious anaemia, type II diabetes mellitus and vitiligo. On examination, she is disorientated and scores 3/10 on the abbreviated mental test (AMT). She is bradycardic at 50 bpm, her blood pressure is 152/92 mmHg and she is hypothermic at 34.9°C. Her blood glucose was 4.1 mmol/L. Which one of the following investigations is most likely to reveal the diagnosis?
- ☐ **a.** Thyroid function tests
- ☐ **b.** ECG
- ☐ **c.** Computed tomography (CT) scan of the head
- ☐ **d.** Echocardiography
- ☐ **e.** Short synacthen test

11 A 38-year-old man presents to the dermatology clinic with intensely itchy elbows and knees. Systemic enquiry reveals past episodes of malabsorption relieved by a wheat-free diet. He is not allergic to any medication and maintains a gluten-free diet. The most likely cause of his itch is:
- ☐ **a.** Atypical eczema
- ☐ **b.** Psoriasis
- ☐ **c.** Dermatitis herpetiformis
- ☐ **d.** Scabies
- ☐ **e.** Polycythaemia rubra vera

12 A 69-year-old man is admitted 3 days after suffering a myocardial infarction (MI). He complains of increasing shortness of breath and on observation is tachypnoeic at rest while sitting up. He is also tachycardic, and his jugular venous pressure (JVP) is raised. Auscultation reveals a systolic murmur. An erect chest X-ray is normal. Which one of the following complications of MI is most likely to be the cause of this man's shortness of breath?
- ☐ **a.** Ventricular septal defect
- ☐ **b.** Recurrent infarction
- ☐ **c.** Aortic regurgitation
- ☐ **d.** Heart failure
- ☐ **e.** Dressler's syndrome

13 A 31-year-old breastfeeding woman is referred complaining of breast pain. On examination, there is evidence of a collection in one of the breasts with overlying erythema and associated pain. An ultrasound scan confirms an abscess. What is the most appropriate management?
- ☐ **a.** Oral flucloxacillin
- ☐ **b.** Incision and drainage of abscess
- ☐ **c.** Needle aspiration
- ☐ **d.** Analgesia and cold compress
- ☐ **e.** Admit for intravenous (IV) antibiotics

14 A 69-year-old man with type II diabetes mellitus is brought to hospital with confusion, drowsiness and aggressive behaviour. He lives with his daughter who noticed that he had become 'not himself' and had checked his blood sugar and found it to be 2.3 mmol/L. Which one of the following is NOT associated with hypoglycaemic states?
- ☐ **a.** Liver failure
- ☐ **b.** Gliclazide
- ☐ **c.** Insulinoma
- ☐ **d.** Addison's disease
- ☐ **e.** Cushing's disease

15 A 45-year-old female librarian was admitted with shortness of breath. Her past medical history consists of inflammatory bowel disease but no cardiac problems. On examination, her apex is laterally displaced and on auscultation a fourth heart sound is audible. A two-dimensional echocardiogram shows a dilated heart with an ejection fraction of 20–25%. The most likely cause of her dilated cardiomyopathy is:
- ☐ **a.** Viral
- ☐ **b.** Alcohol
- ☐ **c.** Outflow obstruction
- ☐ **d.** Congenital
- ☐ **e.** Autoimmune

16 A 42-year-old man presents to his GP with a 2-month history of a painless lump in his neck. He has noticed this lump is slowly growing bigger and as he had been feeling tired with sweats at night he had thought it was a lymph node from a 'head cold'. Recently, he has noticed that he can no longer enjoy wine or beer because they cause him pain. Which one of the following diagnoses is the most likely?

- ☐ **a.** Hodgkin's lymphoma
- ☐ **b.** Infectious mononucleosis
- ☐ **c.** Non-Hodgkin's lymphoma
- ☐ **d.** Polycythaemia rubra vera
- ☐ **e.** Myelodysplastic syndrome

17 The most appropriate diagnostic investigation in a patient presenting with chest pain and a widened mediastinum is:

- ☐ **a.** Four limb blood pressure measurements
- ☐ **b.** Liver function tests (LFTs)
- ☐ **c.** Lateral chest X-ray
- ☐ **d.** CT scan of chest
- ☐ **e.** ECG

18 A young child is brought to her GP by her mother, who has noticed she has developed a rash over her face and neck. On examination, there are multiple small pearly papules with a central umbilicated area of keratin plug distributed randomly over her face and neck. Which one of the following is most likely to be the cause of this rash?

- ☐ **a.** Varicella zoster virus (VZV)
- ☐ **b.** Herpes simplex virus (HSV)
- ☐ **c.** Molluscum contagiosum
- ☐ **d.** Eczema
- ☐ **e.** Pityriasis versicolor

19 Mid ward round, a nurse asks you to review a patient. The patient recently suffered an MI. On assessment, you note that the airway is patent but the patient is acutely short of breath. The first step in your management is:

- ☐ **a.** Contact your senior colleagues for assistance
- ☐ **b.** Perform an arterial blood gas (ABG) analysis
- ☐ **c.** Attach a cardiac monitor
- ☐ **d.** Request a chest X-ray
- ☐ **e.** Complete a primary survey

20 A 23-year-old woman is referred to the breast clinic as she noticed a solitary lump in the upper outer aspect of her left breast. She notes that the lump is not painful and there are no overlying changes to the skin. Which one of the following is the most likely diagnosis?

- ☐ **a.** Fibroadenoma
- ☐ **b.** Ductal carcinoma *in situ* (DCIS)
- ☐ **c.** Invasive ductal carcinoma
- ☐ **d.** Breast cyst
- ☐ **e.** Breast abscess

21 A 45-year-old woman presents to A&E with abdominal pain. She is tested for pregnancy and urinary tract infection and undergoes abdominal examination. She is found to have an enlarged spleen with pain localized to the left upper quadrant. Blood tests reveal a haemoglobin level of 9.8 g/dL with a mean corpuscular volume (MCV) of 92 fL. Her white blood cell count was 26×10^9 and platelet count was 135×10^9. Which one of the following chromosomal translocations is most likely to be found in sufferers of this condition?

- ☐ **a.** t(8;14)
- ☐ **b.** t(9;22)
- ☐ **c.** t(14;21)
- ☐ **d.** t(11;22)
- ☐ **e.** t(4;14)

22 Which one of the following is NOT a clinical finding associated with infective endocarditis?

- ☐ **a.** Osler's nodes
- ☐ **b.** Retinal haemorrhages
- ☐ **c.** Splinter haemorrhages
- ☐ **d.** Clubbing
- ☐ **e.** Erythema nodosum

23 A 58-year-old woman presents to the thyroid clinic to have a check-up for long-term hypothyroidism for which she is taking thyroxine 100 mg od. Her blood results are available in the clinic and demonstrate a high thyroid-stimulating hormone (TSH) and a high thyroxine T4. Which one of the following is most likely to explain these results?

- ☐ **a.** Subclinical hypothyroidism
- ☐ **b.** Sick euthyroid syndrome
- ☐ **c.** Non-compliance and overdosing prior to clinic
- ☐ **d.** Inadequate replacement with thyroxine
- ☐ **e.** Over-replacement with thyroxine

24 An 84-year-old man is urgently referred for increasing swelling of his legs and shortness of breath. On examination, he has oedema up to his groin and has bi-basal inspiratory crepitations up to the mid-zones. He currently takes digoxin and furosemide once daily. You are asked to admit the patient, what changes will you make to his medications?

- ☐ **a.** Add in bumetanide
- ☐ **b.** Change furosemide to IV and double the daily dose
- ☐ **c.** Add an angiotensin-converting enzyme (ACE) inhibitor
- ☐ **d.** Start a beta-blocker
- ☐ **e.** Add in a thiazide diuretic

25 A 35-year-old woman attends A&E with chest pain. Blood tests show a positive troponin and an ECG shows antero-lateral ischaemic changes. Which of the following illegal drugs is associated with this presentation?

- ☐ **a.** Amphetamines
- ☐ **b.** Cocaine
- ☐ **c.** Cannabis
- ☐ **d.** Heroin
- ☐ **e.** Rohypnol

26 A 34-year-old man is referred by the surgical team and seen by a dermatologist for an itchy rash in his elbow creases, which he has been scratching for the past week. On inspection of the rash, he is diagnosed with eczema. Which one of the following patterns is NOT part of the eczema classification?

- ☐ **a.** Atopic eczema
- ☐ **b.** Asteatotic eczema
- ☐ **c.** Discoid eczema
- ☐ **d.** Arthropathic eczema
- ☐ **e.** Varicose eczema

27 Your consultant suggests that you perform a cardiovascular examination on a patient. She is a tall, slim woman wearing glasses who appears otherwise well. What would you expect to find on auscultation?

- ☐ **a.** Systolic murmur at the right upper sternal edge
- ☐ **b.** Diastolic murmur at the right upper sternal edge
- ☐ **c.** Systolic murmur at lower left sternal edge
- ☐ **d.** Systolic murmur at the apex
- ☐ **e.** Diastolic murmur at the apex

28 In patients newly diagnosed with atrial fibrillation on digoxin therapy, which one of the following electrolytes is most important to monitor?
- ☐ **a.** Serum sodium
- ☐ **b.** Serum potassium
- ☐ **c.** Serum calcium
- ☐ **d.** Serum magnesium
- ☐ **e.** None of the above

29 A 54-year-old man presents with pain in his left knee and a red rash on his forearm, elbow and old appendix scar with a white scale that can be rubbed off to leave little spots of bleeding. The nails of his right hand have little roughened depressions. Which one of the following is NOT used in the treatment of this skin disorder?
- ☐ **a.** Topical steroids
- ☐ **b.** Tar
- ☐ **c.** Aqueous cream
- ☐ **d.** Psoralen plus ultraviolet A (PUVA)
- ☐ **e.** Dapsone

30 A 75-year-old man is admitted to hospital following intermittent chest pain for the past 24 hours. His chest pain is central with no radiation but is relieved by glyceryl trinitrate (GTN) spray in 3 minutes. His troponin level is mildly elevated and his ECG shows fixed inverted T waves laterally. He has a past history of peripheral vascular disease. The next stage of his management should include:
- ☐ **a.** An ETT
- ☐ **b.** A thallium cardiac scan
- ☐ **c.** Serial ECGs
- ☐ **d.** CT scan of chest
- ☐ **e.** Coronary angiogram

31 Which one of the following medications is most likely to cause deterioration in thyroid function?
- ☐ **a.** Atenolol
- ☐ **b.** Atorvastatin
- ☐ **c.** Amlodipine
- ☐ **d.** Amiodarone
- ☐ **e.** Acarbose

32 A 69-year-old man presents with gynaecomastia. He has a history of alcohol abuse and drinks approximately 70 units of alcohol per week. Which one of the following is the most likely cause for his gynaecomastia?
- ☐ **a.** Physiological
- ☐ **b.** Liver failure
- ☐ **c.** Kleinfelter's syndrome
- ☐ **d.** Hyperthyroidism
- ☐ **e.** Drugs, including spironolactone

33 A 78-year-old woman is referred for increasingly frequent attacks of angina. She is currently using GTN spray prn, verapamil and enalapril. Her symptoms are becoming more severe and even occurring at rest. Which changes in her medications will improve her symptoms?
- ☐ **a.** Change verapamil to diltiazem and start isosorbide mononitrate
- ☐ **b.** Give regular nitrates
- ☐ **c.** Change ACE inhibitor
- ☐ **d.** Add in beta-blocker
- ☐ **e.** Start digoxin

34 Regarding hyperthyroidism, which one of the following statements is correct?
- ☐ **a.** Thyroxine T3 is more abundantly produced than T4
- ☐ **b.** Eyelid retraction can be used as a rough proxy to monitor therapy
- ☐ **c.** Beta-blockade is always required long term for tachycardia
- ☐ **d.** T4 is more potent than T3
- ☐ **e.** High T4, T3 and TSH levels are seen in thyrotoxicosis

35 An 81-year-old man is admitted to hospital with chest pain and a diagnosis of a non-ST elevation MI is made. Which one of the following is the most appropriate immediate medical management?
- ☐ **a.** Aspirin, warfarin and beta-blocker
- ☐ **b.** Aspirin, clopidogrel, clexane and GTN spray
- ☐ **c.** Clopidogrel, GTN spray, warfarin
- ☐ **d.** Clopidogrel, clexane and warfarin
- ☐ **e.** Clexane, warfarin, beta-blocker and statin

36 A 6-year-old girl is brought to her GP who notices that she is scratching incessantly and has become extremely irritable since starting at a new school. On examination, there are tiny papules with linear tracts surrounded by erythema over the web spaces and fingers of both hands that are intensely itchy. Which one of the following treatments should be instituted?

☐ **a.** Malathion 0.5% cream
☐ **b.** Flucloxacillin 500 mg
☐ **c.** Conservative management
☐ **d.** Topical aqueous cream
☐ **e.** Cold tar

37 A 58-year-old man presents with new-onset chest pain and shortness of breath. ECG shows atrial fibrillation with a rate of 130 bpm. He has no past cardiac history. The most appropriate management is:

☐ **a.** Oxygen, IV digoxin
☐ **b.** Oxygen, beta-blockers
☐ **c.** Oxygen, heparin, warfarin
☐ **d.** Oxygen, heparin, IV amiodarone
☐ **e.** Oxygen, heparin and synchronized direct current (DC) shock

38 A 70-year-old man presents with chest pain. His ECG shows an acute MI with a new left bundle branch block. On admission, he is given 100% oxygen, morphine, metoclopramide, GTN spray and aspirin. On further questioning, you elicit that he suffered a haemorrhagic stroke 1 year ago. The next most appropriate step in management is:

☐ **a.** Coronary artery bypass surgery
☐ **b.** Thrombolytic therapy with streptokinase
☐ **c.** Percutaneous transluminal coronary angioplasty (PTCA)
☐ **d.** Heparin infusion
☐ **e.** Glycoprotein IIb/IIIa inhibitor IV

39 A 45-year-old man presents to hospital complaining of progressive inability to see pedestrians on the sides of the road when he is driving. His wife comments that he has gone up shoe and hat sizes. Which one of the following is the most common pathology associated with this disease?

☐ **a.** Craniopharyngioma
☐ **b.** Hypothalamic glioma
☐ **c.** Pituitary adenoma
☐ **d.** Parasella meningioma
☐ **e.** Metastatic lymphoma

40 Regarding descriptive terms used in dermatology, which one of the following associations is correct?
- ☐ **a.** Macule – a small raised circumscribed area of skin <0.5 cm across
- ☐ **b.** Vesicle – a small collection of fluid within the skin <0.5 cm across
- ☐ **c.** Bulla – a small flat area of circumscribed skin change
- ☐ **d.** Nodule – a small visible and/or palpable lump <0.5 cm across
- ☐ **e.** Weal – a localized collection of pus within the epidermis

41 Which one of the following is NOT a contraindication to thrombolysis following a diagnosis of acute MI?
- ☐ **a.** Previous allergic reaction
- ☐ **b.** Acute pancreatitis
- ☐ **c.** Suspected aortic dissection
- ☐ **d.** Heavy vaginal bleeding
- ☐ **e.** Hypotension

42 Which one of the following facts about DCIS is INCORRECT?
- ☐ **a.** It is a malignant condition
- ☐ **b.** Of breast cancers, it is the most common
- ☐ **c.** It is not capable of metastasizing
- ☐ **d.** It may present with an isolated breast lump
- ☐ **e.** It does not produce nipple discharge

43 Empirical antibiotic therapy for infective endocarditis is:
- ☐ **a.** Flucloxacillin and benzylpenicillin
- ☐ **b.** Benzylpenicillin and gentamycin
- ☐ **c.** Gentamycin and flucloxacillin
- ☐ **d.** Amoxicillin and metronidazole
- ☐ **e.** Cefuroxime and flucloxacillin

44 Which one of the following physical signs is NOT associated with cardiovascular disease?
- ☐ **a.** De Musset's sign
- ☐ **b.** Quincke's sign
- ☐ **c.** Kussmaul's sign
- ☐ **d.** Corrigan's sign
- ☐ **e.** Cullen's sign

45 An 84-year-old woman is brought to hospital after being found collapsed at home. She requires large amounts of fluids to keep her systolic blood pressure above 90 mmHg. She has no fever and her peripheries are cold and clammy. Her medication list includes steroids, amlodipine and aspirin daily, which a neighbour states she has not been taking for some days due to 'stomach flu'. Which one of the following is the most likely explanation for her persistent hypotension?

- ☐ **a.** Intravascular depletion due to vomiting and diarrhoea
- ☐ **b.** Septic shock due to gastrointestinal infection
- ☐ **c.** Haemorrhagic stroke due to hypertension
- ☐ **d.** Vasovagal syncope due to repeated forceful vomiting
- ☐ **e.** Medication-induced adrenocorticoid axis depression

46 A 40-year old man presents to his GP practice with a 3-day history of central chest pain relieved by sitting forward but exacerbated by inspiration or lying flat. He has recently recovered from a viral upper respiratory tract infection and his ECG shows widespread concave upwards ST segment elevation. Examination reveals no positive clinical findings. What is the most appropriate management of this patient?

- ☐ **a.** Non-steroid anti-inflammatory drugs (NSAIDs) and rest
- ☐ **b.** Troponin and creatine kinase (CK) levels
- ☐ **c.** Echocardiogram
- ☐ **d.** Chest X-ray
- ☐ **e.** Referral to A&E

47 Mastectomy is usually the treatment of choice for breast cancer in all of the following situations EXCEPT:

- ☐ **a.** Large tumour >4 cm
- ☐ **b.** Multifocal cancer
- ☐ **c.** Centrally located cancer
- ☐ **d.** Fibroadenoma
- ☐ **e.** Patient choice

48 Which one of the following is NOT a feature of cardiac tamponade?

- ☐ **a.** Bradycardia
- ☐ **b.** Pulsus paradoxus
- ☐ **c.** Hypotension
- ☐ **d.** Raised JVP
- ☐ **e.** Diminished heart sounds

49 Which one of the following statements is INCORRECT?
- ☐ **a.** A bicuspid aortic valve is more likely to calcify than a tricuspid valve
- ☐ **b.** A patent ductus arteriosus (PDA) is not compatible with life
- ☐ **c.** A machinery murmur is heard with PDA
- ☐ **d.** Coarctation of the aorta is associated with Turner's syndrome
- ☐ **e.** Chronic hypothyroidism predisposes to atherosclerosis

50 A 23-year-old man presents to hospital complaining of intermittent headaches, palpitations, sweating, and nausea and vomiting. His blood pressure is 198/124 mmHg and his heart rate is 116 bpm. Routine blood tests are requested along with a 24-hour urine collection for catecholamines. Which one of the following options is the next appropriate step?
- ☐ **a.** CT scan of the abdomen
- ☐ **b.** Surgical intervention
- ☐ **c.** Treatment with phentolamine or phenoxybenzamine
- ☐ **d.** Treatment with esmolol
- ☐ **e.** Renal artery ultrasonography

51 Which one of the following associations is INCORRECT?
- ☐ **a.** Ehlers–Danlos syndrome – mitral valve prolapse
- ☐ **b.** Turner's syndrome – coarctation of aorta
- ☐ **c.** Cushing's syndrome –hypertension
- ☐ **d.** Hypothyroidism – tachycardia
- ☐ **e.** Noonan's syndrome – pulmonary stenosis

52 A 40-year-old woman collapses during an aerobics class and is brought to A&E by ambulance in asystole. She has no past cardiac history of note and has been generally fit and well recently. Which one of the following is the most likely cause of her arrest?
- ☐ **a.** Pulmonary embolus
- ☐ **b.** Hypertrophic obstructive cardiomyopathy
- ☐ **c.** Acute MI
- ☐ **d.** Severe pneumonia
- ☐ **e.** Pneumothorax

53 A 70-year-old man presents to hospital with shortness of breath and pleuritic chest pain. Examination of his back and chest reveals multiple flat segmental brown lesions that are well demarcated and have the appearance of being stuck on to the skin. Which one of the following is the most likely diagnosis?

☐ **a.** Malignant melanoma
☐ **b.** Campbell de Morgan spots
☐ **c.** Keratoacanthoma
☐ **d.** Seborrhoeic keratoses
☐ **e.** Basal cell carcinoma

54 Where in the clotting cascade does warfarin exert its effect?

☐ **a.** Factor 10a
☐ **b.** Factor 2
☐ **c.** Vitamin K
☐ **d.** Vitamin A
☐ **e.** Factor 12

55 A 76-year-old woman has a breast lump that has been present for the past 11 months and has been growing in size. It causes no discomfort. It is 5 cm in diameter, overlying skin ulceration and in-drawing of the nipple on that side. What is the most likely diagnosis?

☐ **a.** Breast cyst
☐ **b.** Breast abscess
☐ **c.** Locally invasive breast cancer
☐ **d.** DCIS
☐ **e.** Mastitis

56 Statins work by competitive inhibition of:

☐ **a.** 3-Hydroxymethylglutaryl coenzyme A (HMG CoA) reductase
☐ **b.** Cytochrome P450
☐ **c.** Succinate coenzyme A (CoA) dehydrogenase
☐ **d.** 2-Peroxide dismutase
☐ **e.** 21-Hydroxylase

57 Which one of the following drugs has both a treatment and diagnostic role in narrow complex tachycardias?

☐ **a.** Atenolol
☐ **b.** Amiodarone
☐ **c.** Adenosine
☐ **d.** Atorvastatin
☐ **e.** Amlodipine

58 A 63-year-old man with poorly controlled type II diabetes mellitus is referred to the dermatology clinic with a history of a darkly pigmented rash under both arms with thickened, rough-textured skin. He also complains of some thickening of the skin over his palms, which making him embarrassed to shake hands. Which one of the following cutaneous manifestations is NOT associated with diabetes?

- ☐ **a.** Necrobiosis lipoidica diabeticorum
- ☐ **b.** Acanthosis nigricans
- ☐ **c.** Lipoatrophy
- ☐ **d.** Granuloma annulare
- ☐ **e.** Pyoderma gangrenosum

59 A patient with known coronary artery disease was seen 1 week ago by one of your colleagues. He presented with abdominal pains and generalized myalgia. Blood tests carried out at the time show deranged LFTs and an elevated CK of 524 IU/L. Which one of his medications is likely to be the cause of his symptoms?

- ☐ **a.** Diltiazem
- ☐ **b.** Simvastatin
- ☐ **c.** Metformin
- ☐ **d.** Diclofenac
- ☐ **e.** Enalapril

60 Which one of the following cardiac rhythms is 'shockable' (unsynchronized DC shock)?

- ☐ **a.** Atrial fibrillation
- ☐ **b.** Ventricular fibrillation
- ☐ **c.** Sinus rhythm
- ☐ **d.** Pulseless electrical activity
- ☐ **e.** Asystole

Extended Matching Questions

Opportunistic infections in HIV/AIDS

a. *Pneumocystis jiroveci* pneumonia
b. Candidiasis
c. Toxoplasmosis
d. Cryptosporidium infection
e. Cryptococcal infection
f. Varicella zoster pneumonitis
g. Cytomegaly virus infection
h. *Mycobacterium avium intracellulare*

The following HIV-positive patients have all presented with opportunistic infections. Please choose the most correct diagnosis from the above list. Each option may be used once, more than once, or not at all.

61 A 34-year-old man presents to hospital with abdominal pain, crampy in nature and associated with loose watery stools. On examination, he is pale, tachycardic and sweaty. He denies eating any seafood recently but has been staying at a friend's farm for the past 2 weeks.

62 A 40-year-old woman presents to hospital with a 3-day history of headache, nausea and lack of appetite. She has been otherwise fit and healthy and describes the headache as not related to any particular time of day but associated with pain on looking at bright lights.

63 A 28-year-old woman presents to her GP with pain on swallowing solid food and a strange taste in her mouth. She describes the pain as retrosternal in nature and associated only with swallowing. It is worse with dry and solid food and less painful with liquids. She denies any significant weight loss.

64 A 45-year-old man is brought to hospital by his friends who are worried that he has been acting 'out of character' recently. Collateral history reveals a gradual change in his behaviour, becoming more confused and agitated over a 2-month period with an episode of shaking of the limbs and arms that was attributed to medication side-effects. On arrival at A&E, he is aggressive, disruptive and would not allow any of the nursing staff to take blood from him.

65 A 32-year-old man was found collapsed at home by his partner
☐ and is brought by ambulance to A&E. On arrival, he is struggling
to breathe and is on an oxygen mask. History from his partner
reveals a gradual onset over the past 2 weeks of increasing shortness of breath and feelings of tiredness after the simplest tasks.
On examination, he is tachypnoeic with a respiratory rate of
34 breaths/minute and on auscultation fine crepitations are
heard in the lower and mid-zones of the lungs.

Chest pain

a. Acute MI
b. Pneumonia
c. Pulmonary embolus
d. Pericarditis
e. Bornholm disease
f. Pneumothorax
g. Gastro-oesophageal reflux disease
h. Aortic dissection

Please select the most suitable option above for each of the following scenarios. each option may be used once, more than once, or not at all.

66 An 87-year-old female nursing home resident has started to complain of chest pain with associated shortness of breath. There are no exacerbating or relieving factors for the pain. She suffers from chronic obstructive pulmonary disease (COPD), which is usually well controlled on inhaled medications.

67 A 30-year-old secretary who has recently recovered from viral chest infection presents to A&E with intermittent chest pain. The chest pain is central in origin with no radiation or any associated symptoms. On examination, the chest pain is recreated by exerting gentle pressure on the sternum.

68 A 68-year-old man has complained of retrosternal chest pain. It is at its worst when he lies flat. He complains of associated nausea but no vomiting. He has coronary artery disease and has recently had a short course of diclofenac for joint pains.

69 A 58-year-old man is brought to A&E by ambulance following an episode of chest pain at work. His colleague that accompanies him to the hospital mentions that he described his central chest pain as if it was tearing through to his back.

70 One week following a total knee replacement, a 63-year-old woman starts to complain of chest pain, right-sided in location and exacerbated by inspiration. It has no radiation or associated symptoms. She had previously complained of a swelling in her right calf that was thought to be related to her joint replacement.

Genitourinary discharge

a. Candidiasis
b. *Trichomonas vaginalis*
c. *Chlamydia trachomatis*
d. Lymphogranuloma venereum
e. *Haemophilus ducreyi*
f. Bacterial vaginosis
g. Gonorrhoea
h. Donovanosis

The following patients have all presented with genitourinary discharge. Please choose the most correct diagnosis from the above list. Each option may be used once, more than once, or not at all.

71 A 33-year-old secretary presents to her GP with an offensive discharge that she noticed 2 days ago. She initially thought it may have been related to her menstrual cycle; however, she denies any previous episodes of discharge. A vaginal swab is taken when it is noticed that the discharge smells fishy; however, the vagina appears normal on speculum examination. Slide microscopy reveals the presence of epithelial clue cells.

72 A 23-year-old man presents to the sexual health clinic with discharge from the penis and a burning sensation on passing urine. He has never had an episode like this before and when questioned he admits to casual sex with multiple partners since breaking up with his girlfriend 1 month ago. On examination, there is a yellowish discharge from the urethra and microscopy shows Gram-negative intracellular diplococci.

73 A 42-year-old man presents to his GP with an itchy rash on his penis. He denies any recent sexual intercourse and has not travelled out of the country for many years. He says that he has had the rash for some time with no ill effect. On examination, the head of the penis has multiple red lesions with cracked and raw skin. His past medical history is remarkable only for osteoarthritis and type II diabetes mellitus treated with diclofenac and metformin.

74 A 34-year-old woman presents to her GP as she and her husband have been trying for their first child for the past year and a half. She is embarrassed and upset to talk about their sexual habits and is frustrated because all her sisters have already borne children. On further questioning, she reveals that she used to work as a prostitute but has 'given that all up now'. An endocervical swab is taken and the organism grown from cell culture is reported as being an obligate intracellular bacterium.

75 A 45-year-old woman presents to her local general practice nurse appointment for a routine smear test. She has not been for regular appointments with the nurse before. While performing the smear test, the nurse notices that the surface of the cervix is dotted with small haemorrhages and that there is an offensive, frothy, yellow-green discharge in the vagina with multiple erythematous areas on the vaginal walls.

Peri-arrest drugs

   a. Atropine
   b. Adrenaline
   c. Amiodarone
   d. Lignocaine
   e. Magnesium sulphate
   f. Adenosine
   g. Verapamil
   h. Flecainide

From the list above, please select the most suitable drug for each of the following scenarios. Each option can be used once, more than once, or not at all.

76 This is the drug of choice in sinus, atrial or nodal bradycardias.
☐ It can also be used in pulseless electrical activity with a rate <60 bpm.

77 Used in the management of torsades de pointes, ventricular
☐ tachyarrhythmias and, occasionally, in acute asthma.

78 Used in refractory ventricular fibrillation or pulseless ventricular
☐ tachycardia.

79 Used in paroxysmal supraventricular tachycardia and narrow
☐ complex tachycardia.

80 Used in atrial fibrillation or supraventricular tachycardias with
☐ an accessory pathway.

Cardiovascular investigations

a. Chest X-ray
b. ECG
c. Echocardiogram
d. ETT
e. Diagnostic coronary angiogram
f. 24-hour tape
g. Cardiac perfusion scan
h. 24-hour blood pressure monitor

From the list above, please select the most appropriate investigation for the following scenarios. Each option can be used once, more than once or not at all.

81 A 58-year-old secretary with a past history of hypertension
☐ presents with intermittent new-onset chest pain. An ECG repeated on admission shows some ST segment depression. Her troponin level is mildly positive. An ETT shows no acute changes.

82 A 74-year-old woman complains of periods of dizziness with oc-
☐ casional associated blackouts. She is on no regular medicines.

83 A 69-year-old woman with a recent diagnosis of atrial fibrilla-
☐ tion enquires about the risks associated with the condition. She is concerned that a cerebrovascular accident is associated with atrial fibrillation and asks about anticoagulation. Which of the above investigations would aid your decision about anticoagulation in this woman?

84 A 68-year-old man who was admitted with troponin-negative
☐ chest pain but T-wave inversion asks about his risks of progressing on to cardiac problems. Which investigation would aid in stratifying his risk?

85 A 72-year-old woman has pulmonary oedema that is medically
☐ treated but she continues to complain of intermittent dizziness and periods of her heart racing. On examination, you note that her heart rate is 60 bpm; however, the observation chart notes that her heart rate is persistently above 100 bpm. Which investigation would provide diagnostic information in this case?

Manifestations of endocrine disease

a. Cushing's syndrome
b. Acromegaly
c. Diabetes mellitus
d. Diabetes insipidus
e. Phaeochromocytoma
f. Syndrome of inappropriate antidiuretic hormone secretion (SIADH)
g. Hypothyroidism
h. Hyperthyroidism
i. Addison's disease

The following patients have all presented with endocrine disease. Please choose the most likely diagnosis from the list above. Each option can be used once, more than once or not at all.

86 A 54-year-old man presents to the renal clinic for regular follow-up post live related kidney transplant. He complains of a feeling of lethargy, weight gain and swelling of his ankles recently. His blood pressure reading is 176/98 mmHg and fasting blood glucose level is 10.2 g/dL. Blood results show a sodium level of 148 mmol/L and a potassium level of 3.5 mmol/L.

87 A 78-year-old woman is brought to hospital by her neighbour who is concerned that she has recently become confused. Abdominal examination reveals a lumpy quality to the abdomen and areas of erythema ab igne on both shins. A keen medical student notes some unusual hair loss over her eyebrows and scalp.

88 A 52-year-old man presents to hospital with shortness of breath and cough productive of green sputum. He complains of feeling weak, thirsty and urinating frequently for the past week and weight loss over the past month. Blood results reveal the following: sodium 147 mmol/L, potassium 4.9 mmol/L, urea 11 mmol/L and plasma osmolality 330 mOsm/L. Urine osmolality is verbally reported as being 'high'.

89 A 42-year-old man presents to his GP with headaches and some recent changes in his vision. On examination, he is a tall and heavy set man who is very tanned. Upon taking a social history he remarks that recently his wedding band has become too tight and is being resized.

90 A 38-year-old man presents to his GP complaining of recurrent anxiety attacks. He describes three or four episodes while he has been out in public when he feels light-headed, has palpitations and a mild tremor and wants to sit down until these feelings subside. Focused questioning reveals he has recently become constipated and he is very anxious that this may be cancer, as his family have a history of 'thyroid and pituitary growths'.

Questions

Single Best Answer Questions

1 A 64-year-old man presents with problems with his chest for the past 10 years. On examination, he has a barrel-shaped chest and there is evidence of use of the accessory muscles of respiration and pursed lip breathing. Which one of the following routine blood results is most likely to be found in this patient?
- ☐ **a.** Lymphopenia
- ☐ **b.** Anaemia
- ☐ **c.** Raised mean corpuscular volume (MCV)
- ☐ **d.** Polycythaemia
- ☐ **e.** Thrombocytopenia

2 A 14-year-old boy is brought to hospital by ambulance having been involved in a road traffic accident. He arrives intubated by the ambulance crew and is hypotensive. A focused assessment with sonography for trauma (FAST) scan demonstrates free fluid in the abdomen from a ruptured spleen. He is scheduled for emergency surgery for exploratory laparotomy and splenectomy. As he is being taken to theatre, his parents arrive and demand that he is not given blood transfusions as he is a Jehovah's Witness and show their cards stating so. Which one of the following actions is the correct course of action?
- ☐ **a.** Refuse to proceed to surgery without blood
- ☐ **b.** Proceed to surgery using crystalloid replacement only
- ☐ **c.** Proceed to surgery as an emergency, using blood as necessary
- ☐ **d.** Reschedule surgery to allow for auto-transfusion
- ☐ **e.** Apply for a court order to allow surgery to proceed

EMQs and SBAs for Medical Finals, Second Edition. Jonathan Bath, Rebecca Morgan and Mehool Patel.
© 2011 John Wiley & Sons, Ltd. Published 2011 by John Wiley & Sons, Ltd.

3 A 65-year-old female presents with a persistent nose bleed for the past 4 hours. She denies any trauma to the local area and has never suffered with this problem in the past. Which one of the following is NOT a known cause of epistaxis?
- ☐ **a.** Hypertension
- ☐ **b.** Trauma
- ☐ **c.** Alcoholic liver disease
- ☐ **d.** Leukaemia
- ☐ **e.** Cannabis use

4 A 16-year-old girl presents to Accident & Emergency (A&E) having taken 35 paracetamol tablets that morning. Examination is unremarkable. Aspartate transaminase (AST), bilirubin, gamma glutamyl transpeptidase (γ-GGT), alkaline phosphatase and alanine transaminase (ALT) are normal. International normalized ratio (INR) is 1.12 with a fibrinogen level <6 g/L and a normal activated partial thromboplastin time (APTT). Which one of the following investigations is the most sensitive indicator of hepatic damage?
- ☐ **a.** AST and ALT
- ☐ **b.** Alkaline phosphatase
- ☐ **c.** INR
- ☐ **d.** Fibrinogen
- ☐ **e.** Albumin

5 A fit 26-year-old woman was admitted to hospital with cellulitis in her left leg and was started on intravenous (IV) antibiotics. She complained of some facial flushing with tingling in her hands and teeth but no shortness of breath or chest tightening. She remained apyrexial throughout. What would your next course of action be?
- ☐ **a.** Consider this to be an anxiety attack and continue treatment with reassurance
- ☐ **b.** Add in erythromycin as current cover is not adequate
- ☐ **c.** Change antibiotics due to allergy
- ☐ **d.** Stop antibiotics, administer steroids and antihistamines
- ☐ **e.** Continue treatment with topical antibiotics

6 A 68-year-old woman is admitted to the ward after an elective hip replacement for osteoarthritis. She develops postoperative pneumonia and appropriate antibiotic therapy commenced. Four days later, she is dehydrated with a low potassium level from profuse diarrhoea and IV fluids are administered. Which one of the following steps is appropriate in the management of this patient?

- ☐ **a.** Administration of IV potassium at a rate of 20 mmol/hour
- ☐ **b.** Administration of oral metronidazole
- ☐ **c.** Administration of oral amoxicillin
- ☐ **d.** Administration of 2 units of blood
- ☐ **e.** Administration of a potassium-sparing diuretic

7 Which one of the following associations is correct?

- ☐ **a.** Acute glaucoma – low intraocular pressure
- ☐ **b.** Conjunctivitis – conjunctival vessels do not blanch on pressure
- ☐ **c.** Iritis – dilated pupil
- ☐ **d.** Subconjunctival haemorrhage – hazy cornea
- ☐ **e.** Acute glaucoma – fixed, dilated pupil

8 A 54-year-old man is brought to hospital by a concerned neighbour who found him collapsed at home, having taken an overdose of medication. He is assessed by the admitting house officer who elicits a history of suicidal ideation, a recent loss of appetite and lack of enjoyment of usual hobbies. The case is discussed with the duty psychiatrist who advises on further management. Which one of the following statements regarding depression is NOT true?

- ☐ **a.** Endogenous depression responds more readily to antidepressants than exogenous (reactive) depression
- ☐ **b.** Females are more likely to take a medication overdose as mode of suicide than males
- ☐ **c.** Lack of a confiding relationship is associated with depression
- ☐ **d.** Antidepressant medication takes action after approximately 2 weeks
- ☐ **e.** Thyroid disease should always be considered in the differential diagnosis of depression

9 A 23-year-old woman presents to hospital feeling nauseated, unwell, with loss of appetite. She is very worried that she is pregnant as she had missed her last period. Systemic review reveals a 2-week history of a painful right knee. On examination, she has a mild yellow tinge to the sclera and an itchy rash over her forearm. The abdomen is very tender over the right upper quadrant but Murphy's sign is negative. Which of the following diagnoses is most likely?

- ☐ **a.** Viral hepatitis
- ☐ **b.** Budd–Chiari syndrome
- ☐ **c.** Cholecystitis
- ☐ **d.** Autoimmune hepatitis
- ☐ **e.** McArdle's disease

10 A 53-year-old man presents to his general practitioner (GP) with a 2-week history of headache and recent blurred vision. Fundoscopy reveals arteriolar narrowing and cotton-wool spots. Some oedema of the optic disc is also reported. Which one of the following conditions is this fundoscopic appearance consistent with?

- ☐ **a.** Diabetic retinopathy
- ☐ **b.** Hypertensive retinopathy
- ☐ **c.** Age-related macular degeneration
- ☐ **d.** Cytomegalovirus (CMV) retinitis
- ☐ **e.** Ankylosing spondylitis

11 A 79-year-old woman with known chronic obstructive pulmonary disease (COPD) has been admitted six times in the past 6 months. Examination reveals tachypnoea and breathing through pursed lips. Arterial blood gas (ABG) studies for assessing domiciliary oxygen requirements are found to be negative and this has been the case on previous admissions. Physiotherapists have noted that her mobility is good. Your team decides that she is medically fit for discharge, what will your next step be?

- ☐ **a.** Discharge to a short-term rehabilitation facility
- ☐ **b.** Ask social services for review with nursing home placement in mind
- ☐ **c.** Keep patient in hospital until she feels ready to leave
- ☐ **d.** Send her home with a GP follow-up immediately
- ☐ **e.** Impress on the patient that she is well and that she has no medical problems requiring attention

12 A 63-year-old woman presents with a month's history of regurgitating food, foul-smelling breath and a sensation of gurgling in her neck when she eats. She describes the regurgitated food as slightly changed but denies any blood or pain when she eats. Which one of the following diagnoses is most likely?

- ☐ **a.** Pharyngeal pouch
- ☐ **b.** Plummer–Vinson syndrome
- ☐ **c.** Chagas' disease
- ☐ **d.** Oesophageal carcinoma
- ☐ **e.** Mallory–Weiss tear

13 A 34-year-old woman is examined in the rheumatology clinic and noticed to have poor vision in the right eye with diplopia. She has a history of cardiac problems and examination of the cardiac system reveals a soft diastolic murmur heard best in the aortic area. Which one of the following diagnoses would this clinical picture be most consistent with?

- ☐ **a.** William's syndrome
- ☐ **b.** Down syndrome
- ☐ **c.** Marfan's syndrome
- ☐ **d.** Turner's syndrome
- ☐ **e.** Reiter's syndrome

14 A 6-year old boy is brought in to A&E with acute difficulty in breathing. He has had a mild fever and audible wheeze and his parents note that he has been more drowsy than usual today. On observation, he is using accessory muscles of respiration and his mother mentions that he had been drooling at home. What is the most likely diagnosis in this case?

- ☐ **a.** Tonsillitis
- ☐ **b.** Acute exacerbation of asthma
- ☐ **c.** Chest infection
- ☐ **d.** Acute epiglottitis
- ☐ **e.** Allergic reaction

15 A 34-year-old man with ulcerative colitis presents in the gastroenterology outpatient clinic with abdominal pain and fatigue. He states the pain has been intermittent for the past 2 weeks and has not settled with simple analgesia. Routine blood tests taken prior to clinic show a markedly raised alkaline phosphatase with mild hyperbilirubinaemia. A right upper quadrant ultrasound has been performed and is abnormal. Which of the following would be the most appropriate next investigation?

- ☐ **a.** CT scan of the abdomen
- ☐ **b.** Endoscopic retrograde cholangiopancreatogram (ERCP)
- ☐ **c.** Colonoscopy
- ☐ **d.** Plain abdominal radiograph
- ☐ **e.** Liver biopsy

16 A 24-year-old man is brought in to hospital by the police after he is found trying to break into an electronics shop because he believed the government was using the television sets to control him. He is agitated on arrival to hospital and demands to be released, saying that it is all part of the government conspiracy keeping him hostage in hospital. You are called by the nurse to assess him, as he was found by the hospital security trying to escape. Which one of the following is the correct course of action?

- ☐ **a.** Admission to hospital under Section 3 of the Mental Health Act
- ☐ **b.** Cuff and restraint under common law
- ☐ **c.** Admission to hospital under Section 4 of the Mental Health Act
- ☐ **d.** Documentation of discharge from hospital against medical advice
- ☐ **e.** Discharge with community psychiatric follow-up

17 A 52-year-old man presents to hospital having had 10 bouts of diarrhoea since the morning and severe abdominal pain. He states that he has severe facial flushes intermittently. On examination, he is slightly anxious and breathless while lying flat. There is peripheral pitting oedema of the ankles and abdominal examination reveals 3-cm bulky hepatomegaly. Cardiac sounds are abnormal with a pansystolic murmur and a raised jugular venous pressure (JVP). Which one of the following investigations is most likely to provide a diagnosis?

☐ **a.** 24-hour urine protein collection
☐ **b.** Plasma osmolality
☐ **c.** 24-hour urine 5-hydroxyindoleacetic acid (5-HIAA)
☐ **d.** Urinary osmolality
☐ **e.** 24-hour urine for 4-hydroxy methyl mandelate (HMMA) (vanillylmandelic acid [VMA])

18 A 32-year-old woman presents to her GP complaining of recurrent episodes of intense discomfort associated with shortness of breath, chest pain and palpitations usually while she is out in public places. The episodes last between 5 and 10 minutes and usually cease on their own. Her past medical history is unremarkable but she tells you that her family have a history of 'heart attacks' and she is worried that her symptoms may be related. Which one of the following is NOT commonly associated with the above condition?

☐ **a.** Irritable bowel syndrome
☐ **b.** Agoraphobia
☐ **c.** Mitral valve prolapse
☐ **d.** COPD
☐ **e.** Age >65 years

19 A 64-year-old woman is seen by her GP for a very red, itchy and painful eye. She describes the eye as having the sensation of there being 'a bit of grit stuck in it'. On further enquiry, she suffers from a dry cough and has trouble eating very dry food as she finds it 'sticks to her mouth and is difficult to swallow'. Which one of the following diagnoses is the most likely?

☐ **a.** Anterior uveitis
☐ **b.** Acute glaucoma
☐ **c.** Subconjunctival haemorrhage
☐ **d.** Sjögren's syndrome
☐ **e.** Retinal vein occlusion

20 A 48-year-old woman presents to hospital complaining of vomiting and diarrhoea after eating chicken fried rice and vegetable spring rolls. On examination, there are no physical signs apart from a previous lower segment Caesarean section in the abdomen. Which one of the following organisms is the most likely infectious agent?

- ☐ **a.** Rotavirus
- ☐ **b.** *Clostridium botulinum*
- ☐ **c.** *Cryptosporidium parvum*
- ☐ **d.** *Bacillus cereus*
- ☐ **e.** *Escherichia coli*

21 A 68-year-old woman with a history of cancer presents to hospital with abdominal pain and distension. On examination, she has a tender distended abdomen with 4-cm smooth hepatomegaly and evidence of fluid shift. The abdominal veins are dilated and there is evidence of caput medusae at the umbilicus. Which one of the following diagnoses is the most likely in this case?

- ☐ **a.** Viral hepatitis
- ☐ **b.** Epstein–Barr virus infection
- ☐ **c.** α1-Antitrypsin deficiency
- ☐ **d.** Wilson's disease
- ☐ **e.** Budd–Chiari syndrome

22 A 67-year-old woman presents to A&E with right-sided chest pain and some shortness of breath. Examination reveals a pleural effusion, which is confirmed on chest X-ray. Aspiration of the fluid identifies <30 g of protein. Which one of the following would NOT be consistent with the above picture?

- ☐ **a.** Hypothyroidism
- ☐ **b.** Liver cirrhosis
- ☐ **c.** Nephrotic syndrome
- ☐ **d.** Pneumonia
- ☐ **e.** Cardiac failure

23 A 26-year-old man presents with diarrhoea with mucus and blood streaks and abdominal pain over a 1-month period. Colonoscopy is arranged and shows multiple areas of cobblestone appearance and aphthous ulceration. Which one of the following statements regarding this disease is correct?

- ☐ **a.** Surgical therapy is likely to be curative
- ☐ **b.** Disease is limited to the terminal ileum and distally
- ☐ **c.** Transmural involvement is seen on histology
- ☐ **d.** Continuous inflammatory change is seen on colonoscopy
- ☐ **e.** Barium follow-through is of no use diagnostically

24 A 56-year-old school teacher visits his GP with sudden-onset unilateral hearing difficulties. He has difficulty hearing both high and low pitch sounds in the affected ear although he comments that there is no associated pain or discharge from the ear. What is the most likely cause for his symptoms?
- ☐ **a.** Otitis media
- ☐ **b.** Otitis externa
- ☐ **c.** Perforated ear drum
- ☐ **d.** Otitis interna
- ☐ **e.** Foreign body in external auditory meatus

25 A 74-year-old woman is referred to A&E with a history of pain and redness in her right eye that is associated with blurred and distorted vision leading her to see 'haloes' around objects. This is worse in the early evening. Which one of the following is the most likely diagnosis?
- ☐ **a.** Endophthalmitis
- ☐ **b.** Acute glaucoma
- ☐ **c.** Retinitis pigmentosa
- ☐ **d.** Retinal detachment
- ☐ **e.** Retinal artery occlusion

26 A 23-year-old man presents to A&E feeling lethargic, passing large amounts of urine and complaining of abdominal pain. Past medical history is remarkable for type I diabetes mellitus. Urine dipstick done on admission show glucose ++, ketones +++ and trace protein. Venous blood gases results show: pH 7.29, HCO_3^- 18 mmol/L with a base excess of −3.4 mmol/L. Which one of the following treatment regimens should be instituted?
- ☐ **a.** Double the usual basal bolus insulin regimen with strict blood glucose monitoring hourly
- ☐ **b.** Start short-acting insulin infusion with 5-L fluid replacement of 0.9% sodium chloride with potassium as required over a 24-hour period
- ☐ **c.** Add a long-acting insulin to the usual basal bolus regimen with 5-L fluid replacement with 0.9% sodium chloride
- ☐ **d.** Start short-acting insulin infusion to reduce blood glucose to less than 15 mmol/L, then restart high-dose oral hypoglycaemic with strict blood glucose measurement
- ☐ **e.** Start a sliding scale of intermediate-acting insulin with 5-L fluid replacement of 0.9% sodium chloride with basal bolus short-acting insulin as required

27 A 43-year-old man presents to clinic with feelings of a lack of enjoyment of his usual hobbies, a feeling of detachment from his family and friends associated with poor sleep, nightmares and irritability. He describes these changes happening a few months ago and states that he has been easily startled and ill at ease ever since. His past medical history is remarkable only for allergic rhinitis and a recent hospital admission for a head injury following a robbery at his home. Which one of the following is the most likely diagnosis?

- ☐ **a.** Acute stress disorder
- ☐ **b.** Depressive disorder
- ☐ **c.** Post-traumatic stress disorder
- ☐ **d.** Schizoid personality disorder
- ☐ **e.** Generalized anxiety disorder

28 A 68-year-old woman presents with pain in her abdomen causing her to vomit. Examination of the abdomen reveals localized tenderness over the left iliac fossa. Routine blood tests show: white cell count 17.3×10^9/L, C-reactive peptide 110 mg/L, urea 6.9 mmol/L, creatinine 118 μmol/L. Which one of the following is a strong indication for emergency surgery?

- ☐ **a.** Faecal peritonitis
- ☐ **b.** Colovesical fistula
- ☐ **c.** Severe ileus
- ☐ **d.** Tender palpable mass
- ☐ **e.** Failure to exclude cancer

29 A university health care centre doctor is called to see a student who has been lethargic and feverish and has been taking ibuprofen. Benzylpenicillin is started empirically to cover for meningitis. A non-blanching rash over his right thigh is noted. In hospital his temperature is recorded at 39.1°C and he has started to vomit. What is the most likely cause of vomiting in this man?

- ☐ **a.** Idiosyncratic reaction to ibuprofen
- ☐ **b.** Allergic reaction to benzylpenicillin
- ☐ **c.** Neurogenic (central) reaction
- ☐ **d.** Systemic inflammatory response to infection
- ☐ **e.** Non-steroidal anti-inflammatory drug (NSAID) irritation to gastric mucosa

30 A 43-year-old man with known alcoholic liver disease presents to hospital with a distended abdomen, pain and yellow discoloration to his skin and sclera. Regarding portal–systemic venous anastomoses in portal hypertension, which one of the following associations is NOT correct?

☐ **a.** Left gastric with azygous leading to oesophageal varices
☐ **b.** Para-umbilical with inferior epigastric leading to caput medusae
☐ **c.** Superior to middle/inferior rectal leading to rectal varices
☐ **d.** Splenic with left gastric leading to splenic varices
☐ **e.** Retroperitoneal and phrenic leading to diaphragmatic varices

31 A 59-year-old man presents to hospital with progressive deterioration in visual acuity over a period of weeks such that he had trouble focusing on even the closest of objects and had had to stop driving completely. Which one of the following has NOT been associated with the development of posterior subcapsular cataract?

☐ **a.** Obesity
☐ **b.** Steroids
☐ **c.** Hypertriglyceridaemia
☐ **d.** Hypertension
☐ **e.** Hypoglycaemia

32 A 78-year-old man presents to hospital after not passing a stool for 3 days. A careful history from his daughter reveals he has lost 8 kg in weight over the past 2 months. Which of the following tumour markers might be expected to be raised in this disease?

☐ **a.** Carcino-embryonic antigen (CEA)
☐ **b.** Cancer antigen 15-3 (CA 15-3)
☐ **c.** Alpha-fetoprotein (AFP)
☐ **d.** Neurone specific enolase (NSE)
☐ **e.** Human chorionic gonadotropin (hCG)

33 A 45-year-old woman is admitted electively to hospital for an open cholecystectomy. On the fourth day post-surgery she starts to complain of abdominal pain with fever, nausea and a tender abdomen. Routine blood tests show a high white cell count and a bilirubin of 32 μmol/L. Which one of the following is the next diagnostic investigation to perform?

☐ **a.** Ultrasound liver and gallbladder
☐ **b.** Hepatobiliary iminodiacetic acid (HIDA) scan
☐ **c.** Plain abdominal radiograph
☐ **d.** Computed tomography (CT) scan of the abdomen
☐ **e.** ERCP

34 A 62-year-old man is brought to hospital complaining of pain in his abdomen after a laparoscopic cholecystectomy 1 week ago. He has been experiencing rigors and his friends say that his skin has changed colour. The abdomen is tender in the right upper quadrant. He is pyrexic at 38.2°C with a systolic blood pressure of 165/68 mmHg. Which one of the following most accurately describes the clinical picture?

- ☐ **a.** Reynolds' pentad
- ☐ **b.** Fitz–Hugh–Curtis syndrome
- ☐ **c.** Leriche's syndrome
- ☐ **d.** Wernicke–Korsakoff syndrome
- ☐ **e.** Charcot's triad

35 A 23-year-old Jewish man presented to A&E after the sudden onset of abdominal cramping and complaining of a sudden desire to defecate. On further questioning, he admits to noticing some mucus accompanying the stool and has passed occasional small amounts of fresh blood. Which one of the following is the most likely diagnosis?

- ☐ **a.** Pseudomembranous colitis
- ☐ **b.** Ischaemic colitis
- ☐ **c.** Ulcerative colitis
- ☐ **d.** Angiodysplasia
- ☐ **e.** Haemorrhoids

36 A 60-year-old man presents to his GP complaining of feeling tired all the time. On examination, there is a faint bronzed appearance to the skin, the sclera are slightly yellow-tinged and there are non-blanching red lesions on the upper body. Cardiac examination reveals a third heart sound and tachycardia with mild pitting oedema to both ankles. The abdomen is soft but tender in the right upper quadrant with a 2-cm palpable liver edge. Routine blood tests demonstrate raised bilirubin, AST and ALT with a random blood glucose of 14 mmol/L. Haematinics done at a routine check-up 1 month ago demonstrated a raised serum ferritin with a raised serum iron and decreased total iron binding capacity (TIBC). Which one of the following investigations would be LEAST useful in confirming the diagnosis?

- ☐ **a.** Magnetic resonance imaging (MRI) scan
- ☐ **b.** Fasting transferrin saturation
- ☐ **c.** Liver biopsy
- ☐ **d.** Liver ultrasound scan
- ☐ **e.** C28Y mutation screen

37 A 25-year-old woman who works as a waitress presents with unsteadiness in carrying heavy loads and customers have been having trouble understanding her speech. On examination she is noted to have a tremor and dysarthria. Careful examination of the eye reveals an area of pigmentation at the junction between cornea and sclera. Which one of the following investigations is the most discriminative in making the diagnosis?

- ☐ **a.** Four vessel neck angiography
- ☐ **b.** Serum bilirubin and liver enzymes
- ☐ **c.** Thyroid function tests
- ☐ **d.** Serum copper and caeruloplasmin
- ☐ **e.** Peripheral blood film and vitamin B12 levels

38 A 63-year-old man is brought to hospital by ambulance following a fall at home. He lives alone and is unaccompanied to hospital. On arrival, he is assessed by the emergency staff and appears confused and disorientated but moving all four limbs and communicating, albeit inappropriately. His urine dipstick is positive for leucocytes, nitrites and protein. He scores 3/10 on the abbreviated mental test (AMT) and is uncooperative with physical examination, pulling out his IV lines and trying to leave the hospital. Which one of the following medications would be of most benefit in managing this patient?

- ☐ **a.** Haloperidol
- ☐ **b.** Lorazepam
- ☐ **c.** Memantine
- ☐ **d.** Olanzapine
- ☐ **e.** Sertraline

39 A 30-year-old man complains of severe lower-right-sided abdominal pain. On administration of a bolus dose of normal saline intravenously, he states that his pain feels much better. Which one of the following options explains this phenomenon?

- ☐ **a.** He has borderline personality disorder
- ☐ **b.** His pain is psychogenic
- ☐ **c.** He is responding to a placebo
- ☐ **d.** His pain is somatic in origin
- ☐ **e.** His electrolyte abnormalities are corrected

40 A 67-year-old diabetic man is seen by his GP for follow-up of glycaemic control and monitoring. Screening fundoscopy is undertaken, which demonstrates changes consistent with those seen in proliferative diabetic retinopathy. Which one of the following complications is associated with this condition?

- ☐ **a.** Retinal detachment
- ☐ **b.** Aqueous haemorrhage
- ☐ **c.** Retinal vein thrombosis
- ☐ **d.** Optic neuritis
- ☐ **e.** Bitemporal hemianopia

41 A 60-year-old female patient makes an appointment with her GP to discuss her recently depressed mood. She describes early morning waking, a reduced libido and a reduced enjoyment of hobbies. She has recently been started on a new medication. Which of the following drugs is most likely to be the cause of her depressed mood?

- ☐ **a.** NSAIDs
- ☐ **b.** Oral hypoglycaemic drugs
- ☐ **c.** Antihypertensive drugs
- ☐ **d.** Calcium supplements
- ☐ **e.** Digoxin

42 An 80-year-old male returns to his GP for a routine appointment following having some blood tests taken for a general health screen. Which one of the following results is abnormal for this patient?

- ☐ **a.** Mild glucose intolerance
- ☐ **b.** Increased autoantibody production
- ☐ **c.** Raised alkaline phosphatase
- ☐ **d.** Reduced creatinine clearance
- ☐ **e.** Increase in haemoglobin concentration

43 A 74-year-old man complains of shortness of breath and chest pain. On examination, there are signs of a left lower lobe pneumonia and an irregular pulse with a rate of 146 beats/minute (bpm). His temperature is 37.9°C, blood pressure is 124/86 mmHg and oxygen saturations are 99% on 10 L oxygen. Which one of the following management options is correct?

- ☐ **a.** Digoxin 500 μg every 12 hours, then digoxin maintenance
- ☐ **b.** Digoxin one-off stat dose, then anticoagulation
- ☐ **c.** Beta-blocker one-off stat dose, then digoxin maintenance
- ☐ **d.** Beta-blocker one-off stat dose, then anticoagulation
- ☐ **e.** Digoxin 500 μg every 12 hours, then beta-blocker maintenance

41

44 A 56-year-old homeless man presents with abdominal pain and mild shortness of breath. Chest X-ray demonstrates a right-sided pleural effusion and the abdominal X-ray shows an absent psoas shadow. What is the most useful next investigation to aid in diagnosis?

☐ **a.** Pleural tap
☐ **b.** Serum glucose
☐ **c.** Serum amylase
☐ **d.** Transoesophageal echocardiogram
☐ **e.** Endoscopy

45 A 24-year-old man presents to his GP with an itchy rash on the head of his penis. He denies any dysuria or urethral discharge but does say that he has noticed he needs to urinate more frequently and has been feeling lethargic and very thirsty. On examination of the glans penis there are multiple areas of underlying erythema with a whitish layer to them. Which one of the following investigations is likely to confirm the underlying diagnosis?

☐ **a.** Blood glucose level
☐ **b.** Erythrocyte sedimentation rate (ESR)
☐ **c.** Urine analysis
☐ **d.** Human T-cell lymphotropic virus (HTLV-1 and -2) assay
☐ **e.** Full blood count

46 A 43-year-old woman is brought to hospital by her husband after he found she had taken an overdose of her medication in her bathroom. Her past medical history is remarkable for hypertension and depression. She denies taking any medication overdose, stating that her husband is simply worrying unnecessarily. On examination, she is drowsy with dilated pupils and sluggish reflexes. A tachycardia is clinically evident and electrocardiography is performed that demonstrates a prolonged PR and QT interval. Which one of the following medications is most likely responsible for her symptoms?

☐ **a.** Tranylcypromine
☐ **b.** Amitriptyline
☐ **c.** Digoxin
☐ **d.** Atenolol
☐ **e.** Sertraline

47 A 45-year-old obese woman presents to her GP with a sensation of food sticking in her throat when she has a meal, associated with some pain. She states that the sensation is worse with solids and dry food, with no problems drinking liquids. She endorses a long history of proton pump inhibition with marginal effect. Which one of the following diagnoses is the most likely cause for her dysphagia?

☐ **a.** Systemic sclerosis
☐ **b.** Reflux oesophagitis stricture
☐ **c.** Radiation oesophagitis
☐ **d.** Oesophageal carcinoma
☐ **e.** Oesophageal candidiasis

48 A 52-year-old man presents to his GP with bilateral symmetrically enlarged breasts. His past medical history is remarkable for gastro-oesophageal reflux disease and angina. Which one of the following medications is most likely responsible for gynaecomastia in this man?

☐ **a.** Atenolol
☐ **b.** Gaviscon
☐ **c.** Cimetidine
☐ **d.** Enalapril
☐ **e.** Aspirin

49 An 18-month-old boy is brought to hospital by his mother who is worried that he looks 'cross-eyed'. She describes a history in her family of eye problems and says that she thinks her father had his right eye taken out at a young age. On clinical examination of the eye, there is a white reflective reflex in the left eye with obvious divergent squint. Which one of the following is the most likely diagnosis?

☐ **a.** Congenital cataract
☐ **b.** Endophthalmitis
☐ **c.** Retinoblastoma
☐ **d.** Ocular tuberculosis
☐ **e.** Retinopathy of prematurity

50 A 52-year-old businessman presents with bright red blood per rectum that is apparent on the toilet paper and can be seen in the toilet bowl after straining at stool. Digital rectal examination reveals soft fluctuant masses felt at 11, 3 and 7 o'clock with the patient in the lithotomy position and a few spots of fresh red blood on the glove. Which one of the following is the most likely diagnosis in this man?

☐ **a.** Rectosigmoid carcinoma
☐ **b.** Anal fissure
☐ **c.** Angiodysplasia
☐ **d.** Inflammatory bowel disorder
☐ **e.** Internal haemorrhoids

51 A 28-year-old man is seen by his GP for a vaccination prior to travel abroad. During the consultation, he is preoccupied with the forms that are being filled in, requesting to have copies of all documentation and becoming increasingly worried that the government will find out about his trip abroad. When asked about friends and family contacts he becomes agitated and denies having any close friends, saying that they would just spy on him. Which one of the following is the most likely diagnosis?

☐ **a.** Antisocial personality disorder
☐ **b.** Schizotypal personality disorder
☐ **c.** Schizoid personality disorder
☐ **d.** Dependent personality disorder
☐ **e.** Avoidant personality disorder

52 A 74-year-old woman presents to her GP with a lack of energy and weight loss. Routine blood tests show: haemoglobin 7.4 g/dL, MCV 72 fL, AST 140 IU/L, ALT 212 IU/L. Which one of the following investigations would NOT form part of the investigational work-up?

☐ **a.** Liver biopsy
☐ **b.** CT scan of abdomen
☐ **c.** Chest radiography
☐ **d.** Colonoscopy
☐ **e.** Oesophagogastroduodenoscopy (OGD)

53 A 54-year-old man is brought into A&E by ambulance, having collapsed at home. He is short of breath on arrival and drowsy, with a tachycardia of 130 bpm. He has been passing very dark stools for the past couple of days and had taken some aspirin for the pain. Examination reveals a drop in blood pressure of 25 mmHg from lying to sitting and digital rectal examination reveals dark offensive stool. Blood tests reveal: urea 11.3 mmol/L, haemoglobin 8.5 g/dL, with normal electrolytes and creatinine. Which one of the following is the most appropriate course of action?

☐ **a.** Referral to surgeons for an emergency laparotomy
☐ **b.** 2-unit blood transfusion and colonoscopy
☐ **c.** 2-L normal saline bolus and urgent upper gastrointestinal endoscopy
☐ **d.** Coeliac arteriography
☐ **e.** Proton pump inhibition and routine endoscopy

54 A 35-year-old woman presents to hospital over a 2-month period complaining of abdominal pain in her left lower quadrant with abdominal distension and progressive shortness of breath. A transvaginal ultrasound is performed, which demonstrated a cystic mass in the left ovary reported as most likely a benign mass. On examination, the abdomen is distended with evidence of shifting dullness. Which one of the following eponymous syndromes describes this clinical picture?

☐ **a.** Jarisch–Herxheimer reaction
☐ **b.** Meigs' syndrome
☐ **c.** Fitz–Hugh–Curtis syndrome
☐ **d.** Peyronie's disease
☐ **e.** Raynaud's syndrome

55 A 34-year-old woman presents to A&E complaining of severe generalized abdominal pain associated with weakness of both legs. A sample of urine for dipstick was dark in colour but was negative for blood, protein or nitrites on testing. On examination, the abdomen is soft but tender over the suprapubic region and neurological examination reveals markedly reduced sensation in the distal lower limbs but normal tone, power and co-ordination. She repeatedly states that no documentation must be taken, as the government has been spying on her. Which one of the following investigations would be most useful in making the diagnosis?

   ☐ **a.** 24-hour urinary protein collection
   ☐ **b.** Thyroid function tests (TFTs)
   ☐ **c.** Urinary porphobilinogen levels
   ☐ **d.** CT scan of the abdomen
   ☐ **e.** Urinary metadrenalines (HMMA/VMA)

56 Regarding dementia, which one of the following is NOT a recognized feature of this condition?

   ☐ **a.** Fluctuating level of consciousness
   ☐ **b.** Sundowning effect
   ☐ **c.** Mood changes
   ☐ **d.** Personality changes
   ☐ **e.** Potentially reversible

57 An elderly man is admitted to hospital following a fall and fractured neck of femur. The nursing staff notice that recently he has lost control of his bowels and is incontinent of watery, foul-smelling stools up to four times a day. Physical examination reveals a distended abdomen with active bowel sounds and digital rectal examination reveals hard faeces. An abdominal radiograph shows a patchy ground glass appearance throughout the distribution of the colon. Which one of the following is the most likely cause?

   ☐ **a.** Faecal impaction
   ☐ **b.** Cholesterol embolus
   ☐ **c.** Sigmoid volvulus
   ☐ **d.** Cauda equina syndrome
   ☐ **e.** *Clostridium difficile* infection

58 Regarding motor innervation to ocular structures, which one of the following associations is NOT correct?

- ☐ **a.** Levator palpebrae superioris – sympathetic nervous system
- ☐ **b.** Lateral rectus muscle – abducens nerve
- ☐ **c.** Superior oblique – trochlear nerve
- ☐ **d.** Lacrimal glands – parasympathetic nervous system
- ☐ **e.** Medial rectus muscle – abducens nerve

59 A 45-year-old man is shot in the abdomen and is taken to surgery, requiring massive blood transfusion. His recovery is complicated by poorly controlled abdominal sepsis. Total parenteral nutrition (TPN) was instituted and continued throughout his prolonged hospital stay. His liver enzymes are elevated on routine blood tests. Which one of the following is the most likely explanation for the derangement in liver enzymes?

- ☐ **a.** Blood transfusion reaction
- ☐ **b.** Parenteral-nutrition-related cholestasis
- ☐ **c.** Unrecognized biliary leak
- ☐ **d.** Hepatitis secondary to blood transfusion
- ☐ **e.** Sedation-related side-effect

60 A 69-year-old man is admitted to A&E 7 days after suffering a myocardial infarction (MI). He complains of increasing shortness of breath and on observation was tachypnoeic at rest sitting up. On examination, there is evidence of a systolic murmur and raised JVP. An erect chest radiograph is normal. Which one of the following complications of MI is most likely to be the cause of this man's shortness of breath?

- ☐ **a.** Ventricular septal defect
- ☐ **b.** Recurrent infarction
- ☐ **c.** Aortic regurgitation
- ☐ **d.** Heart failure
- ☐ **e.** Dressler's syndrome

Extended Matching Questions

Lower gastrointestinal bleeding

a. Angiodysplasia
b. Osler–Weber–Rendu syndrome
c. Colorectal carcinoma
d. Internal haemorrhoids
e. Drug-induced bleeding
f. Mesenteric embolus
g. Inflammatory bowel disease
h. Diverticulitis
i. Inherited coagulopathy
j. Rectal polyp

The following patients have all suffered from bleeding from the lower gastrointestinal tract. Please choose the most correct diagnosis from the above list. Each option may be used once, more than once, or not at all.

61 A 43-year-old man presents with bright red rectal bleeding. He
☐ denies any pain and states that it came on suddenly, with no warning. He has not had any change in bowel habit and does not take any regular medication. Past medical history is remarkable for a total knee replacement 5 years ago and an inpatient admission under the ear, nose and throat (ENT) surgeons for a severe nose bleed as a child.

62 A 62-year-old woman presents with rectal bleeding on passing
☐ stools. Bleeding is seen on the toilet paper and in the toilet bowl. She states that she has had a few episodes of small fresh bleedings but denies any weight loss or diarrhoea. She describes a feeling of something descending in the rectum when she strains at stool and often feels the urge to defecate but without success. In fact, she suffers from constipation and is due to see her GP for a repeat prescription for senna and lactulose as she has run out.

63 A 67-year-old man presents with rectal bleeding with no warn-
☐ ing or associated change in bowel habit. He has experienced episodes of bleeding like this in the past, which usually settle on their own. Referred by his GP to hospital for the last serious episode of rectal bleeding, he underwent colonoscopy, which demonstrated a small vascular abnormality.

64 A 54-year-old man presents to the dermatology clinic with a history of multiple red lesions on his nose and around his mouth. He has been suffering recurrent nose bleeds intermittently since he was a child and has had the lesions as long as he can remember. Past medical history is remarkable only for an aspirin allergy that caused severe rectal bleeding. On examination, there are multiple, small red lesions that blanch on pressure distributed over the face, lips, nose and mouth.

65 A 67-year-old man collapses in the street and is brought to A&E. He has recently been started on digoxin and atenolol for an episode of shortness of breath and palpitations and was due for an anticoagulation clinic appointment to commence on warfarin. He complains of abdominal pain and rectal bleeding and had passed fresh blood per rectum in A&E. Clinically, he exhibits signs of shock and requires fluid resuscitation and blood transfusion.

Diseases of the hand

a. Dupuytren's contracture
b. Scleroderma
c. Paronychia
d. Nail bed haematoma
e. Radial nerve injury
f. Lower brachial plexus root injury
g. Ulnar nerve injury
h. Scaphoid fracture
i. Glomus tumour
j. Carpal tunnel syndrome
k. Ganglion cyst

The following patients have all presented with diseases of the hand. Please choose the most likely diagnosis from the above list. Each option may be used once, more than once, or not at all.

66 A 35-year-old keen gardener presents to her GP with a swollen left index finger. She states that it has caused her throbbing pain for the past 2 weeks and came on after she cut her finger on some rose thorns. There is swelling, redness and tenderness surrounding the nail itself on the left index finger only.

67 A 43-year-old man presents with an extremely painful mass under one of the nails of his right hand. He states that he has become more aware of the mass over the past month. There is a bluish hue to the mass with lifting of the nail bed.

68 A 31-year-old woman is brought in to A&E after cutting herself with a knife following a break-up with her partner. On examination of her hand, there are multiple lacerations on the wrist by the base of the thumb. She complains of an inability to extend her wrist.

69 A 13-year-old boy falls on to concrete while roller skating. He is seen by the out-of-hours GP and is found to have a tender swollen base of the thumb with tenderness in the anatomical snuffbox. He has weakness on making a pincer grip but has normal abductor pollicis brevis function.

70 A 54-year-old man who is seen regularly in the endocrinology clinic presents with the complaint that during the night he wakes up with tingling and numbness in his hands that is only relieved by shaking them out. On further questioning, he has otherwise been fit and well but states that in recent years he has gone up many shoe sizes and cannot now fit into his favourite hat.

Treatment of psychiatric disorders

a. Olanzapine
b. Sertraline
c. Cognitive behavioural therapy
d. Electroconvulsive therapy (ECT)
e. Eye movement desensitization and reprocessing (EMDR)
f. Temazepam
g. Reduction in caffeine intake
h. Haloperidol
i. Lithium

The following patients have all presented with a psychiatric disorder. Please choose the most appropriate treatment from the above list. Each option may be used once, more than once, or not at all.

71 A 34-year-old woman is brought to hospital by a friend who is concerned that recently she has been acting bizarrely, for example going on shopping trips every other day and spending money in the local betting shop, which she never used to do. She has also been socializing more often than usual and had been throwing house parties every weekend.

72 A 42-year-old aid worker presents to his GP with a 5-week history of inability to sleep, a feeling of being on edge and easily startled, and nightmares of persecution and violence. He had previously returned from an aid mission overseas where he had to be evacuated due to unsafe conditions.

73 A 24-year-old man who has recently arrived in the UK is referred to the acute psychiatric clinic by his GP who is concerned that he has been experiencing auditory hallucinations telling him that the immigration officials have been monitoring his activities and are planning to use him as a spy. He became agitated when confronted about these thoughts and claims that people are stealing ideas from his head.

74 A 43-year-old woman presents to her GP complaining of feeling a sense of overwhelming fear associated with shortness of breath and a racing heart beat when she is asked to give a presentation or speak in front of a large number of people. She says she does not take any illicit drugs and has been teetotal for years.

75 A 67-year-old woman is brought to A&E by her neighbour who
☐ has been increasingly worried about her behaviour. She is un-
kempt and was found by her neighbour at home in her chair
where she had not moved for 3 days. She has been on antidepressant medication in the past, started by her GP. Psychiatric
assessment in hospital revealed a low mood with deep suicidal
ideation and morbid delusions.

Causes of hepatomegaly

a. Congestive cardiac failure
b. Riedel's lobe
c. Gaucher's disease
d. Leukaemia
e. Metastatic disease
f. Hodgkin's disease
g. Viral hepatitis
h. Amyloid
i. Alcoholic hepatitis
j. Budd–Chiari syndrome

The following patients have all presented with hepatomegaly. Please choose the more correct diagnosis from the above list. Each option may be used once, more than once, or not at all.

76 A 45-year-old man is due to join a new company as a finance
☐ director. Prior to his contract starting, he has a medical check-up at his GP. He states that he feels in good health although he has been tired recently, which he attributes to the stress of changing firms. As part of the routine examination, he has blood tests and is examined clinically. On examination of the abdomen there is a 2-cm smooth and non-tender enlarged mass in the right upper quadrant. The rest of the examination is normal.

77 A 54-year-old patient, who has been seen regularly for many
☐ years in the rheumatology clinic for management of rheumatoid arthritis, presents to hospital with a 2-week history of lethargy, progressive shortness of breath and facial swelling. She has noticed a vague discomfort under her right ribs and states that she feels her body has become more swollen recently. Additionally, she has not been able to use her hands so much recently, although she is convinced that this is not due to her rheumatoid disease flaring up. Abdominal examination reveals mild tenderness in the flanks and a 3-cm smooth non-tender mass in the right upper quadrant.

78 A 73-year-old man presents to hospital complaining of an in-
☐ ability to open his bowels for the past 2 days. He states that he
has not been feeling bright for the past month and has been
feeling nauseated and anorexic. Further questioning reveals a
10-kg weight loss over the past 2 months and he puts this down
to not eating like he used to as a young man. On examination
of the abdomen, there is a 4-cm craggy non-tender liver edge.
Digital rectal examination reveals an empty rectum and a firm
3-cm poorly defined mass on palpation.

79 A 65-year-old woman presents to hospital with shortness or
☐ breath, reduced exercise tolerance and gross peripheral oedema.
Echocardiography a year ago confirmed a poorly functioning left
ventricle with an ejection fraction of 35% and right ventricle
hypertrophy. On examination of the cardiovascular system, she
has a raised JVP of 9 cm of H_2O, a third heart sound, systolic
murmur heard best at the right lower sternal edge and tachycardia with marked bilateral pitting oedema to the knee. Abdominal examination reveals a distended abdomen with a 3-cm
mildly tender liver edge.

80 A 45-year-old man presents to A&E with falls and confusion. He
☐ is admitted to the medical wards and started on Pabrinex and vitamin B12 by IV infusion and is written up for chlordiazepoxide
(Heminevrin) in a reducing dose over 4 days. On examination,
he is malnourished and there is a faint jaundice detectable in
the skin and sclera. Abdominal examination is difficult as the
patient is not co-operative but you notice there is pain in the
right upper quadrant and a very tender 2-cm smoothly enlarged
liver edge.

Substance abuse

    a. Cocaine
    b. Amphetamines
    c. Lysergic acid diethylamide (LSD)
    d. Phencyclidine (PCP)
    e. Benzodiazepines
    f. Opioids
    g. Alcohol
    h. Barbiturates
    i. Marijuana

The following patients have all presented with signs and symptoms of substance abuse. Please choose the most likely substance of abuse from the above list. Each option may be used once, more than once, or not at all.

81 A 43-year-old business man presents to hospital after going for some drinks with colleagues from work. He is restless, stating that he does not need to be in hospital and asking when he can go home. On examination, he is tachycardic at 120 bpm with dilated pupils. While you are examining him, he starts to have episodic chest pain.

82 A 52-year-old man is admitted to hospital as he was found wandering the streets confused and 'talking to himself'. He is well known to the local hospitals, attending frequently with malnutrition and chest infections. On examination, he has heavily injected conjunctivae, appears to be hearing voices and does not readily make eye contact. He is somnolent and exhibits a lack of interest in food or drink when brought to him.

83 A 62-year-old woman is brought to hospital having suffered a fall in the street. On arrival, she is disorientated and complaining of chest pain. An electrocardiogram (ECG) performed demonstrates a prolonged QT interval and U waves. On examination, she exhibits a lateral gaze palsy and is very unsteady on her feet.

84 A 32-year-old woman is found collapsed in a nearby residential estate and is brought to A&E. She is unconscious and paramedics are securing an endotracheal tube with 100% oxygen on arrival at hospital. Her blood pressure is 90/55 mmHg on her left arm and her temperature is 34.7°C. An ABG reading taken in hospital shows pH 7.31, pO_2 15 kPa and pCO_2 6.3 kPa.

85 A 17-year-old high-school student is brought to hospital by
☐ his parents who were concerned about his recent strange behaviour. He was found in his room unable to move his legs and
complaining that his room was all blurry. On arrival at hospital, he is sweating, agitated and violent with a blood pressure of
195/89 mmHg. Neurological examination reveals no pyramidal
abnormality but is remarkable for a florid vertical nystagmus.

Management of diarrhoeal illnesses

a. Oral metronidazole
b. Fluid rehydration and insulin infusion
c. Phosphate enema
d. Systemic steroids, with or without mesalazine
e. Carbimazole and beta-blockade
f. Synthetic pancreatic enzymes (Pancrex)
g. Oral rehydration therapy
h. Proton-pump inhibition, with or without endoscopy
i. Psychiatric counselling
j. IV cefuroxime and metronidazole

The following patients have all presented with diarrhoeal illnesses. Please choose the more correct diagnosis from the above list. Each option may be used once, more than once, or not at all.

86 A 26-year-old woman presents to A&E with increased stool frequency, passing up to six motions a day. She feels very weak and states that she has been passing blood mixed with the stool, mucus and loose stools since yesterday evening. She denies any recent foreign travel and has been married for the past 2 years with no extramarital partners. It is noted by an observant onlooker that she has a very tender red eye and, on review of systems, she complains of a pain in her knee that she has noticed over the past few days.

87 A 64-year-old man has been recently admitted to hospital with a chest infection and treated on IV clarithromycin and amoxicillin for suspected community-acquired pneumonia. A week into his course of antibiotics he started complaining to the nursing staff about an inability to hold his stool with faecal incontinence that he has never had before. The nursing staff note that the stools are offensive and slightly green tinged.

88 A 32-year-old known diabetic presents to hospital complaining of polyuria, polydipsia, diarrhoea and fatigue. He had recently come back from a backpacking holiday in Europe and thinks he may have caught something there as he has been exhibiting coryzal features and a productive cough of green sputum for the past 3 days. Blood glucose measurement shows a glucose of 27.6 g/dL with significant dehydration, ketones ++ in the urine with a venous gas measurement recording pH 7.31 and a slightly reduced bicarbonate.

89 A 45-year-old man presents to his GP complaining of recent
☐ changes in his weight, mood and bowel habit. He has noticed
that over the past few months he has become increasingly heat
intolerant such that taking his son sledging in the snow caused
him to sweat profusely and he could wear no more than a pair
of shorts and a t-shirt. His wife states he has lost about 6 kg of
weight over the past month and he attributes this to regular
bouts of loose stools up to five times a day over the same period.

90 A 16-year-old girl is brought to hospital by her mother with di-
☐ arrhoea and recent rapid weight loss. Her mother tells you that
she has noticed that her daughter has become more withdrawn
at school and has been spending more time in her room these
days. When enquiring about eating habits, her mother states
that she has been eating good healthy amounts but is always
keen to leave the table when she is done and will not wait for
the rest of the family to finish. On examination, the girl is un-
derweight for her height and has noticeable blistering over the
knuckles on both hands. She has some soft swellings at the base
of the jaw and these are non-mobile and diffuse in character.

PAPER 3

Questions

Single Best Answer Questions

1 Which one of the following signs or symptoms is consistent with a *severe* asthma attack?

- ☐ **a.** Silent chest, peak expiratory flow rate (PEFR) <33% of predicted
- ☐ **b.** Tachycardia >110 beats/minute (bpm), PEFR <50% of predicted
- ☐ **c.** Exhaustion, hypotension
- ☐ **d.** $PaCO_2$ normal or high on arterial sampling
- ☐ **e.** Completing sentences, respiratory rate 15 breaths/minute

2 A 7-year-old boy is taken to hospital for excruciating sudden-onset lower abdominal pain and vomiting. His temperature is 38.0°C and he denies any diarrhoea. Examination of his ears, nose, throat and chest is normal. In this case, which one of the following must you be sure to check?

- ☐ **a.** Rovsing's sign
- ☐ **b.** Scrotal examination
- ☐ **c.** Rectal examination
- ☐ **d.** Full blood count
- ☐ **e.** Abdominal X-ray

3 A 33-year-old woman presents to hospital on return from a skiing holiday. Her ski got caught in the snow causing her to fall over and the ski did not release from her foot. You make a diagnosis of a ruptured Achilles tendon. What would be your management plan?

- ☐ **a.** Surgical Achilles tendon repair
- ☐ **b.** Above knee backslab
- ☐ **c.** Below knee cast with foot in neutral position
- ☐ **d.** Below knee cast with foot in equinus position
- ☐ **e.** Discharge with general practitioner (GP) follow-up

EMQs and SBAs for Medical Finals, Second Edition. Jonathan Bath,
Rebecca Morgan and Mehool Patel.
© 2011 John Wiley & Sons, Ltd. Published 2011 by John Wiley & Sons, Ltd.

4 An adolescent boy presents to his school doctor with bilateral tender and swollen breasts. He has become increasingly self-conscious of late and has been avoiding physical education classes. On examination, there are tender soft masses in the lower quadrants of both breasts. Which one of the following is the most appropriate next step in managing this patient?

- ☐ **a.** Urgent referral to social services
- ☐ **b.** Reassure the patient that this is normal
- ☐ **c.** Needle aspiration and send fluid for culture and cytology
- ☐ **d.** Referral to a breast surgeon for excision and biopsy
- ☐ **e.** Short course of oral prednisolone and 2-week review

5 A new non-invasive test for the influenza virus is produced by a pharmaceutical company based on a study of 1340 individuals The data are published in an infectious disease journal that you are reading in your spare time and is given in table format below:

	Disease	
Test	Positive	Negative
Positive	580	150
Negative	140	450

Which one of the following statements regarding statistical aspects of the new test is correct?

- ☐ **a.** The sensitivity of the test is $(580/(580 + 140)) = 80.1\%$
- ☐ **b.** The positive predictive value of the test is $580/(580 + 140) = 80.1\%$
- ☐ **c.** There were 150 false negatives in the test
- ☐ **d.** A high specificity will predict a low false-negative rate
- ☐ **e.** This test should be used as a screening test for influenza?

6 Two hours after a football game in which a 34-year-old man was struck with the ball in the groin, he is brought to hospital with a swelling in the scrotum that has not resolved with application of an ice-pack. On examination there is a small, hard lump in the right testis with the left testis lying slightly higher than the right. The testicular adnexae are firm but non-tender. These findings are suggestive of:

- ☐ **a.** Torsion of the hydatid of Morgagni
- ☐ **b.** Epididymo-orchitis
- ☐ **c.** Testicular cancer
- ☐ **d.** Spermatocele
- ☐ **e.** Scrotal haematoma

7 A 57-year-old woman complains of acute-onset shortness of breath. She suffers from well-controlled asthma. Which one of the following is NOT a reasonable differential diagnosis for an acute exacerbation of asthma?

☐ **a.** Anaphylaxis
☐ **b.** Pneumothorax
☐ **c.** Upper respiratory tract obstruction
☐ **d.** Massive pulmonary embolus
☐ **e.** Upper respiratory tract infection

8 A 43-year-old man comes to hospital with severe pain and tenderness in the left flank. A provisional diagnosis of ureteric obstruction by a renal calculus is made. An intravenous urogram (IVU) taken shortly after admission to hospital would be most likely to show:

☐ **a.** Reduced size of left kidney
☐ **b.** Reduced size of right kidney
☐ **c.** Perfusion defect in the left pelvicalyceal region
☐ **d.** Bladder residual post-micturition
☐ **e.** Delayed excretion by left kidney

9 A 72-year-old Afro-Caribbean man presents to his GP after problems initiating micturition. He has taken to wearing a pad during the day and finds that he has to use the toilet frequently at night, with occasional urinary accidents and post-void dribbling. Which one of the following should be performed as a first line?

☐ **a.** Suprapubic catheterization
☐ **b.** Blood glucose evaluation
☐ **c.** Anti-dsDNA antibody evaluation
☐ **d.** Prostate-specific antigen (PSA) evaluation
☐ **e.** Ultrasound scan of the renal tract

10 A 43-year-old man presents to his GP with a 1-week history of a painful swollen left knee. On examination, the left knee is painful in all ranges of movement and is warm to touch. There is evidence of a boggy diffuse swelling and routine blood tests reveal a neutrophilia, raised white cell count and pyrexia. Which one of the following investigations is the most important to perform?

☐ **a.** Blood cultures
☐ **b.** Joint aspiration
☐ **c.** Serum urate levels
☐ **d.** Magnetic resonance imaging (MRI) knee
☐ **e.** Skyline views of the knee

11 A 25-year-old woman presents to Accident and Emergency (A&E) after a sudden onset of shortness of breath. She has a past medical history of asthma and dysmenorrhoea and takes the oral contraceptive pill regularly. On examination, she is a tall thin woman, tachypnoeic, and has a pulse of 122 bpm, blood pressure of 94/56 mmHg and a raised jugular venous pressure (JVP). Electrocardiography (ECG) demonstrates sinus tachycardia. Which one of the following options is the most appropriate?

☐ **a.** Carotid massage with cardiac monitoring

☐ **b.** Needle aspiration in the second intercostal space anterior chest

☐ **c.** Slow intravenous (IV) frusemide infusion

☐ **d.** Computed tomography (CT) scan with pulmonary angiography

☐ **e.** IV heparin

12 In patients with tibial plateau fractures, which one of the following nerves is most likely to be damaged as a result of the injury?

☐ **a.** Common peroneal nerve

☐ **b.** Tibial nerve

☐ **c.** Sciatic nerve

☐ **d.** Femoral nerve

☐ **e.** Lateral cutaneous nerve of thigh

13 Which one of the following is NOT a true cause of haematuria?

☐ **a.** Glomerulonephritis

☐ **b.** Ureteric stone

☐ **c.** Schistosomiasis

☐ **d.** Rifampicin

☐ **e.** Malaria

14 A 31-year-old woman is admitted to hospital with nausea, bilious vomiting and generalized abdominal pain. She has previously undergone a laparoscopic bilateral tubal ligation. Abdominal X-ray performed on admission demonstrates dilated loops of the small bowel. Which one of the following is the most likely cause of the radiological findings?

☐ **a.** Meckel's diverticulum

☐ **b.** Intussusception

☐ **c.** Adhesions

☐ **d.** Stricture due to ulcerative colitis

☐ **e.** Gastrocolic fistula due to Crohn's disease

15 An 87-year-old man is admitted to hospital for shortness of breath and coughing up blood-stained sputum. A chest radiograph demonstrates a ring-shadow in the right upper lobe with histological diagnosis of cancer. One of the daughters approaches you and urges you not to inform her father of the cancer diagnosis. Which one of the following is the correct course of action?

☐ **a.** Comply with her wishes to not let her father know the diagnosis on grounds of compassion

☐ **b.** Only disclose the diagnosis to the father is he asks directly

☐ **c.** Allow the grieving period to come to a close and let his GP break the diagnosis once out of hospital

☐ **d.** State that you understand the delicate situation but inform the patient of his diagnosis if he wishes, as it is his right to know

☐ **e.** Ask the family to break the diagnosis to their father at an appropriate time

16 A 73-year-old woman presents to the on-call surgical team complaining of right-sided abdominal pain radiating down to the groin. On examination, she has tenderness on palpation of the renal angle. Urine dipstick is positive for leucocytes, nitrites, glucose and blood. Observations include a temperature of 38.3°C, heart rate of 106 bpm and blood pressure of 98/64 mmHg. Which one of the following is the most appropriate management for this patient?

☐ **a.** Oral antibiotics and follow-up with her GP

☐ **b.** IV antibiotics and IV fluids

☐ **c.** Catheterization

☐ **d.** Prescription for oral analgesia

☐ **e.** Diuretics and IV fluids

17 A 34-year-old man is brought in by his colleagues with acute dyspnoea. Regular medications include salbutamol inhaler and antihistamines for allergic rhinitis. On examination, there is evidence of stridor and some peri-oral swelling. What is the most important next step in managing this patient?

☐ **a.** Nebulized salbutamol

☐ **b.** Intramuscular (IM) adrenaline

☐ **c.** IV hydrocortisone

☐ **d.** Insertion of a laryngeal mask airway

☐ **e.** Endotracheal intubation

18 A 27-year-old man has injured his left hand by punching a wall following a fight with his girlfriend. He notes that the hand is swollen and he is not quite able to form a fist due to the pain and swelling. Neurovascular supply is intact. X-ray shows a mid-shaft 5th metacarpal fracture that appears to be rotated on the true lateral view. How would you manage this case?

☐ **a.** Below elbow backslab and clinic follow-up
☐ **b.** Sling for support and outpatient physiotherapy
☐ **c.** Admit for open reduction and internal fixation of fracture
☐ **d.** Admit for analgesia and physiotherapy
☐ **e.** GP review in 1 week

19 In estimating the prevalence of disease in a small town, the public health statistician gathers population data, including epidemiological data regarding the number of cases and deaths over the past year. There are currently 20 000 people who suffer from a disease. There were 250 deaths over the past year attributed to this disease and 500 new cases were diagnosed in the same period. Information regarding deaths was further broken down into those occurring due to natural causes and those due to violent crime or homicide, of which there were 135 and 28, respectively. The population of the town is estimated from voting records to be 140 000. Which one of the following correctly describes the prevalence of the disease?

☐ **a.** 250/20 000
☐ **b.** 500/140 000
☐ **c.** 500/20 000
☐ **d.** 20 000/140 000
☐ **e.** 250/140 000

20 A 22-year-old man is brought into hospital following a high-speed road traffic accident where he is able to tell you that he was the driver. On initial assessment, he is found to have marked facial injury, chest injury consistent with steering wheel impact and multiple areas of subcutaneous emphysema. He is tachycardic, hypotensive with respiratory distress and further respiratory examination reveals a displaced trachea to the left side of the chest. Which of the following is the next step in management?

☐ **a.** Endotracheal intubation
☐ **b.** Needle thoracocentesis of the right chest
☐ **c.** Insert a nasopharyngeal airway
☐ **d.** Insert a chest drain with underwater seal
☐ **e.** Perform an emergency cricothyroidotomy

21 A 49-year-old man is involved in a high-speed road traffic accident where he was the passenger. He is complaining of a lot of left upper quadrant abdominal pain but has stable vital signs on presentation to A&E and is taken for a CT scan that demonstrates a shattered spleen with obvious free fluid in the abdomen, possible aortic injury just distal to the left subclavian artery and clear lung fields. In the CT scanner he becomes hypotensive with systolic blood pressure of 84 mmHg and complains of pain consistent with peritonitis on physical examination. Which of the following is the most appropriate next step?

- ☐ **a.** Exploratory laparotomy
- ☐ **b.** Thoracoabdominal incision
- ☐ **c.** Immediate angiography
- ☐ **d.** Immediate intubation in A&E
- ☐ **e.** Immediate infusion of cross-matched blood

22 Postoperatively, in the Intensive Care Unit (ICU), you are concerned that the patient in the previous question is oozing from the wound site and through all the injury dressings. A set of emergency blood tests for full blood count, biochemistry and coagulation screen taken prior to surgery is normal. Which one of the following is the correct course of action?

- ☐ **a.** Administration of 4 units of fresh frozen plasma and 2 pools of platelets
- ☐ **b.** Exploratory laparotomy to control bleeding
- ☐ **c.** Routine blood tests for coagulation screen and full blood count
- ☐ **d.** Administration of 4 units of packed red cells to replace loss
- ☐ **e.** Urgent haemophilia A and B screen with a 10-mg vitamin K injection

23 A 71-year-old woman is admitted for advanced stage cervical cancer. She is noted to have lower abdominal pain and confusion. Serum creatinine is elevated and a renal ultrasound has been ordered. What is the likely cause of her renal failure?

- ☐ **a.** Fluid dehydration from cancer cachexia
- ☐ **b.** Pyelonephritis
- ☐ **c.** Hypercalcaemic nephropathy
- ☐ **d.** External involvement of the urinary system
- ☐ **e.** Tumour lysis syndrome

24 Which one of the following would be most likely to be seen in association with acute pancreatitis?

- ☐ **a.** Jaundice
- ☐ **b.** Pseudocyst formation
- ☐ **c.** Hypercalcaemia
- ☐ **d.** Bowel necrosis
- ☐ **e.** Raised albumin

25 A 23-year-old man presents to hospital with back pain and trouble performing at his basketball practices. On examination, the only positive findings are of a reduced range of movement in back flexion and tenderness over the left Achilles tendon. Which one of the following diagnoses is correct?

- ☐ **a.** Early-onset rheumatoid arthritis
- ☐ **b.** Left-sided prolapsed lumbar disc
- ☐ **c.** Right-sided prolapsed lumbar disc
- ☐ **d.** Ankylosing spondylitis
- ☐ **e.** Facet-joint arthritis

26 A 63-year-old man presents with right-sided intermittent chest pain and shortness of breath. He has a past medical history of severe Parkinson's disease and is cared for by his wife. On auscultation, he has inspiratory crepitations at the right base but no other findings. Which one of the following is the most likely cause for his symptoms?

- ☐ **a.** Atypical pneumonia
- ☐ **b.** Aspiration pneumonia
- ☐ **c.** Reflux disease
- ☐ **d.** Levodopa toxicity
- ☐ **e.** Parkinson's disease associated heart failure

27 Which one of the following causes of scrotal swellings is painless?

- ☐ **a.** Torsion of the testis
- ☐ **b.** Epididymis
- ☐ **c.** Testicular cancer
- ☐ **d.** Orchitis
- ☐ **e.** Hydrocele

28 A 65-year-old known diabetic recently diagnosed with chronic renal failure presents to his GP with acute onset of pain, reduced sensation and a pale right leg. On examination, the skin on his leg is cool and the pallor is emphasized by raising his leg. These symptoms and signs are characteristic of which one of the following conditions?

☐ **a.** Arterial occlusion
☐ **b.** Venous insufficiency
☐ **c.** Cellulitis
☐ **d.** Reduced circulating volume
☐ **e.** Vasculitis

29 A patient with longstanding lung fibrosis is admitted for assessment of increasing levels of home oxygen. An arterial blood gas (ABG) taken on 35% oxygen via facemask shows: pH 7.41, PaO_2 11.1 kPa, $PaCO_2$ 5.4 kPa, bicarbonate 26 mmol/L. Which one of the following is most appropriate in this case?

☐ **a.** Reduce oxygen to 28% and repeat ABG
☐ **b.** Increase oxygen to 40% and repeat ABG
☐ **c.** 35% is adequate oxygen for this patient
☐ **d.** Increase oxygen to 60% and reassess
☐ **e.** Repeat ABG measurement on air

30 A 58-year-old man was admitted to hospital complaining of lower back pain. He was afebrile and had a limited straight leg raise to 30 degrees. Hip movements were good bilaterally. X-rays of his lumbar spine revealed no cause for his symptoms. His past medical history includes a pneumonectomy for a malignant mesothelioma. Which one of the following investigations will provide the best diagnostic information?

☐ **a.** Blood cultures
☐ **b.** Bone scan
☐ **c.** MRI spine
☐ **d.** Lumbar puncture
☐ **e.** CT spine

31 A 24-year-old man is brought in to A&E by ambulance following a road traffic accident. He is confused and combative with a Glasgow Coma Scale (GCS) of 11/15. A CT scan of chest, abdomen and pelvis is performed, revealing multiple long bone and rib fractures and a small amount of free fluid in the abdomen and pelvis. Clinically, he is globally tender over the abdomen with a blood pressure of 90/60 mmHg and pulse of 120 bpm. Which one of the following is the correct next step in management?

☐ **a.** Urgent orthopaedic referral to exclude fat embolus
☐ **b.** IV noradrenaline for hypotension
☐ **c.** Rapid sequence intubation and ventilation
☐ **d.** Emergency exploratory laparotomy
☐ **e.** Fluid resuscitation and repeat urgent CT abdomen

32 You review a 76-year-old man who has the following clinical signs: unilateral ↓ chest expansion, ↓ breath sounds, ↓ percussion note. Which one of the following clinical conditions would provide these clinical signs?

☐ **a.** Pneumothorax
☐ **b.** Fibrosis
☐ **c.** Consolidation
☐ **d.** Pleural effusion
☐ **e.** Extensive collapse/lobectomy/pneumonectomy

33 A 51-year-old woman presents to A&E with episodes of coughing up blood over a 2-week period. Further questioning reveals a history of weight loss, frequent cough and a feeling of tiredness and malaise. Routine blood tests taken in hospital reveal: erythrocyte sedimentation rate (ESR) 70 mm/hour, sodium 135 mmol/L, potassium 5.3 mmol/L, creatinine 167 μmol/L, urea 9.3 mmol/L, haemoglobin 10.2 g/dL and a mild neutrophilia. Which one of the following investigations is most likely to be positive?

☐ **a.** Antineutrophil cytoplasmic antibody (ANCA)
☐ **b.** Antiglomerular basement membrane
☐ **c.** Anti-Scl 70
☐ **d.** Antimitochondrial antibodies
☐ **e.** Rheumatoid factor

34 A 56-year-old man is seen by his GP for a single episode of haematuria. His GP decides to refer him to the urologist for cystoscopy. What is the most likely cause of this man's haematuria?

- [ ] **a.** Prostate cancer
- [ ] **b.** Bladder cancer
- [ ] **c.** Renal cell carcinoma
- [ ] **d.** Benign prostatic hypertrophy
- [ ] **e.** Prostatism

35 A 37-year-old woman is admitted to hospital at 2 a.m. following a fall out of her first-floor bedroom window. The circumstances surrounding the accident are unclear but on arrival to hospital she is immobilized in a hard collar and sandbags and has a GCS of 15. Her injuries include a left-sided distal radial fracture and a fractured left iliac wing. She denies any pain in her thoracic and lumbar spine during a log roll examination and a rectal examination is found to be unremarkable. Examination of her cervical spine elicits no bony tenderness and good flexion and extension without development of any paraesthesia or pain. Antero-posterior, lateral and peg views of her cervical spine show no evidence of any fractures, subluxations or dislocations. How should we proceed?

- [ ] **a.** Remove hard collar and three-way immobilization
- [ ] **b.** Keep only hard collar on
- [ ] **c.** Keep hard collar and three-way immobilization *in situ* and organize CT of the cervical spine to confirm the X-ray findings
- [ ] **d.** Remove hard collar but organize CT of cervical spine urgently
- [ ] **e.** Get flexion and extension cervical spine views.

36 Which of the following flow volume loops would represent a normal appearance?

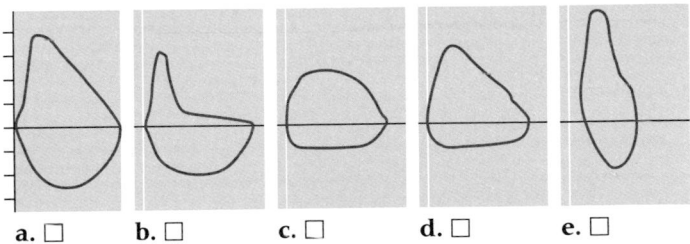

a. ☐   b. ☐   c. ☐   d. ☐   e. ☐

37 A 48-year-old ex-secretary presents to clinic with a 2-week history of tingling over her fingers and hands and numbness over the palms of her fingers and thumbs, apart from the little fingers on both hands. On examination, there are multiple bilateral joint deformities and tapping over the volar aspect of the wrist exacerbates her symptoms. Which one of the following management options should be considered next?
- ☐ **a.** Intra-articular steroid injection
- ☐ **b.** Carpal tunnel decompression
- ☐ **c.** Nerve conduction studies
- ☐ **d.** Plain radiographs of both wrists/hands
- ☐ **e.** Wrist splinting

38 A 75-year-old woman presents with abdominal pain and confusion. Creatinine is 457 μmol/L, sodium 140 mmol/L and potassium 4.7 mmol/L. She is catheterized and has been anuric for the past 12 hours. An urgent ultrasound scan of the kidneys and bladder reveals hydroureter and hydronephrosis with 40 ml bladder volume. Which one of the following is the most appropriate next step?
- ☐ **a.** Insertion of suprapubic catheter
- ☐ **b.** 5-day course of IV cefuroxime
- ☐ **c.** 3 L of IV fluids over 12 hours
- ☐ **d.** Urgent decompressive bilateral nephrostomy
- ☐ **e.** Urgent renal referral with dialysis

39 Which one of the following signs is NOT an early sign of compartment syndrome?
- ☐ **a.** Pain in the affected limb on passive movements
- ☐ **b.** Pallor
- ☐ **c.** Tension of the muscle group
- ☐ **d.** Loss of pulse
- ☐ **e.** Paraesthesiae

40 A 67-year-old diabetic man complains of abdominal pain after eating. Over the past few months he has lost approximately 7 kg, which he attributes to a reduced appetite due to fear of the ensuing pain after eating. Examination of his vascular system reveals absent distal pulses bilaterally in both legs. Which of the following is most likely to be the cause of his problem?
- ☐ **a.** Neoplastic
- ☐ **b.** Inflammatory
- ☐ **c.** Congenital
- ☐ **d.** Psychogenic
- ☐ **e.** Ischaemic

41 A research fellow is assessing the effectiveness of a new surgical therapy for melanoma and recruits newly diagnosed melanoma sufferers to the study. He randomizes the total participants to either the existing treatment or the novel treatment arm and performs the standard operation for melanoma excision on the first group ($n = 420$). He also performs the newly proposed therapy on the second group ($n = 390$). The treatment arms are double-blinded (both to him and the patients). Six months after the surgery the patients are seen in clinic to assess for recurrence rates. The following data are obtained:

	Disease present	Disease absent
Standard treatment	80	340
Novel treatment	60	330

Which one of the following investigations would be the most suitable for investigating the effect of the novel treatment?
- ☐ **a.** Mann–Whitney U test
- ☐ **b.** Paired *t*-test
- ☐ **c.** Positive-predictive value
- ☐ **d.** Odds ratio
- ☐ **e.** Chi-squared test

42 A 78-year-old man with no history of respiratory disease is diagnosed with a community-acquired pneumonia. Which one of the following is the commonest cause of a community-acquired pneumonia?
- ☐ **a.** *Haemophilus influenzae*
- ☐ **b.** *Mycoplasma*
- ☐ **c.** *Moraxella catarrhalis*
- ☐ **d.** *Streptococcus pneumoniae*
- ☐ **e.** *Staphylococcus aureus*

43 Which one of the following is NOT associated with the Glasgow criteria for predicting the severity of acute pancreatitis?
- ☐ **a.** pO_2 <8 kPa
- ☐ **b.** Glucose >10 mmol/L
- ☐ **c.** Urea <10 mmol/L
- ☐ **d.** Age >55 years
- ☐ **e.** Albumin <32 g/L

44 Following a motorbike accident, a 38-year-old man complains of shoulder pain. Other injuries include abrasions over his shins and face but no fractures. He is reluctant to move his arm due to pain and it is being held in internal rotation. Antero-posterior X-ray views show no obvious fractures or displacement. What should be the next step in your management or investigation of this man?

- ☐ **a.** Apply a broad arm sling and regular analgesia
- ☐ **b.** Request a lateral X-ray of the shoulder
- ☐ **c.** Ultrasound shoulder to investigate for a soft tissue injury
- ☐ **d.** Fracture clinic appointment in a couple of days
- ☐ **e.** Shoulder arthroscopy to investigate for rotator cuff injury

45 Assuming no contraindications, which one of the following antimicrobials would be the most appropriate choice for a community-acquired pneumonia?

- ☐ **a.** Erythromycin
- ☐ **b.** Cefalexin
- ☐ **c.** Amoxicillin
- ☐ **d.** Co-amoxiclav
- ☐ **e.** Metronidazole

46 Which one of the following relationships is correct?

- ☐ **a.** Femoral hernia – high incidence of strangulation in females
- ☐ **b.** Ventral hernia – most common in neonates
- ☐ **c.** Direct hernia – herniates into the scrotal sac
- ☐ **d.** Pantaloon hernia – hernia protrudes either side of femoral artery
- ☐ **e.** Indirect hernia – herniates through the superficial ring only

47 Which one of the following modalities represents the most useful indicator of the severity of disease in a rheumatoid arthritis sufferer?

- ☐ **a.** Serial radiographs of hands and wrists
- ☐ **b.** Commencement of biological agents
- ☐ **c.** Ability to dress and care for oneself
- ☐ **d.** Number of visits to hospital
- ☐ **e.** Length of treatment with steroids

48 A 70-year-old man, recently returned from holiday, presents with flu-like symptoms. He is becoming increasingly short of breath and his chest X-ray shows a bi-basal consolidation. Which one of the following organisms is most likely to be the causative agent?

☐ **a.** *Legionella*
☐ **b.** *Mycoplasma pneumoniae*
☐ **c.** *Chlamydia pneumoniae*
☐ **d.** *Pneumococcus*
☐ **e.** *Staphylococcus aureus*

49 You are on call and are asked to review an X-ray by A&E staff. The patient is an 8-year-old child who has banged her elbow on a door frame. She has mild bruising and swelling over the affected elbow but a good range of movement. Which one of the following growth plates would you expect still to be visible on her elbow X-ray?

☐ **a.** Capitulum and lateral epicondyle only
☐ **b.** Medial and lateral epicondyles only
☐ **c.** Trochlear, olecranon and lateral epicondyle
☐ **d.** Capitulum and trochlear
☐ **e.** Olecranon, lateral and medial epicondyles

50 A 37-year-old man presents to A&E complaining of the worst groin pain that he has ever experienced. He does not have fever and thinks the pain may be due to a football-related injury. He is unable to sit down during the consultation and walks around constantly. The pain is worse on urinating and is only on the left side. Dipstick reveals microscopic haematuria. What is the most likely diagnosis?

☐ **a.** Pyelonephritis
☐ **b.** Bladder cancer
☐ **c.** Ureteric calculus
☐ **d.** Renal cell carcinoma
☐ **e.** Prostatism

51 A 75-year-old man undergoes a cholecystectomy for recurrent bouts of gallstones. Ten days after the surgery, he develops pain and swelling of the right parotid gland. Which one of the following is most likely to be the cause of the parotid swelling?

☐ **a.** Haemorrhage into the parotid gland
☐ **b.** *Staphylococcus aureus* infection
☐ **c.** Trauma to the gland during surgery
☐ **d.** Stone formation and obstruction of the parotid duct
☐ **e.** Mumps infection

52 A 32-year-old woman presents to hospital with sudden-onset weakness in her left leg and arm, with an obvious facial droop on the left hand side. Past medical history is remarkable only for four miscarriages and peptic ulcer disease. Which one of the following is the most likely diagnosis?

- ☐ **a.** Systemic sclerosis
- ☐ **b.** Marfan's syndrome
- ☐ **c.** Dermatomyositis
- ☐ **d.** Antiphospholipid syndrome
- ☐ **e.** Reiter's syndrome

53 A 67-year-old woman recently completed a course of antibiotics for a hospital-acquired pneumonia. She has developed a swinging fever and still has a productive cough with foul-smelling sputum. She notes occasional haemoptysis. Chest X-ray shows a walled cavity. Which one of the following is the most likely diagnosis?

- ☐ **a.** Lung cancer
- ☐ **b.** Pulmonary embolus
- ☐ **c.** Recurrent infection
- ☐ **d.** Lung abscess
- ☐ **e.** Empyema

54 A 37-year-old man is a driver involved in a road traffic accident. On examination, he is found to have point tenderness over the lower left ribs and tachycardia and falling blood pressure, among other signs of hypovolaemic shock. Breath sounds are normal bilaterally. These findings are most likely to be due to which one of the following?

- ☐ **a.** Rupture of liver capsule
- ☐ **b.** Rupture of spleen
- ☐ **c.** Cardiac contusions
- ☐ **d.** Abdominal aortic transection
- ☐ **e.** Haemothorax secondary to pulmonary contusions

55 A 36-year-old woman presents to her GP with widespread muscle aches, left-sided chest pain and cough, and a rash on her face that has appeared over the past month. She is a known epileptic and has been taking medication for many years. Which one of the following medications is NOT associated with drug-induced lupus?

- ☐ **a.** Isoniazid
- ☐ **b.** Hydralazine
- ☐ **c.** Phenytoin
- ☐ **d.** Procainamide
- ☐ **e.** Prednisolone

56 A 58-year-old man is referred to A&E with recurrent pneumonia. He has been complaining of a persistent cough for 2 weeks with copious sputum and occasional haemoptysis. An erect chest X-ray shows cystic shadows. Which one of the following is the most likely diagnosis?

- ☐ **a.** Lung cancer
- ☐ **b.** Bronchiectasis
- ☐ **c.** Pulmonary fibrosis
- ☐ **d.** Pneumonia
- ☐ **e.** Pulmonary embolus

57 An otherwise fit and well 41-year-old woman sustained an ankle fracture by falling over at home and she thinks that she may have inverted her ankle. She can dorsiflex her foot to 90 degrees and plantarflex to 30 degrees but all movements are painful. X-rays show an isolated fracture of the distal fibula above the syndesmosis with no talar shift. Which of the following is the most appropriate management of this injury?

- ☐ **a.** Apply a backslab to the leg and give regular analgesia
- ☐ **b.** Admit for internal fixation
- ☐ **c.** Place in a walking cast
- ☐ **d.** Apply a cylinder cast and bring back to fracture clinic
- ☐ **e.** Discharge with crutches for 6 weeks

58 You are asked to review a chest X-ray for a colleague. You notice a round opacity which of the following is NOT one of your differential diagnoses?

- ☐ **a.** Tuberculosis
- ☐ **b.** Aspergilloma
- ☐ **c.** Lung cancer
- ☐ **d.** Sarcoidosis
- ☐ **e.** Carcinoid tumour

59 Regarding antiphospholipid syndrome, which one of the following autoantibodies is most strongly associated with this condition?

- ☐ **a.** Anticardiolipin antibodies
- ☐ **b.** Antinuclear antibodies
- ☐ **c.** Antireticulin antibodies
- ☐ **d.** Anti-Ro antibodies
- ☐ **e.** ANCA

60 A 74-year-old man is 1 day post-transurethral resection of the prostate (TURP) for benign prostatic hyperplasia. On inspecting the catheter for potential blockage, it is discovered that there is a tight constricting band just proximal to the glans penis, which is swollen and pale. What abnormality does this man have?

- ☐ **a.** Phimosis
- ☐ **b.** Paraphimosis
- ☐ **c.** Epispadias
- ☐ **d.** Hypospadias
- ☐ **e.** Peyronie's disease

Extended Matching Questions

Shortness of breath
- **a.** Atelectasis
- **b.** Lung cancer
- **c.** Aspiration pneumonia
- **d.** Pneumothorax
- **e.** Exacerbation of asthma/chronic obstructive pulmonary disease (COPD)
- **f.** Pulmonary embolus
- **g.** Congestive cardiac failure
- **h.** Pleural effusion

For each of the following questions, please select the most suitable answer from the selection above. Each option may be used once, more than once, or not at all.

61 A postoperative patient is recovering from a total hip replacement. He has a history of COPD. He has developed a temperature of 38.5°C and has noticed a dry cough. What is the most likely cause for his shortness of breath?

62 You are called to a cardiac arrest. Review of the charts reveals that the patient has been on warfarin to treat a pulmonary embolus. Prior to arresting, he had complained of increasing shortness of breath but responded reasonably well to oxygen and bronchodilators. What is the likely cause for this man's demise?

63 You review an elderly patient on the ward. He appears to be slumped in his chair and has slurred speech. He has developed a cough and low-grade temperature. What is the most likely diagnosis in this case?

64 A 49-year-old woman with a 30-pack year history of smoking is referred to A&E as her GP is concerned she has a pleural effusion. This is confirmed on chest X-ray. What is the likely diagnosis?

65 A 74-year-old woman presents with dyspnoea, gradually worsening over the past few days. She admits a productive cough but no chest pain. She has not used her bronchodilators and inhaled steroids for 5 days. Examination reveals tachypnoea, widespread wheeze and crepitations in the left upper zone. What is the likely diagnosis?

Rheumatological conditions

a. Gout
b. Rheumatoid arthritis
c. Osteoarthritis
d. Pseudogout
e. Septic arthritis
f. Ankylosing spondylitis
g. Polymyalgia rheumatica
h. Psoriatic arthropathy

The following patients have all presented with rheumatological problems. Please choose the most correct diagnosis from the above list. Each option may be used once, more than once, or not at all.

66 A 27-year-old woman presents to her GP with pain and swelling □ in her joints, particularly the small joints of the hands. She has noticed this discomfort for the past month but has no other symptoms other than a bit of malaise and non-specific feeling of 'not being herself'. She had put these symptoms down to having a young child. She takes the combined oral contraceptive pill but no other medications and suffers from no other illnesses.

67 A 47-year-old builder complains of pain in his foot. On ex- □ amination, there is evidence of redness and discomfort in the right hallux, although there is no evidence of ulceration or skin changes. Social history reveals an intake of alcohol in the region of 40 units/week, often in binges, and a diet rich in red meat.

68 A 63-year-old woman returns to the rheumatology clinic with □ pain in the joints of the hands and some loss of function. The ring finger on her right hand has become shortened in length; all other fingers are normal although there is a degree of ulnar deviation. Current medications include topical steroids, tar and regular light therapy.

69 A 23-year-old man presents to his GP with an increasing pain □ in his lower back and stiffness that is worse in the mornings. He has noticed some intermittent pain in his knees and increasing pain in the soles of his feet towards the end of the day. Spine X-ray reveals squaring of the vertebrae.

70 A 74-year-old woman has suffered with increasing pain in her hip for a number of years, which she tolerates with non-steroidal anti-inflammatory drugs (NSAIDs). Recently, she has noticed squaring of the thumb joint on her left hand and the pain in her hip is becoming more problematic and more troublesome towards the end of the day.

Hip pain

  a. Irritable hip
  b. Fractured neck of femur
  c. Slipped upper femoral epiphysis
  d. Hip dislocation
  e. Peri-prosthetic fracture
  f. Congenital dislocation of the hip
  g. Perthes' disease
  h. Septic arthritis

For each of the following questions, please select the most suitable answer from the selection above. Each option may be used once, more than once, or not at all.

71 A 78-year-old overweight woman with a history of osteoarthritis of the right hip and a total hip replacement presents to A&E. She complains of pain on the lateral aspect of her right leg and in her right groin and has been unable to weight bear since the morning when she fell over and landed on her right hip. On examination, you note that her leg is shortened and internally rotated while being held in an adducted position. The neurovascular supply to the leg is intact.

72 A 7-year-old boy is referred to orthopaedics for hip pain, which has gradually developed over the past 4 hours. His mother notes that over the same time period he has developed a limp, is not keen on moving his leg and is insisting on being carried everywhere. Plain X-rays show no obvious problem and an ultrasound of the affected hip shows a collection of fluid. He is afebrile and otherwise well and his hip does not feel hot.

73 An 87-year-old nursing home resident sustained a fall a week ago and has complained of hip pain since. During the past week, he has been treated with regular analgesia and despite this has experienced difficulty in weight bearing due to pain. On examination, his GP noted that his leg was found to be shortened and externally rotated with tenderness on palpation of the groin and greater trochanter. Straight leg raise was limited due to pain and internal rotation caused severe pain.

74 A 49-year-old woman presents to A&E 6 weeks after insertion
☐ of a hip resurfacing prosthesis. She describes the hip as 'not ever
being quite right' since the operation. In the 2 days prior to presentation, she noticed increasingly bad pain in her right hip (the
same side as prosthesis) that radiates into her groin. The pain is
preventing her from weight bearing; while lying supine all hip
movements are possible passively to some degree, although they
are limited by pain.

75 A 78-year-old man complains of left-sided hip pain for the past
☐ 6 hours that is becoming increasingly painful to the point that
he is unable to weight bear. He has a fever of 38°C, with pain
on palpation of the hip joint and virtually no movement in any
direction in the hip. Past medical history includes a right total
hip replacement 3 years ago. He is referred to the on-call orthopaedic team and blood results show: white blood cell count
17.1×10^9/L, C-reactive protein 56 mg/L, ESR 24 mm/hour.
What is the likely diagnosis?

Causes of upper abdominal pain

a. Hepatitis
b. Cholecystitis
c. Cystic liver disease
d. Lower lobe pneumonia
e. Ruptured spleen
f. Diabetic ketoacidosis
g. Myocardial infarction (MI)
h. Subphrenic collection

The following patients have all presented with abdominal complaints. Please choose the most correct diagnosis from the above list. Each option may be used once, more than once, or not at all.

76 A 42-year-old haemophiliac presents to hospital with pain in the right upper quadrant and a mild yellow tinge to the skin. He complains of feeling nauseated with poor appetite and feels very tired at work. Examination reveals a smoothly enlarged tender liver edge 4 cm from the right costal margin.

77 A 63-year-old nursing home resident is brought in by ambulance to hospital as the nursing staff are worried that she has become increasingly confused with upper abdominal pain and fever. She is normally nil by mouth due to a stroke and fed via a percutaneous endoscopic gastrostomy (PEG) tube; however, one of the nursing staff had noticed some regurgitation of feeds earlier this week.

78 A 31-year-old man presents to A&E with severe upper abdominal pain. Focused history taking reveals he has recently suffered 'a bad cold' and has been not been able to take his regular medication recently due to feeling nauseated. From his medical notes he is under regular yearly review in the retinopathy eye clinic and is seen regularly by the renal physicians. Routine investigations reveal pH 7.21, PaO_2 14 kPa and $PaCO_2$ 3.8 kPa.

79 A 43-year-old woman is seen in the general surgery clinic and admitted to hospital with abdominal pain associated with vomiting and nausea. On examination, she is obese and has tenderness over the right upper quadrant. An ultrasound of the abdomen was requested and during the investigation she is noticed to catch her breath when the probe is placed over the right upper quadrant. Blood tests reveal a raised white cell count and C-reactive peptide.

80 A 64-year-old woman is 6 days post-laparoscopic liver cyst fen-
☐ estration. She is complaining of pain over the right upper quadrant and has been spiking fevers throughout the night. Over
the next couple of days she repeatedly develops high swinging
fevers and pain in the right shoulder tip.

Seronegative arthritides

a. Reiter's syndrome
b. Enteropathic arthropathy
c. Rheumatoid arthritis
d. Ankylosing spondylitis
e. Reactive arthritis
f. Scleroderma
g. Psoriatic arthropathy
h. Enthesopathy

The following patients have all presented with rheumatological problems. Please choose the most correct diagnosis from the above list. Each option may be used once, more than once, or not at all.

81 A 31-year-old business man presents to his GP complaining of
☐ an ache in his right knee with an inability to weight bear for the past week. He denies any history of trauma and recent travel history is remarkable only for a 12-hour flight to Thailand a few weeks previously. He denies any previous episodes of joint problems. On examination, he is reluctant to remove his trousers when examining the knee and you notice he has a very tender, sore left eye.

82 A 53-year-old man presents to the rheumatology clinic for reg-
☐ ular follow-up. He undergoes regular light therapy and his only medications are topical tar and ibuprofen for chronic back pain. On examination, he has pitting of his nails on two of the digits on one hand with an asymmetrical oligoarthritis affecting the small joints of both hands.

83 A 20-year-old man presents with a pain in his left foot associ-
☐ ated with walking and standing. He works in an office as a sales clerk and denies any particularly strenuous exercise recently. On examination, when asked to demonstrate the site of pain he has particular difficulty bending over to touch his foot. Further questioning reveals a similar episode of pain affecting the 'tendon at the back of his right ankle' last year.

84 A 22-year-old man presents to his GP with a 2-month history of pain and stiffness in his back associated with a reduced range of movement. He noticed this while stretching before a football game. He is anxious during the consultation and tells you that he is worried as he has been experiencing a tight sensation around his chest associated with pain that sometimes happens in the morning. Schober's test is markedly reduced.

85 A 34-year-old woman presents to hospital with multiple episodes of loose stools associated with some mucus and blood. History taking reveals a history of weight loss, fluctuating diarrhoea and previous hospital admission for a severely painful red eye. She has been investigated previously at her GP surgery for back pain and swollen joints.

Respiratory investigations

   a. Pulmonary function tests
   b. Chest X-ray
   c. ABG
   d. CT chest
   e. Ventilation–perfusion (V/Q) scan
   f. Computed tomographic pulmonary angiography (CT-PA)
   g. PEFR
   h. Full blood count

From the above list, please choose the most appropriate investigation for each of the scenarios below. Each option may be used once, more than once, or not at all.

86 A 17-year-old known asthmatic presents with acute-onset □ shortness of breath. She has never been hospitalized due to asthma. She usually takes regular salbutamol and beclomethasone inhalers.

87 A 76-year-old has been admitted to hospital with pneumonia. □ He has acutely desaturated to 85% but is not complaining of worsening shortness of breath. He had a chest X-ray earlier that day that showed a lobar pneumonia.

88 A 27-year-old with known Marfan's disease presents with new-□ onset shortness of breath. He denies a cough but has noticed a small amount of right-sided chest pain.

89 A 51-year-old has noticed a mild chest pain, which she thought □ would resolve with time. Two days later, the pain is worsening and she has developed shortness of breath. On examination, her saturations on room air are 89%, but her chest is clear.

90 A 41-year-old man is referred to the respiratory clinic for in-□ vestigation of his worsening dyspnoea and dry cough. In addition, clinically he has finger clubbing and fine end inspiratory crackles.

PAPER 4

Questions

Single Best Answer Questions

1 A 26-year-old man suffers a severe headache. The headache is the worst pain he has ever experienced. He also mentions that he feels unsteady and drunk. He describes the pain as being occipital in location, of rapid onset and continuous. There are no focal neurological signs. What is the next step in investigation of this man's headache?
- ☐ **a.** Magnetic resonance imaging (MRI) scan brain
- ☐ **b.** Computed tomography (CT) scan of head
- ☐ **c.** Lumbar puncture
- ☐ **d.** Blood cultures
- ☐ **e.** Admit for neurological observations and regular analgesia

2 A 31-year-old vegan woman attends her general practitioner (GP) practice complaining of fatigue. Her GP is concerned about her dietary content and requests blood tests. Which one of the following is NOT a recognized feature of iron-deficiency anaemia?
- ☐ **a.** Koilonychia
- ☐ **b.** Angular stomatitis
- ☐ **c.** Dysphagia
- ☐ **d.** Peripheral neuropathy
- ☐ **e.** Tongue atrophy

3 Which one of the following is NOT typically seen in nephrotic syndrome?
- ☐ **a.** Proteinuria
- ☐ **b.** Hypoalbuminaemia
- ☐ **c.** Oedema
- ☐ **d.** Hypercholesterolaemia
- ☐ **e.** Haematuria

EMQs and SBAs for Medical Finals, Second Edition. Jonathan Bath, Rebecca Morgan and Mehool Patel.

4 A 10-year-old boy presents to Accident and Emergency (A&E) with acute generalized abdominal pain and fatigue. A family history reveals a cousin that suffers from sickle cell disease. Which one of the following clinical features is NOT consistent with a diagnosis of sickle cell disease?

☐ **a.** Pallor

☐ **b.** Splenomegaly

☐ **c.** Bone pain

☐ **d.** Vesicular rash

☐ **e.** Gallstones

5 Relatives of a 70-year-old woman are concerned that she appears to be increasingly confused. Clinically, she has slurred speech, bilateral past pointing and trunkal ataxia with no evidence of nystagmus. Routine blood tests reveal no cause for these symptoms. Where is this woman's lesion most likely to be located?

☐ **a.** Bilateral basal ganglia

☐ **b.** Left temporo-parietal lobe

☐ **c.** Cerebellar vermis

☐ **d.** Left lateral cerebellar lobe

☐ **e.** Left-sided frontal lobe

6 A 4-year-old child is brought to his GP by his mother who is concerned about poor weight gain. He is at the 15th centile for height and weight and his past medical history includes admissions to hospital for recurrent chest infections and an episode of gastroenteritis. Developmental parameters are normal except for slightly reduced hearing in the right ear, which is slightly erythematous. Which one of the following pathologies is likely in this child?

☐ **a.** Periodic acid Schiff (PAS) positive macrophages on intestinal film

☐ **b.** Cobblestoned appearance on barium enema

☐ **c.** Single amino acid defect in a chloride-channel transporter

☐ **d.** Double bubble on abdominal X-ray

☐ **e.** Abnormal bone marrow cytology

7 A 45-year-old man with known chronic renal failure secondary to diabetic nephropathy presents to A&E with shortness of breath, cough productive of green sputum and swollen ankles. Routine biochemistry is taken and reveals worsening of renal failure with a potassium level of 6.8 mmol/L. Which one of the following treatment options for hyperkalaemia is correct as first-line therapy?

☐ **a.** Calcium resonium 15 g mixed with water
☐ **b.** Kayexalate
☐ **c.** Calcium gluconate, then insulin/dextrose infusion
☐ **d.** Haemodialysis
☐ **e.** Fluid restriction and potassium-poor diet

8 A 70-year-old man is admitted to hospital with new-onset left-sided weakness. He has a history of coronary artery disease, for which he takes warfarin, but examination reveals no other findings of note. Which one of the following investigations is the most important to obtain?

☐ **a.** Carotid duplex scan
☐ **b.** Echocardiogram
☐ **c.** CT scan of the brain
☐ **d.** International normalized ratio (INR)
☐ **e.** Electrocardiogram (ECG)

9 A 14-year-old girl presents to her GP distressed and upset. She tells you that she was in a relationship with an older boy and that they had been engaging in sexual intercourse. She has recently become worried that is pregnant as they have been having unprotected sex and an over-the-counter pregnancy test confirmed this. She begs you not to tell her mother and to refer her to a family planning clinic for an abortion. Which one of the following is NOT the correct course of action?

☐ **a.** Referral to a family planning clinic
☐ **b.** Counselling her about contraceptive options
☐ **c.** Offering her a sexually transmitted infection screen
☐ **d.** Informing her parents, as she is a legal minor
☐ **e.** Advocating her discussing the pregnancy with her parents

10 A 24-year-old woman presents with progressive seizure-like jerking movements of all extremities. On admission, her Glasgow coma score (GCS) is 14/15, as she is slightly confused. An MRI scan revealed areas of reduced density bilaterally at the basal ganglia. Routine blood tests revealed abnormal liver function tests (LFTs) but nothing else of note. Which one of the following is the most likely diagnosis?

☐ **a.** Early-onset Parkinson's disease
☐ **b.** Wilson's disease
☐ **c.** Glycogen storage disorder
☐ **d.** Porphyria
☐ **e.** Lead poisoning

11 A 5-year-old girl is brought to her GP as she has become increasingly tired and pale. She intermittently suffers with fevers that are not controlled with paracetamol. On clinical examination, she appears pale and has a widespread purpuric rash, which blanches on pressure. Blood tests reveal a low platelet count and a leucopenia. What is the most likely diagnosis in this case?

☐ **a.** Bacterial meningitis
☐ **b.** Acute lymphocytic leukaemia (ALL)
☐ **c.** Chronic myeloid leukaemia (CML)
☐ **d.** Acute myeloid leukaemia (AML)
☐ **e.** Viral encephalitis

12 A 34-year-old man presents to hospital with episodes of severe nose bleeds and of 'coughing up blood'. While taking a history, you notice that he has been gaining weight over the past month, producing small amounts of concentrated urine and has been experiencing progressive swelling of the ankles associated with itch. Which one of the following investigations is indicated in the first instance?

☐ **a.** Autoantibody screen
☐ **b.** Endoscopy
☐ **c.** Renal biopsy
☐ **d.** 24-hour urine protein collection
☐ **e.** Chest CT scan

13 Which of the following immunizations represents the correct combination that an infant should receive at 2 months of age according to the current UK schedule?
- ☐ **a.** Bacille Calmette Guerin (BCG)/*Haemophilus*/meningitis C
- ☐ **b.** Meningitis C/tetanus/*Haemophilus*/diphtheria
- ☐ **c.** Pertussis/tetanus/diphtheria/polio/measles, mumps and rubella (MMR)
- ☐ **d.** Diphtheria/tetanus/pertussis/*Haemophilus*/polio and pneumococcal
- ☐ **e.** Pneumococcal/meningitis C/diphtheria/tetanus/pertussis

14 A 50-year-old man presents with headache and tenderness over his scalp. Focused questioning reveals he also suffers with muscular aches and has been a bit slow of late. Which one of the following diagnoses is LEAST likely in this man?
- ☐ **a.** Superficial temporal arteritis
- ☐ **b.** Migraine
- ☐ **c.** Tension headache
- ☐ **d.** Viral meningitis
- ☐ **e.** Cluster headache

15 Regarding renal disease and urinalysis results, which one of the following associations is correct?
- ☐ **a.** Glucose – starvation
- ☐ **b.** Bilirubin – haemolytic anaemia
- ☐ **c.** Red cell casts – glomerulonephritis
- ☐ **d.** Cystine crystals – gout
- ☐ **e.** Nitrites – high-carbohydrate, low-protein diet

16 Which one of the following facts about chronic leukaemia is INCORRECT?
- ☐ **a.** Chronic lymphocytic leukaemia (CLL) is a chronic incurable condition
- ☐ **b.** Ionizing radiation is a known cause of CML
- ☐ **c.** CLL cells contain the Philadelphia chromosome
- ☐ **d.** Early disease prognosis for CLL is 8–10 years
- ☐ **e.** CLL is a malignant disease of B-lymphocytes.

17 A 30-year-old woman presents with a 24-hour history of worsening headaches. The headaches are constant, with no relieving factors and associated nausea. On examination, there are no peripheral neurological signs but you note papilloedema on fundoscopy. Which one of the following options is NOT a cause of this sign?

☐ **a.** Meningitis
☐ **b.** Benign intracranial hypertension
☐ **c.** Cerebellar haemangioblastoma
☐ **d.** Hyperparathyroidism
☐ **e.** Malignant hypertension

18 A 50-year-old man presents to his GP for an annual medical check-up. An elevated blood pressure and raised creatinine and urea are found. Renal ultrasonography is performed as an outpatient, the results of which demonstrate enlarged kidneys. Which one of the following conditions is NOT associated with renal enlargement?

☐ **a.** Amyloidosis
☐ **b.** Congenital single kidney
☐ **c.** Chronic renal failure
☐ **d.** Polycystic kidney disease
☐ **e.** Renal cell carcinoma

19 A 25-year-old man presents to his GP complaining of feeling very hot at night and of slight weight loss. Examination reveals a unilateral cervical mass. The mass is in the anterior compartment of the neck. It is not tethered to the skin and does not move on swallowing or protrusion of the tongue. What is the most likely diagnosis in this case?

☐ **a.** Hodgkin's lymphoma
☐ **b.** Sarcoidosis
☐ **c.** Tuberculosis
☐ **d.** Anxiety
☐ **e.** ALL

20 The daughter of an 81-year-old widower is concerned that he does not seem to be himself. She notes that he is becoming increasingly forgetful; for example, leaving the taps running or the oven on when it is not in use. In the case of Alzheimer's disease, which one of the following is INCORRECT?

☐ **a.** A CT brain scan will be normal
☐ **b.** Dysphasia may be the presenting feature
☐ **c.** Brisk reflexes and up-going plantars are often seen
☐ **d.** There may be a relevant family history
☐ **e.** Depression is commonly seen

21 A 13-year-old boy falls on to concrete while roller-skating. He is seen by the out-of-hours GP and is found to have a tender swollen base of the thumb with tenderness in the anatomical snuffbox. He has weakness on making a pincer grip but has normal abductor pollicis brevis function. Which one of the following is the most likely diagnosis?

- ☐ **a.** Paronychia
- ☐ **b.** Nail bed haematoma
- ☐ **c.** Radial nerve injury
- ☐ **d.** Lower brachial plexus root injury
- ☐ **e.** Scaphoid fracture

22 A 78-year-old woman is scheduled to have a low colonic resection for colonic carcinoma. Postoperatively, her urine output has been sluggish and blood results taken at the end of the second postoperative day demonstrate: urea 12.3 mmol/L and creatinine 172 μmol/L. Which one of the following is the most likely cause of renal failure in this woman?

- ☐ **a.** Analgesic nephropathy
- ☐ **b.** Dehydration
- ☐ **c.** Renal metastases
- ☐ **d.** Postsurgical rhabdomyolysis
- ☐ **e.** Urinary retention

23 A 36-year-old multiparous woman presents to the Emergency Gynaecology Unit after an episode of vaginal bleeding. She is 31 weeks' gestation and her vital signs are within normal limits and physical examination is unremarkable. Which one of the following is the most likely diagnosis?

- ☐ **a.** Cervical cancer
- ☐ **b.** Placenta praevia
- ☐ **c.** Abruptio placentae
- ☐ **d.** Placenta accreta
- ☐ **e.** Chorioamnionitis

24 A 31-year-old bank clerk presents with an acute-onset, sharp headache. She denies any history of trauma. Examination is unremarkable and observations are stable. Her GP refers her to the on-call medical team for review. Which diagnosis is her GP particularly concerned about?

- ☐ **a.** Bacterial meningitis
- ☐ **b.** Tension headache
- ☐ **c.** Subarachnoid haemorrhage
- ☐ **d.** Subdural haemorrhage
- ☐ **e.** Benign raised intracranial pressure

25 Which one of the following associations is INCORRECT?

- ☐ **a.** Trichomonas – yellow discharge
- ☐ **b.** Chlamydia – chronic cervicitis
- ☐ **c.** Gonorrhoea – urethritis
- ☐ **d.** *Gardnerella vaginalis* – white discharge
- ☐ **e.** Atrophic vaginitis – yellow discharge

26 Which one of the following statements about abdominal aortic aneurysm (AAA) is INCORRECT?

- ☐ **a.** More common in males than females.
- ☐ **b.** 10% have associated popliteal aneurysm
- ☐ **c.** A diameter >4 cm requires operative intervention
- ☐ **d.** Renal failure is a known postoperative complication of AAA repair
- ☐ **e.** 5% risk of rupture when aneurysm reaches 6 cm diameter

27 A 73-year-old woman with end-stage renal failure undergoes haemodialysis three times a week at a local satellite dialysis centre. Which one of the following complications has NOT been associated with long-term dialysis?

- ☐ **a.** Carpal tunnel syndrome
- ☐ **b.** Bleeding tendency
- ☐ **c.** Bone fractures
- ☐ **d.** Aluminium toxicity
- ☐ **e.** Reversal of renal function

28 A 20-week pregnant primigravida contacts her midwife for advice about a painful left leg. The leg began to swell 2 days earlier and is now painful to walk on. Clinically, there is a discrepancy of 7 cm between the diameter of both calves. What is the likely diagnosis in her case?

- ☐ **a.** Cellulitis
- ☐ **b.** Fat embolus
- ☐ **c.** Deep vein thrombosis
- ☐ **d.** Ischaemic limb
- ☐ **e.** Varicose veins

29 A 78-year-old woman has developed a facial asymmetry, which was not mentioned in her initial clerking. On your review, she notes that this has been there for some time and her GP was investigating the cause prior to her admission into hospital. Which one of the following is NOT known to cause a lower motor neurone facial weakness?

- ☐ **a.** Head injury
- ☐ **b.** Sarcoidosis
- ☐ **c.** Guillain–Barre syndrome
- ☐ **d.** Lyme disease
- ☐ **e.** Medullary infarction

30 A 23-year-old woman has attended A&E complaining of a high fever, diarrhoea and vomiting. She has noticed a headache and occasional muscle aches. Her menstrual cycle is regular, lasting for 5 days a month and her most recent period finished 5 days ago. On examination, she appears dehydrated and is hypotensive. What is the most likely diagnosis in her case?

- ☐ **a.** Viral gastroenteritis
- ☐ **b.** Bowel ischaemia
- ☐ **c.** Dysmenorrhoea
- ☐ **d.** Pregnancy
- ☐ **e.** Toxic shock syndrome

31 A 42-year-old woman presents to hospital with confusion and back pain. Past medical history reveals a modified radical mastectomy 3 years ago. Blood tests reveal a creatinine level of 192 μmol/L. Serum corrected calcium is 3.12 mmol/L. Metastatic malignancy is strongly suspected. Which one of the following investigations should NOT be performed immediately in the work-up?

- ☐ **a.** Staging contrast CT scan
- ☐ **b.** Liver ultrasound
- ☐ **c.** Breast examination
- ☐ **d.** Mammography
- ☐ **e.** Thoracic spine radiographs

32 A 14-year-old girl presents to her GP with severe cramping abdominal pain and bloody diarrhoea for the past 2 weeks. Oral ulcers are noted on examination, which are painful. Her family history includes a grandfather who had a colostomy for a gastrointestinal problem. What is the most likely cause for her symptoms and signs?

- ☐ **a.** Crohn's disease
- ☐ **b.** Ulcerative colitis
- ☐ **c.** Henoch–Schönlein purpura
- ☐ **d.** *Shigella* infection
- ☐ **e.** *Giardia* infection

33 You review a 25-year-old with headache. Clinically, these sound like tension headaches and neurological examination is perfectly normal apart from small pupils, which are equal and reactive to light and accommodation. In which one of the following conditions are small pupils characteristic?

- ☐ **a.** Holmes–Adie syndrome
- ☐ **b.** Acute retrobulbar neuritis
- ☐ **c.** Amitriptyline overdose
- ☐ **d.** Pontine haemorrhage
- ☐ **e.** Syphilis

34 A 70-year-old woman presents to her GP with vague aches and pains. Other symptoms include polyuria and constipation. An X-ray shows two crush fractures of her lumbar vertebrae. Blood tests taken show: calcium 2.96 mmol/L, phosphate 0.9 mmol/L and a normal albumin level. What is the likely diagnosis?

- ☐ **a.** Myeloma
- ☐ **b.** Myelofibrosis
- ☐ **c.** Myelodysplasia
- ☐ **d.** Adrenal tumour
- ☐ **e.** Prolapsed lumbar disc

35 A 17-year-old girl has lower abdominal pain, she has some associated nausea but no vomiting. She notes some dyspareunia and admits to having had unprotected sexual intercourse. She has a low-grade fever and confirms a smelly vaginal discharge. Which of the following is the most likely diagnosis in this case?

- ☐ **a.** Endometriosis
- ☐ **b.** Ruptured ovarian cyst
- ☐ **c.** Pelvic inflammatory disease
- ☐ **d.** Uterine fibroids
- ☐ **e.** Mittelschmerz pain

36 A 67-year-old woman is admitted under the care of the general surgeons with abdominal pain and vomiting. An intravenous (IV) contrast CT scan is arranged as an inpatient, which confirms the diagnosis of pancreatitis. Two days post-admission her creatinine is noted to have doubled. Which one of the following medications is likely responsible?

- ☐ **a.** Atenolol
- ☐ **b.** Metformin
- ☐ **c.** Simvastatin
- ☐ **d.** Paracetamol
- ☐ **e.** Aspirin

37 A 12-year-old boy presents to his GP with several days of generalized tiredness, painful joints (particularly the knees), nodular swelling over his elbows and associated low-grade fever with a mild rash on his chest. Weeks earlier he had complained of a sore throat that was managed supportively. Which of the following is the most likely diagnosis?

- ☐ **a.** Rheumatic fever
- ☐ **b.** Rheumatoid arthritis
- ☐ **c.** Reiter's syndrome
- ☐ **d.** Scarlet fever
- ☐ **e.** Systemic lupus erythematosus

38 A 79-year-old woman is seen by her GP for her annual blood tests. Her full blood count shows a macrocytic anaemia with a normal vitamin B12 and folate level, low platelet count and a neutropenia. Blood film showed abnormal looking cells. Bone marrow analysis confirms hypercellularity and dysplasia. What is the likely diagnosis in this case?

- ☐ **a.** Myeloma
- ☐ **b.** Myelofibrosis
- ☐ **c.** ALL
- ☐ **d.** CLL
- ☐ **e.** Myelodysplasia

39 A 65-year-old hypertensive patient has been referred with a spastic paraparesis. Which one of the following conditions would be consistent with that clinical finding?

- ☐ **a.** Neuropraxia
- ☐ **b.** Spondylosis of the lumbosacral spine
- ☐ **c.** Motor neurone disease
- ☐ **d.** Syringomyelia
- ☐ **e.** Meningioma

40 A 54-year-old man with a history of the nephrotic syndrome presents to A&E with abdominal pain and haematuria. The pain is in his left flank with radiation to the front and his face and legs have become swollen. Clinical examination reveals a very tender left flank with evidence of fullness in the same region. His blood pressure is 180/78 mmHg and a D-dimer of 7580 ng/mL. Which of the following is the most likely diagnosis?

☐ **a.** Pyelonephritis
☐ **b.** Addisonian crisis
☐ **c.** Pancreatitis
☐ **d.** Renal vein thrombosis
☐ **e.** Pulmonary embolus

41 Which one of the following facts about carcinoma of the cervix is INCORRECT?

☐ **a.** 90% are adenocarcinoma
☐ **b.** Associated with human papilloma virus
☐ **c.** Common presentation is intermenstrual vaginal bleeding
☐ **d.** Cervical erosions may be seen on speculum examination
☐ **e.** The disease may not present until the advanced stage

42 Which one of the following associations is INCORRECT?

☐ **a.** Hyponatraemia and central pontine myelinolysis
☐ **b.** Hyperthyroidism and tremor
☐ **c.** Hypernatraemia and seizures
☐ **d.** Hypoglycaemia and hemiparesis
☐ **e.** Hypercalcaemia and muscle cramps

43 A 5-year-old boy is brought to see his GP by his parents as they are concerned that he seems to tire easily and complains of pain in his legs. He prefers to stay indoor and watch television rather than playing outdoors with other children. On physical examination, he looks well. His blood pressure readings are discrepant in his right and left arms and his legs are mottled in colour. Which one of the following findings is UNLIKELY to be present in this boy?

☐ **a.** Reduced lower extremity pulses
☐ **b.** Cyanosis of the toes
☐ **c.** A bicuspid aortic valve on echocardiography
☐ **d.** Rib notching on chest X-ray
☐ **e.** Left ventricular hypertrophy on ECG

44 A 75-year-old woman presents to hospital with chest pain and mild shortness of breath. She describes a 3-day history of a cough productive of green sputum and is diagnosed with lower respiratory tract infection. Which one of the medications below is the most likely precipitant of deterioration in renal function?

- ☐ **a.** Amoxicillin
- ☐ **b.** Clarithromycin
- ☐ **c.** Paracetamol
- ☐ **d.** Diclofenac
- ☐ **e.** Sodium docusate

45 A 48-year-old man presents to his GP complaining of tiredness, headaches and visual disturbance. Having excluded any hard neurological symptoms, his GP organizes blood tests that show a haemoglobin level of 20 g/dL. He smokes 30 cigarettes a day and has done so for many years. Which one of the following is UNLIKELY to be the cause of his symptoms?

- ☐ **a.** Chronic obstructive pulmonary disease (COPD)
- ☐ **b.** Gaisbock's syndrome
- ☐ **c.** Polycythaemia rubra vera
- ☐ **d.** Dehydration
- ☐ **e.** Ischaemic heart disease.

46 A 97-year-old woman has been complaining of a cold, painful leg for the past 6 hours with mottled skin and absent pulses below the femoral artery on the affected side. Of note her past medical history includes atrial fibrillation for which she is not anticoagulated. What diagnosis was the GP concerned about in this woman?

- ☐ **a.** Buerger's disease
- ☐ **b.** Femoral artery embolus
- ☐ **c.** Arterial insufficiency
- ☐ **d.** Abdominal aortic aneurysm
- ☐ **e.** Venous ulceration

47 A 57-year-old man presents with reduced power in his dominant hand. Examination reveals no other neurological symptom apart from wasting and weakness in the thenar and hypothenar muscles of his affected hand. Which one of the following conditions would NOT account for these signs?

- ☐ **a.** Peripheral motor neuropathies
- ☐ **b.** Syringomyelia
- ☐ **c.** Ulnar nerve lesion at the elbow
- ☐ **d.** Amyotrophic lateral sclerosis
- ☐ **e.** Osteoarthritis of cervical and thoracic spine

48 A 58-year-old man who has been followed up in the renal clinic for chronic renal failure for many years is listed for cadaveric renal transplantation and managed expectantly with haemodialysis three times weekly. Which one of the following is an ABSOLUTE contraindication to renal transplantation?

☐ **a.** Severe depression
☐ **b.** Excised skin cancer
☐ **c.** Heart failure
☐ **d.** Recent urinary tract infection
☐ **e.** Chronic hepatitis C

49 Which one of the following physiological changes is well known to occur during pregnancy?

☐ **a.** Increase in cardiac output by 30%
☐ **b.** Increase in blood volume by 30%
☐ **c.** Slight drop in haemoglobin
☐ **d.** Increased oesophageal sphincter pressure resulting in heartburn
☐ **e.** Increased venous pressure in the pelvis

50 An 18-month-old boy has tetralogy of Fallot. His symptoms include irritability, cyanosis and tachypnoea. He has suffered one episode of syncope. Which one of the following is the best treatment for these episodes?

☐ **a.** Reassuring the parents that these episodes will resolve themselves
☐ **b.** Lifting the lower extremities above the level of the heart
☐ **c.** Dropping the legs off the side of the bed.
☐ **d.** Bringing his knees up to his chest
☐ **e.** Making the child adopt the Trendelenburg position

51 A 37-year-old man is brought in by ambulance to hospital after suffering an industrial accident where he was trapped underneath an iron girder. A radiographic screen of his limbs reveals bilateral complex fractures of tibia and fibula and extensive soft tissue swelling. Post-admission blood tests demonstrate deranged renal function with a creatinine level of 196 μmol/L and he is very oliguric. What is the most likely diagnosis?

☐ **a.** Renal contusion
☐ **b.** Rhabdomyolysis
☐ **c.** Cholesterol embolus
☐ **d.** Acute interstitial nephritis
☐ **e.** Urethral rupture

52 Regarding the above case, which of the following investigations would be most useful to perform next?
- ☐ **a.** Creatine kinase (CK)
- ☐ **b.** Renal ultrasound scan
- ☐ **c.** 24-hour urine protein collection
- ☐ **d.** Bence–Jones protein
- ☐ **e.** Renal artery Doppler scans

53 Which one of the following is NOT a risk factor for ectopic pregnancy?
- ☐ **a.** Pelvic inflammatory disease
- ☐ **b.** Pelvic surgery/adhesions
- ☐ **c.** Intrauterine contraceptive device (IUCD)
- ☐ **d.** Progesterone-only pill
- ☐ **e.** Previous Caesarean section

54 Which one of the following facts about Creutzfeldt–Jakob disease is INCORRECT?
- ☐ **a.** Caused by a slowly mutating virus
- ☐ **b.** A typical presentation would involve a progressive dementia
- ☐ **c.** Has been shown to be transmissible by surgery
- ☐ **d.** Rises from a conformational change in a prion protein
- ☐ **e.** Can be tested for with tonsil biopsies

55 Which of the following associations are INCORRECT?
- ☐ **a.** Crohn's disease and iron-deficiency anaemia
- ☐ **b.** Myelodysplasia and macrocytic anaemia
- ☐ **c.** Pregnancy and normocytic anaemia
- ☐ **d.** Thalassaemia and macrocytic anaemia
- ☐ **e.** Hypothyroidism and macrocytic anaemia

56 A 63-year-old man is admitted to hospital after suffering a transient ischaemic attack. On examination, he has no residual neurological findings and no cardiovascular findings of note. Which would be the most useful investigation in this scenario to determine the cause of the event?
- ☐ **a.** MRI scan brain
- ☐ **b.** Chest X-ray
- ☐ **c.** Abdominal ultrasound scan
- ☐ **d.** Carotid Doppler scan
- ☐ **e.** ECG

57 During your final year objective structured clinical examination you are asked to examine the neurology of a patient's upper limb. You suspect a lesion of the median nerve. Which one of the following facts about the median nerve is INCORRECT?

☐ **a.** Supplies the muscles of the thenar eminence

☐ **b.** Contains fibres of C6 and C7

☐ **c.** Passes around the lateral epicondyle

☐ **d.** Provides sensory supply to the lateral 3½ digits of the hand

☐ **e.** May become trapped in the carpal tunnel

58 Which one of the following facts about primary postpartum haemorrhage is INCORRECT?

☐ **a.** ≥500 ml blood lost per vagina in the first 12 hours after delivery

☐ **b.** Commonest cause is retained products of conception

☐ **c.** Other causes include intrauterine infection

☐ **d.** Bleeding may be treated with IV oxytocin

☐ **e.** Vaginal bleeding 1–6 weeks after delivery is considered postpartum haemorrhage

59 A 2-week-old male infant is brought into A&E by his parents because of persistent vomiting. They state that he forcibly vomits almost immediately after eating and the vomit appears to be partially digested food. On examination, there is a small, non-tender, palpable mass in the epigastrium. Which one of the following investigations is most likely to be diagnostic?

☐ **a.** CT scan of the abdomen

☐ **b.** Barium swallow

☐ **c.** Abdominal ultrasound scan

☐ **d.** Abdominal X-ray

☐ **e.** Laparoscopy

60 During a walk-in clinic in General Practice you are asked to see a patient who has been complaining of headaches, palpitations and occasional blurred vision. You take the blood pressure while listening to the history and find a reading of 185/98 mmHg. Which one of the following renal conditions is NOT usually associated with hypertension?

☐ **a.** Renal artery stenosis

☐ **b.** Recurrent urinary tract infections

☐ **c.** Polycystic kidney disease

☐ **d.** Glomerulonephritis

☐ **e.** Severe acute pyelonephritis

Extended Matching Questions

Abdominal pain

a. Intussusception
b. Pyloric stenosis
c. Hirschsprung's disease
d. Midgut volvulus
e. Appendicitis
f. Nephroblastoma
g. Inguinal hernia
h. Constipation

The following patients have all presented with abdominal pain. Please choose the most correct diagnosis from the above list. Each option may be used once, more than once, or not at all.

61 A 9-year-old girl is brought to see her GP by her mother. She has been complaining of passing heavily blood-stained urine, which her mother believes represents early menarche. On further questioning, the girl also complains of left-sided abdominal pain that is constant but has gradually been worsening over the past few weeks. She denies any constitutional symptoms and generally feels well. On examination, she has a mass in her left flank.

62 A 4-year-old boy is brought to A&E by his father for abdominal pain. He has passed one stool that appeared to be quite abnormal; his father likens it to redcurrant jelly. He feels nauseated but has not vomited. On examination, he has a palpable mass in his right lower quadrant.

63 A 3-year-old boy is brought to his GP with new-onset severe abdominal pain in the past 4 hours. On examination, abdominal distension is noted. His mother states that the boy has been having a lot of very green-coloured vomiting.

64 A 6-week-old infant is brought to see his GP as he is suffering from frequent episodes of projectile vomiting. His mother is nervous as she has not had any other children and he appears to be hungry immediately after vomiting unaltered milk.

65 A 14-year-old girl is sent home from school after complaining of abdominal pain. She describes the pain as being increasingly constant in the right iliac fossa and has some associated diarrhoea and nausea. On examination, she is found to be febrile and have tenderness in the right iliac fossa with some guarding.

Dementia

a. Alzheimer's dementia
b. Creutzfeldt–Jakob disease
c. Multi-infarct dementia
d. Frontotemporal dementia
e. Human immunodeficiency virus (HIV) dementia
f. Alcohol-related dementia
g. Lewy body dementia
h. Pseudo-dementia

The following patients have all presented with dementia. Please choose the most correct diagnosis from the above list. Each option may be used once, more than once, or not at all.

66 A 65-year-old man with a past history of stroke and transient
☐ ischaemic attack is brought to his GP by his wife. She is worried that he has become more forgetful and he has difficulty focusing on conversations.

67 A 68-year-old man is brought to A&E having fallen and broken
☐ his hip. He is confused and upon talking to a relative a history of tremors and long-standing hypertension is gained. Mini-mental state examination yields a score of 21. His relative states that he often seems to hallucinate and become restless.

68 A 61-year-old woman is found wandering at night in her dress-
☐ ing gown and brought in to hospital by the police. A mini-mental state examination reveals a score of 18. Her memory is declining and her behaviour has become more aggressive.

69 A 58-year-old recently widowed woman is brought to hospital
☐ by her relatives. She was found at home lying in bed in a poor state of hygiene. Her mini-mental state examination score was 24 and during the test she became very agitated and tearful.

70 A 31-year-old man from Botswana is brought to A&E by the
☐ police. He was found at 2 a.m. wandering the street outside his house holding a knife. He believes that somebody is poisoning him and he complains of a 'flu-like illness'. On examination, he is slim with poor nutrition and vital signs reveal a low-grade pyrexia.

Contraceptives

    a. Combined oral contraceptive pill
    b. Progesterone-only pill
    c. IUCD
    d. Depo-provera intramuscular (IM) injection
    e. Abstinence
    f. Low-dose oestrogen combined contraceptive
    g. Emergency contraceptive pill
    h. Contraceptive patch

Please select one of the contraceptive solutions listed above for each clinical vignette. Each option may be used once, more than once, or not at all.

71 A 16-year-old girl attends her GP complaining of worsening dysmenorrhoea and worsening vaginal bleeding. She denies any risk factors for venous thrombosis.

72 A 37-year-old clinically obese woman, who is a heavy smoker, has no past history of venous thrombosis. She works as an office clerk but is well known to be forgetful. She has defaulted from cervical screening due to inadequate samples being taken repeatedly.

73 A 21-year-old woman normally uses the combined oral contraceptive pill. She has recently suffered with a diarrhoeal illness, which has resolved. She had sex with her regular partner the night before but has not missed any pills.

74 A 22-year-old medical student is diagnosed with hypertension at a regular 'pill check'. She wants a regular contraceptive solution.

75 A 37-year-old multiparous woman wants to discuss contraceptive options. She has used combined oral contraceptives in the past, but since having her last child has decided that she wants a more reliable option.

Causes of haematuria
a. Prostatic hyperplasia
b. Renal cell carcinoma
c. Schistosomiasis
d. Bladder carcinoma
e. Tuberculosis
f. Urinary tract infection
g. Glomerulonephritis
h. Renal contusion
i. Renal vein thrombosis

The following patients have all presented with haematuria. Please choose the most likely diagnosis from the list above. Each option can be used once, more than once or not at all.

76 A 63-year old Afro-Caribbean man presents to his GP with problems passing urine for the past 2 months. He has been noticing that he has to get up to go to the toilet frequently and when he has been, he feels that he needs to go again 'less than 5 minutes afterwards'. He is distressed because he has recently discovered blood in his urine and is worried he has cancer.

77 An 82-year-old woman is brought to hospital by her carer who discovered she had been passing frank blood in the urine that was not associated with any pain. The carer was unsure how long this had been going on for. The patient is not taking any anticoagulation and had otherwise been fit and well. An occupational history revealed that she had worked for many years in the dye industry.

78 A 43-year-old man presents to hospital with abdominal pain, haematuria and symptoms of dysuria. He states that these symptoms have been getting progressively worse over a month's period after a water sports holiday in Egypt. He also describes an itchy papular rash over his lower legs.

79 A 78-year-old woman is brought to hospital by her worried neighbours as she has been acting 'not herself' and has been found wandering around in the evening in just her nightgown and slippers. On examination, she has an abbreviated mental test (AMT) score of 3/10, is found to be pyrexic and has tenderness over her suprapubic region. A urine sample is reddish-orange in colour.

80 A 34-year-old man presents to hospital after suffering a fall while under the influence of alcohol. He is inebriated on arrival and unable to give a full history apart from that of falling from the standing position on to his right flank. He is in pain and clutching his back and when he rolls to his left side you notice some bruising over his lower right posterior ribs. He is incontinent and the nursing staff notice his urine is very dark red.

Theme: relevant milestones

a. 0–3 months
b. 3–6 months
c. 6–9 months
d. 9–12 months
e. 12–18 months
f. 18–24 months
g. 2–5 years
h. 5–10 years

For the scenarios shown below, please choose the correct age from the list above. Each option can be used once, more than once, or not at all.

81 A healthy child with heart rate of 95–140 beats/minute (bpm), a
☐ respiratory rate of 25 breaths/minute, and a systolic blood pressure of 90 mmHg.

82 The child sits unaided.
☐

83 First dose of diphtheria, tetanus, pertussis, polio, *Haemophilus*
☐ *influenza B* and meningitis C vaccination is administered in accordance with the normal vaccination schedule in the UK.

84 Persistent runny nose, mild fever, shortness of breath with asso-
☐ ciated dry cough and wheeze. On examination, accessory muscles are being used and there are fine end inspiratory crackles on the chest.

85 Able to follow movements with eyes.
☐

Headaches

a. Tension headache
b. Subarachnoid haemorrhage
c. Subdural haemorrhage
d. Extradural haemorrhage
e. Cavernous sinus thrombosis
f. Meningitis
g. Sinusitis
h. Cluster headache

The following patients have all presented with headache. Please choose the most likely diagnosis from the list above. Each option can be used once, more than once or not at all.

86 A 37-year-old man presents to his GP complaining of headache. ☐ The pain is mainly behind his left eye and in his forehead and his eye on that side appears to bulge and has limited range of movements.

87 A 47-year-old woman is suffering with right-sided weakness ☐ and fluctuations in her levels of consciousness. She is known to suffer with epilepsy and has been having an increased number of fits recently.

88 A 48-year-old office worker presents with a 3-month history ☐ of pain that she describes as a band around her head. These episodes are worse during the afternoon and evening and are exacerbated by stress.

89 A 35-year-old woman suddenly notices an almighty headache. ☐ It is located in the occipital region and she describes it as the worst pain she has ever experienced. She has associated nausea but no vomiting and starts to complain of neck stiffness.

90 A 17-year-old boy presents with a headache. He has suffered ☐ with a recent flu-like infection but has recovered. His eyes feel like they are bulging and the main bulk of the pain is behind his eyes bilaterally. There is no neurological deficit but you notice pain on palpation over the maxilla bilaterally.

Questions

Single Best Answer Questions

1 A 33-year-old man presents with upper abdominal pain and vomiting. Blood tests demonstrate a raised white cell count and an amylase level of 300 IU/L. Of the following differentials, which one is the LEAST likely to be correct?
- ☐ **a.** Pancreatitis
- ☐ **b.** Perforated duodenal ulcer
- ☐ **c.** Ruptured abdominal aortic aneurysm (AAA)
- ☐ **d.** Transverse colon diverticulitis
- ☐ **e.** Diabetic ketoacidosis

2 Which one of the following is NOT a recognized complication of lung cancer?
- ☐ **a.** Hyponatraemia
- ☐ **b.** Superior vena cava obstruction
- ☐ **c.** Hoarse voice
- ☐ **d.** Horner's syndrome
- ☐ **e.** Pulmonary oedema

3 A 41-year-old homeless man with a previous history of drug abuse is brought in to Accident and Emergency (A&E) after suffering a seizure. During the assessment, he suffers a further generalized tonic–clonic seizure that lasts around 2 minutes and is terminated with administration of rectal diazepam. Which one of the following is NOT a cause of generalized tonic–clonic seizures?
- ☐ **a.** Alcohol abuse
- ☐ **b.** Hypoglycaemia
- ☐ **c.** Glioma
- ☐ **d.** Antidepressant overdose
- ☐ **e.** Subdural haemorrhage

EMQs and SBAs for Medical Finals, Second Edition. Jonathan Bath, Rebecca Morgan and Mehool Patel.
© 2011 John Wiley & Sons, Ltd. Published 2011 by John Wiley & Sons, Ltd.

4 Regarding clinical signs of abdominal disease, which one of the following is associated with bowel perforation?

- ☐ **a.** Rovsing's sign
- ☐ **b.** Murphy's sign
- ☐ **c.** Rigler's sign
- ☐ **d.** Kerr's sign
- ☐ **e.** Trousseau's sign

5 A 54-year-old man presents with raised urea and creatinine levels and blood pressure of 165/92 mmHg. Abdominal palpation reveals a suprapubic dome-shaped mass that is dull to percussion. Computed tomography (CT) scan of the abdomen reveals a poorly defined peri-aortic mass and a bladder volume estimated to be 1.5 L. Which one of the following drugs is most likely responsible for this presentation?

- ☐ **a.** Gold
- ☐ **b.** Paracetamol
- ☐ **c.** Acyclovir
- ☐ **d.** Rosiglitazone
- ☐ **e.** Methysergide

6 Causes of type I respiratory failure include all of the following EXCEPT:

- ☐ **a.** Pneumonia
- ☐ **b.** Pulmonary embolus
- ☐ **c.** Acute asthma
- ☐ **d.** Acute respiratory distress syndrome
- ☐ **e.** Pulmonary fibrosis

7 A 45-year-old woman attends her general practitioner (GP) practice due to worsening headaches. She is concerned about migraines as she has a positive family history and her symptoms do not resolve with simple analgesia. Which one of the following is NOT a known risk factor for migraine?

- ☐ **a.** Caffeine withdrawal
- ☐ **b.** Cheese
- ☐ **c.** Oral contraceptives
- ☐ **d.** Travel
- ☐ **e.** Depression

8 A 55-year-old woman is 2 days post-fenestration of liver cysts. She complains of pain in the abdomen, nausea and malaise. Routine blood tests taken postoperatively show: bilirubin 135 μmol/L, gamma-glutamyl transpeptidase (γ-GGT) 210 IU/L, aspartate transaminase (AST) 150 IU/L and a slightly elevated white cell count. Which of the following is the most likely explanation?

- ☐ **a.** Biliary sepsis
- ☐ **b.** Propofol hepatotoxicity
- ☐ **c.** Common bile duct ligation
- ☐ **d.** Bile leak
- ☐ **e.** Cholecystitis

9 According to the British Thoracic Society, which one of the following is NOT a major criterion for a pulmonary embolus?

- ☐ **a.** Abdominal malignancy
- ☐ **b.** Recent hip replacement
- ☐ **c.** Oral contraceptive pill
- ☐ **d.** Previous venous thromboembolism
- ☐ **e.** Immobility

10 A 46-year-old woman recently returned from visiting her relatives in Bangladesh. Shortly after her return, she developed a fever, lost 7 kg in weight and complains of an ache in her left flank. On examination, she is tender in the renal angle and a mid-stream urine result demonstrates a sterile pyuria. Which one of the following should be undertaken in the management of this woman?

- ☐ **a.** Treat for a fungal pyelonephritis
- ☐ **b.** Treat empirically with a 7-day course of antibiotics
- ☐ **c.** Intravenous urogram (IVU)
- ☐ **d.** Chest X-ray
- ☐ **e.** Cystoscopy

11 A 47-year-old business man is caught in a fire in an enclosed space and suffers severe burns to his upper body, face and neck. He is assessed to have 35% burns to the upper body, which extend from front to back; however, they are not painful to touch and are white in colour. Which one of the following complications of this type of injury is especially important to recognize?

- ☐ **a.** Respiratory distress
- ☐ **b.** Bacterial infection
- ☐ **c.** Loss of peripheral pulses
- ☐ **d.** Severe dehydration
- ☐ **e.** Acute stress ulceration

12 A 17-year-old girl presents to A&E after suffering a witnessed blackout. She denies any aura and her friend who was with her at the time denied any seizure-like activity. Which one of the following investigations would be the LEAST useful in this case?

☐ **a.** Electrocardiogram (ECG)
☐ **b.** Serum glucose
☐ **c.** Echocardiogram
☐ **d.** Full blood count
☐ **e.** CT brain scan

13 Which of the following is NOT consistent with a diagnosis of a pulmonary embolus?

☐ **a.** Normal chest X-ray
☐ **b.** Arterial blood gas (ABG) $\downarrow$ PaO_2, $\uparrow$ $PaCO_2$
☐ **c.** ECG – tachycardia $S_IQ_{III}T_{III}$
☐ **d.** Hypotension
☐ **e.** Unilateral calf swelling

14 A 57-year old man presents to his GP generally feeling tired and complaining of generalized weakness. On examination, his GP notices a waddling gait and bilateral proximal myopathy in his lower limbs. Which one of the following is NOT a causes of proximal myopathy?

☐ **a.** Hypercalcaemia
☐ **b.** Steroid use
☐ **c.** Alcoholism
☐ **d.** Syphilis infection
☐ **e.** Myasthenia gravis

15 A 79-year-old obese woman underwent a laparoscopic cholecystectomy for complicated gallstone disease 5 days ago. She returns to A&E with dyspnoea and chest pain. Observations record blood pressure of 110/60 mmHg, pulse 106 beats/minute (bpm) and saturations of 92% on 4 L of oxygen. Which one of the following postoperative complications is the most likely diagnosis?

☐ **a.** Pulmonary embolus
☐ **b.** Postoperative atelectasis
☐ **c.** Myocardial infarction (MI)
☐ **d.** Left ventricular failure
☐ **e.** Diaphragmatic injury

16 You are called to the ward to see a 55-year-old otherwise healthy postoperative patient who has undergone a difficult open sigmoid colectomy 2 days earlier. The Foley catheter was removed in the morning; however, the nurses are concerned that he has not passed urine for the past 4 hours. Which of the following is the next step in management?

- ☐ **a.** 1 L normal saline bolus
- ☐ **b.** Renal ultrasound
- ☐ **c.** Foley catheterization
- ☐ **d.** Urine electrolytes
- ☐ **e.** 20 mg of intravenous (IV) furosemide

17 Which one of the following is NOT a known cause of pneumothoraces?

- ☐ **a.** Asthma
- ☐ **b.** Lung abscess
- ☐ **c.** Connective tissue disorder
- ☐ **d.** Pulmonary embolus
- ☐ **e.** Spontaneous

18 Which one of the following is LEAST useful in investigating the above complication?

- ☐ **a.** Computed tomography with pulmonary angiography (CT-PA)
- ☐ **b.** Fibrin degradation product (D-dimer)
- ☐ **c.** ABG
- ☐ **d.** ECG
- ☐ **e.** Chest X-ray

19 A 78-year-old man presents complaining of deteriorating eyesight. He has had surgery to remove cataracts in the past. While mapping out his visual fields you note that he has a deficit in the lateral aspect of his right eye and the medial aspect of his left visual field. In both cases his central field of vision remains. Where is the lesion?

- ☐ **a.** Optic chiasm
- ☐ **b.** Left optic tract
- ☐ **c.** Lower fibres of optic radiation (temporal lobe)
- ☐ **d.** Right optic nerve
- ☐ **e.** Optic radiation posterior parietal lobe

20 On diagnosing a pulmonary embolus, which one of the following represents the most appropriate treatment regime?

- ☐ **a.** Aspirin, low molecular weight heparin and warfarin
- ☐ **b.** Low molecular weight heparin and warfarin
- ☐ **c.** Aspirin, clopidogrel and warfarin
- ☐ **d.** Aspirin and warfarin
- ☐ **e.** Unfractionated heparin and warfarin

21 A 53-year-old man presents to A&E complaining of a warm, tender swelling in the right groin associated with nausea, vomiting and constipation. On examination, there is a tender, 2-cm swelling that is irreducible. On examination intraoperatively, the mass is medial to the inferior epigastric artery and above the inguinal ligament. Which one of the following correctly describes this mass?

- ☐ **a.** Spigelian hernia
- ☐ **b.** Indirect inguinal hernia
- ☐ **c.** Direct inguinal hernia
- ☐ **d.** Femoral hernia
- ☐ **e.** Ventral hernia

22 Which one of the following facts about multiple sclerosis is NOT true?

- ☐ **a.** It has a relapsing/remitting course
- ☐ **b.** 97% of multiple sclerosis patients have oligoclonal bands in cerebrospinal fluid (CSF)
- ☐ **c.** Clinical picture is caused by demyelination in the central nervous system
- ☐ **d.** Good treatments are available
- ☐ **e.** Symptoms are worsened by immersion in a hot bath

23 A 54-year-old man presents to hospital with lethargy, shortness of breath and complaining of itching all over. His previous notes state that he is well known to the renal physicians for chronic renal failure secondary to diabetic nephropathy. He has been taking pain medication for chronic back pain. On examination, there is bilateral pitting oedema to the mid-thigh and he is short of breath with a respiratory rate of 30 breaths/minute. Which one of the following medications has most likely precipitated this admission?

- ☐ **a.** Erythropoietin
- ☐ **b.** Frusemide
- ☐ **c.** Ibuprofen
- ☐ **d.** Pioglitazone
- ☐ **e.** Chlorpheniramine

24 A young child presents with regurgitation of food and vomiting occurring frequently after meals. The mother is worried that the child has failed to progress along the normal centile chart and finds that the vomiting is worse when the child lies horizontal after mealtimes. Further investigation reveals a moderate congenital diaphragmatic hernia. Which one of the following statements regarding diaphragmatic hernias is correct?

- [ ] **a.** Traumatic right-sided defects are more common than left-sided defects
- [ ] **b.** Large central hernias may present as respiratory distress in neonates
- [ ] **c.** Hernias through the foramen of Morgagni are usually significant
- [ ] **d.** Congenital hiatal hernias almost always require surgical treatment
- [ ] **e.** Traumatic diaphragmatic hernias are usually treated conservatively

25 A 70-year old man presents to A&E with what clinically appears to be a large pleural effusion. A sample is aspirated using an aseptic technique and its analysis shows straw-coloured fluid, protein 35 g/L and no blood. Which one of the following conditions would be consistent with this analysis?

- [ ] **a.** Constrictive pericarditis
- [ ] **b.** Cirrhosis of the liver
- [ ] **c.** Hypothyroidism
- [ ] **d.** Bronchogenic carcinoma
- [ ] **e.** Nephrotic syndrome

26 A 10-year-old boy is brought to hospital by his mother who is worried that he has been passing very dark smoky urine and has a swollen face. On further questioning, his mother tells you that he had been fine up until a nasty bout of 'flu' that he caught from school just over a week ago that required a few days off school. Which of the following diagnoses is the most likely?

- [ ] **a.** Minimal change glomerulonephritis
- [ ] **b.** Post-streptococcal glomerulonephritis
- [ ] **c.** Henoch–Schönlein purpura
- [ ] **d.** Berger's disease (immunoglobulin A [IgA] nephropathy)
- [ ] **e.** Rapidly progressive glomerulonephritis

27 A 37-year-old school teacher undergoes a lumbar puncture for a history highly suggestive of a bacterial meningitis. Which one of the following findings on analysis of CSF would rule against a diagnosis of bacterial meningitis?

☐ **a.** Normal CSF pressure
☐ **b.** Moderately/severely raised protein level
☐ **c.** >50 polymorphs
☐ **d.** Low glucose
☐ **e.** Raised opening CSF pressure

28 Regarding factors associated with peptic ulcer disease, which one of the following is NOT considered to be a risk factor for ulceration?

☐ **a.** Pregnancy
☐ **b.** Male sex
☐ **c.** Head injury
☐ **d.** Severe burns
☐ **e.** Steroids

29 A 78-year-old woman with a history of chronic obstructive pulmonary disease (COPD) is being reviewed for domiciliary oxygen. She has noticed increasing breathlessness of late, both on exertion and intermittently at rest. ABG on air shows pH 7.4, pO_2 7.3 kPA and pCO_2 4.8 kPA. What would be your next step in the assessment?

☐ **a.** Increase her oxygen to 2 L/minute and repeat ABG in 1 hour
☐ **b.** Discharge her as she does not require domiciliary oxygen
☐ **c.** Try 1 L/minute oxygen and repeat ABG in 1 hour
☐ **d.** Re-check ABG on air after 1 hour
☐ **e.** Ask patient to mobilize and then re-check ABG

30 A 54-year-old man with chronic renal failure is seen at his regular follow-up with his GP. His blood pressure is 145/78 mmHg and he has a normocytic anaemia (haemoglobin, 9.5 g/dL), with urea 11.4 mmol/L and creatinine 145 μmol/L. Which one of the following is NOT associated with chronic renal failure?

☐ **a.** Anorexia
☐ **b.** Nausea
☐ **c.** Restless legs
☐ **d.** Hypokalaemia
☐ **e.** Hyperphosphataemia

31 A 51-year-old man is referred by his GP for acutely worsening back pain and an inability to pass urine. Which one of the following investigations is most likely to be diagnostic?

☐ **a.** Thoracolumbar spine X-rays

☐ **b.** Magnetic resonance imaging (MRI) spine

☐ **c.** Bloods, including erythrocyte sedimentation rate (ESR) and C-reactive protein

☐ **d.** CT scan head

☐ **e.** Nerve conduction studies

32 A 25-year-old Afro-Caribbean office worker has been referred to the respiratory clinic for investigation of dry cough, mild chest pain and reduced exercise tolerance. A chest X-ray shows bilateral hilar lymphadenopathy. Which one of the following is the most likely diagnosis?

☐ **a.** Sarcoidosis

☐ **b.** Tuberculosis

☐ **c.** Asthma

☐ **d.** Pulmonary fibrosis

☐ **e.** Malignancy

33 A 15-year-old boy is admitted for pain in the right iliac fossa associated with nausea and vomiting for 2 days with signs of peritonism. Twelve hours postoperatively the nursing staff are worried, as the child is vomiting. On examination, the abdomen is soft but appropriately tender. He has been allowed to eat and drink but has not managed to keep anything down. Which one of the following is most likely to have occurred?

☐ **a.** Small bowel obstruction

☐ **b.** Anastomotic leak

☐ **c.** Adverse reaction to anaesthetic agent

☐ **d.** Acute stress ulceration

☐ **e.** Postoperative ileus

34 On seeing the patient in the above case, you arrive at a diagnosis and decide on further management of the vomiting. Which one of the following options should be considered in the first instance?

☐ **a.** Nasogastric tube insertion for oral intake

☐ **b.** Erect chest X-ray

☐ **c.** Abdominal X-ray

☐ **d.** Antiemetic medication

☐ **e.** Proton pump inhibitor

35 Which one of the following associations is INCORRECT?

☐ **a.** Pulmonary fibrosis – fine end inspiratory crackles

☐ **b.** Extrinsic allergic alveolitis – type I respiratory failure

☐ **c.** Pulmonary embolus – hypoxia

☐ **d.** Cystic fibrosis – fine crepitations

☐ **e.** Pneumonectomy – reduced breath sounds

36 A 43-year-old woman presents to hospital with shortness of breath, malaise and bilateral pitting oedema to the knees. She is treated for acute renal failure and started on a diuretic that acts at the thick ascending limb of the loop of Henlé. Which one of the following diuretics acts at this particular site?

☐ **a.** Acetazolamide

☐ **b.** Mannitol

☐ **c.** Frusemide

☐ **d.** Bendrofluazide

☐ **e.** Spironolactone

37 An 11-year-old girl is diagnosed with type I diabetes mellitus following investigation for polyuria and polydipsia. Her family are particularly concerned that she may develop neurological complications in later life. Which one of the following is NOT known to be associated with diabetes?

☐ **a.** Third nerve palsy

☐ **b.** Bilateral pupillary abnormalities

☐ **c.** Transient hemiparesis

☐ **d.** Headaches

☐ **e.** Autonomic neuropathy

38 Which one of the following states is NOT an indication for renal replacement therapy (dialysis)?

☐ **a.** Refractory metabolic acidosis

☐ **b.** Oliguria

☐ **c.** Severe hyperkalaemia

☐ **d.** Uraemic symptoms

☐ **e.** Drug ingestion

39 Causes of fibrosing alveolitis include all of the following EXCEPT which option?

☐ **a.** Cryptogenic

☐ **b.** Rheumatoid arthritis

☐ **c.** Sjögren's disease

☐ **d.** Ulcerative colitis

☐ **e.** *Aspergillus*

40 A 56-year-old woman presents to her GP complaining of a transient intense stabbing pain over her left cheek and forehead. She notes that she always has the pain on the left side and it is exacerbated by touching the skin. Which one of the following conditions is most likely to account for her symptoms?

- ☐ **a.** Trigeminal neuralgia
- ☐ **b.** Cluster headache
- ☐ **c.** Parotitis
- ☐ **d.** Temporal arteritis
- ☐ **e.** Otitis media

41 A 15-year-old boy is referred to the renal clinic by his GP with a history of worsening haematuria. His mother has been worried as he has been finding it more difficult to cope at school and has been falling behind in his schoolwork. He also seems to be less attentive of late sitting close to the television on his own with the volume up loud. Which one of the following conditions fits most closely with the clinical history?

- ☐ **a.** Alport's syndrome
- ☐ **b.** Anderson–Fabry disease
- ☐ **c.** Goodpasture's syndrome
- ☐ **d.** Wegener's granulomatosis
- ☐ **e.** Von Hippel–Lindau syndrome

42 A 76-year-old man is referred by his GP to hospital due to recent weight loss, a high blood glucose reading of 18 mmol/L and yellow discoloration of the skin and sclera. Examination reveals a cachectic habitus. Which one of the following diagnoses is the most likely?

- ☐ **a.** Pancreatic adenocarcinoma
- ☐ **b.** Cholangiocarcinoma
- ☐ **c.** Choledocholithiasis
- ☐ **d.** Hepatitis
- ☐ **e.** New-onset diabetes mellitus

43 Recurrent pleural effusions may be caused by malignant mesothelioma. Which one of the following facts about mesothelioma is NOT true?

- ☐ **a.** Occurs in both pleura and peritoneum
- ☐ **b.** The period between exposure and development of cancer is approximately 40 years
- ☐ **c.** Pleural mesothelioma is more common on the right than the left side
- ☐ **d.** Prognosis is approximately 2 years
- ☐ **e.** Incidence is more common in females than males

44 An 80-year-old woman presents to A&E with confusion and pain in her back. Routine blood tests demonstrate: calcium 3.1 mmol/L, alkaline phosphatase 249 IU/L, urea 12 mmol/L, creatinine 317 μmol/L and haemoglobin 10.7 g/dL. Plain lumbosacral radiographs were taken after eliciting point tenderness over the lower vertebrae and demonstrated punched-out lytic lesions. Which one of the following is the most likely diagnosis?

☐ **a.** Paget's disease
☐ **b.** Sarcoidosis
☐ **c.** Hyperparathyroidism
☐ **d.** Myeloma
☐ **e.** Osteosarcoma

45 A 73-year-old man is brought to his GP by his wife as his gait has been deteriorating for some time and he is now shuffling and having difficulty initiating movements. Which one of the following characteristics is associated with Parkinson's disease?

☐ **a.** Waddling
☐ **b.** Wide base
☐ **c.** High stepping
☐ **d.** Difficulty initiating movements
☐ **e.** Falls

46 Which one of the following is NOT routinely considered as part of a renal screen in the investigation of new-onset renal failure?

☐ **a.** Complement
☐ **b.** Renal ultrasound
☐ **c.** Caeruloplasmin and serum copper
☐ **d.** Antineutrophil cytoplasmic antibodies (ANCA)
☐ **e.** Bence–Jones protein

47 An 82-year-old man presents with progressive shortness of breath, paroxysmal nocturnal dyspnoea and orthopnoea over the past 3 weeks. He is a heavy smoker and drinks moderate amounts of alcohol. Clinical examination reveals tachypnoea and tachycardia. Dullness of the percussion note of the right hemithorax is elicited with reduced breath sounds to the right mid-zone in addition to bibasal crepitations. Which one of the following should be carried out next?

☐ **a.** Echocardiography
☐ **b.** Chest X-ray
☐ **c.** Pleural tap and drainage
☐ **d.** IV clarithromycin and amoxicillin
☐ **e.** ECG

48 Which one of the following is NOT a clinical feature of sleep apnoea?
- □ **a.** Recurrent cough
- □ **b.** Daytime somnolence
- □ **c.** Reduced libido
- □ **d.** Morning headache
- □ **e.** Reduced cognitive performance

49 A few hours following a football match, a 15-year-old boy who had been hit on the left side of his head by a football has gradually become drowsy. He is complaining of a headache. What is the likely diagnosis?
- □ **a.** Subdural haemorrhage
- □ **b.** Extradural haemorrhage
- □ **c.** Subarachnoid haemorrhage
- □ **d.** Intracranial venous thrombosis
- □ **e.** Cerebrovascular accident

50 A 58-year-old woman presents to hospital with headache, blurred vision and palpitations. Family history is remarkable for two of her family members suffering from strokes at a young age. Routine observations record a blood pressure reading of 194/110 mmHg. Routine blood tests demonstrate creatinine 172 μmol/L and haemoglobin 9.8 g/dL. Which one of the following investigations in indicated in the first line?
- □ **a.** Renal ultrasound
- □ **b.** CT scan of the head
- □ **c.** Renal biopsy
- □ **d.** 24-hour urinary metanephrines (vanillylmandelic acid – VMA)
- □ **e.** Carotid and vertebral artery Doppler scans

51 A 78-year-old woman admitted with a urinary tract infection has become increasingly confused. She has been found to have a fluctuating level of consciousness and is disorientated in time and place. She intermittently becomes very noisy and agitated. What is the likely cause for her symptoms?
- □ **a.** Dementia
- □ **b.** Delirium
- □ **c.** Schizophrenia
- □ **d.** Depression
- □ **e.** Cerebral mass

52 A 65-year-old patient with increasing shortness of breath is diagnosed with heart failure. Causes of cor pulmonale include all of the following EXCEPT:

☐ **a.** Pulmonary fibrosis
☐ **b.** Primary pulmonary hypertension
☐ **c.** Sickle cell disease
☐ **d.** Enlarged adenoids in children
☐ **e.** Acute asthma

53 In the case above, chest radiography confirms a pleural effusion and pleural tap and drainage is performed. Pleural fluid analysis reveals a murky dark brown fluid with a protein content of 45 g/dL and heavy lymphocytic involvement. Which of the following is the LEAST likely diagnosis?

☐ **a.** Tuberculosis
☐ **b.** Malignancy
☐ **c.** Rheumatoid arthritis
☐ **d.** Liver failure
☐ **e.** Systemic lupus erythematosus (SLE)

54 A 5-year-old boy is referred to the paediatric nephrology clinic by his GP. His father states that his son has been passing dark urine. On examination, there is a painless mass in the right flank and a urine sample performed at the clinic shows frank haematuria. Which one of the following investigations should be obtained next?

☐ **a.** CT scan of the abdomen
☐ **b.** Exploratory laparotomy
☐ **c.** Bilateral renal biopsies
☐ **d.** Albumin/creatinine ratio
☐ **e.** Chest X-ray

55 A 34-year-old man is admitted to hospital short of breath and is diagnosed with a chest infection and treated with amoxicillin and clarithromycin. Shortly after commencement of antibiotic therapy, he is found on the ward to be passing only 10 mL/hour via his urinary catheter although he is well hydrated. Urinalysis reveals proteinuria and eosinophils. Which one of the following diagnoses is the most likely?

☐ **a.** Ascending urinary tract infection
☐ **b.** Haemolytic uraemic syndrome
☐ **c.** Drug-induced interstitial nephritis
☐ **d.** Cholesterol embolus
☐ **e.** Acute tubular necrosis

56 You diagnose a peripheral neuropathy in a 73-year-old man. Which one of the following is NOT a known cause of a peripheral neuropathy?

☐ **a.** Diabetes

☐ **b.** Vitamin B12 deficiency

☐ **c.** Hereditary

☐ **d.** Alcohol

☐ **e.** Paracetamol overdose

57 A 44-year-old man is brought in to A&E by helicopter, having fallen from a third-floor building. On arrival, he has a Glasgow coma scale (GCS) of 4/15 and is intubated and ventilated. Neurological examination reveals unequal pupils and an urgent CT scan of the head is performed, which demonstrates mid-line shift and a left-sided convex enhancing area. Which one of the following is the next most appropriate course of action?

☐ **a.** IV mannitol to reduce intracranial pressure

☐ **b.** Conservative management with 30 degree head-up nursing

☐ **c.** IV thiopentone to reduce intracranial pressure

☐ **d.** Urgent neurosurgical evacuation of extradural haematoma

☐ **e.** Urgent coiling of burst aneurysm under neuroradiological guidance

58 A 40-year-old man presents with acute shortage of breath. Clinically, he is becoming more dyspnoeic. You note use of accessory muscles and tracheal deviation to the left hand side. On the right, you note increased resonance on percussion, reduced breath sounds and reduced chest expansion on that side. What is the next step in your management?

☐ **a.** Chest X-ray

☐ **b.** ABG

☐ **c.** Insert large bore cannula into second intercostal space on right hand side

☐ **d.** Insert chest drain

☐ **e.** Administer bronchodilators

59 A 78-year-old man presents to his GP with a swelling in his scrotum associated with a dragging sensation. On examination, there is a mass in the left hemiscrotum that transmits a cough impulse and is described like a 'bag of worms'. Which of the following is the most likely diagnosis?

☐ **a.** Testicular carcinoma
☐ **b.** Bladder carcinoma
☐ **c.** Nephroblastoma (Wilms' tumour)
☐ **d.** Renal cell carcinoma
☐ **e.** Prostate carcinoma

60 You review a male patient who is 'off his legs'. The history is poor but clinically, he has vague lower limb weakness and seems a little confused. His neighbour has brought his medications, which are atenolol and losartan. On examination, you note that he has bilateral pin-point pupils. Which one of the following would account for his pupils?

☐ **a.** Pontine haemorrhage
☐ **b.** Frontal lobe infarct
☐ **c.** Atenolol overdose
☐ **d.** Cerebellar mass
☐ **e.** Multiple sclerosis

Extended Matching Questions

Acute abdomen

a. Appendicitis
b. Pancreatitis
c. Diverticulitis
d. Intussusception
e. Sigmoid volvulus
f. Perforated peptic ulcer
g. Ruptured abdominal aortic aneurysm
h. Basal pneumonia
i. Rectosigmoid carcinoma
j. Appendiceal carcinoid

The following patients have all presented with abdominal complaints. Please choose the most correct diagnosis from the above list. Each option may be used once, more than once, or not at all.

61 A 15-year-old boy presents to his GP with a 2-day history of vomiting, nausea and loss of appetite. On examination, he is generally tender but more so over the right side of his abdomen. Blood tests reveal low-grade pyrexia, high white cell count and raised C-reactive protein.

62 A 65-year-old woman is brought to hospital complaining of bright red blood in her stools. On examination, she is tender in the left iliac fossa with a hard non-fluctuant mass palpable in the same region. Tests reveal a high white cell count, C-reactive protein level of 135 mg/L and temperature of 37.9°C.

63 A 72-year old-man presents to A&E with a history of weight loss, confusion and abdominal pain. His nursing home states that he has not opened his bowels for 2 days and has become increasingly unwell over the past few weeks. Blood results reveal haemoglobin 7.2 g/dL, mean corpuscular volume (MCV) 74.3 fL, urea 9.4 mmol/L and creatinine 155 μmol/L.

64 A 45-year-old stockbroker presents to hospital complaining of severe abdominal pain. He states that he was watching the morning news when he first experienced the pain. On examination, his abdomen is tense with absent bowel sounds and is very tender over the epigastrium.

65 A 57-year-old woman is brought to hospital by ambulance with abdominal pain. She has vomited and has been very constipated since yesterday. Past medical history reveals high blood pressure and cholesterol, treated with atenolol and simvastatin. On examination, she is sitting forward on the bed and in pain. Clinically, the abdomen is exquisitely tender over the epigastrium. Chest examination reveals reduced breath sounds in the left base.

Glomerulonephritides

  a. Minimal change disease
  b. Immunoglobulin A (IgA) nephropathy (Berger's disease)
  c. Focal segmental glomerulosclerosis
  d. Post-streptococcal glomerulonephritis
  e. Rapidly progressive glomerulonephritis
  f. Membranous glomerulonephritis
  g. Wegener's granulomatosis
  h. Henoch–Schönlein purpura
  i. SLE

The following patients have all presented with renal disease. Please choose the most likely option from the list above. Each option can be used once, more than once, or not at all.

66 A 10-year-old boy is brought to A&E with a rash over his buttocks associated with abdominal pain and vomiting. He is accompanied by his mother and stepfather. His mother had left him with his stepfather for a long weekend but was called to come back from holiday as he had started to have some bloody stools associated with the rash. Social services had been notified on arrival to hospital.

67 A 30-year-old man presents to hospital complaining that his urine has been very dark recently, resembling coffee at worst. He has been under the weather recently and has taken a few days off work with a very sore throat and coryzal symptoms. Urine dipstick in hospital returns highly positive for blood and protein. He is admitted for supportive management and is scheduled for a renal biopsy, which shows mesangial proliferation with a positive immunofluorescence pattern.

68 A 5-year-old boy is brought to hospital by his father who is worried that he has been listless. His father is not sure why his GP suggested he should come to A&E and is keen to 'get some tablets and go home'. On examination, the child is tired and irritable and has some swelling around his eyes. Carefully considered renal biopsy is remarkable only for some podocyte fusion on electron microscopy.

69 A 40-year-old woman is admitted to A&E with a history of
☐ arthralgia, facial rash, chest pain and neuropsychiatric symptoms. Initially, she undergoes urine dipstick, simple blood tests,
ECG, porphyria and sickle screens and troponin levels. She is
found to have renal failure with poor urine output and a decision to perform a renal biopsy is taken, which demonstrates
wire-loop lesions on light microscopy.

70 A 28-year-old man presents with shortness of breath, haemop-
☐ tysis, swollen legs and face and haematuria. Clinically, he
exhibits signs of renal failure and his blood results show a
glomerular filtration rate of 8 mL/minute (severe). He is admitted to hospital and rapidly deteriorates over a matter of
weeks requiring emergency renal replacement therapy. An autoantibody screen returns positive for antiglomerular basement
membrane and renal biopsy demonstrates a florid necrotizing
glomerulonephritis with crescent formation.

Upper gastrointestinal bleeding

a. Mallory–Weiss tear
b. Oesophageal varices
c. Barrett's oesophagus
d. Gastritis
e. Peptic ulceration
f. Boerhaave's syndrome
g. Gastric carcinoma
h. Aortoenteric fistula
i. Cricopharyngeal carcinoma
j. Oesophageal carcinoma

The following patients have all presented with haematemesis. Please choose the most correct diagnosis from the above list. Each option may be used once, more than once, or not at all.

71 A 64-year-old woman presents to A&E with a month's history of progressive difficulty in swallowing, especially for solid food with associated regurgitation of food. She has noticed when she vomits that there are often bright red streaks of blood mixed with the food. Recently, she has been complaining that her dresses seem to be too big for her.

72 A 34-year-old accountant presents to A&E on a Friday night with a history of vomiting, severe retching and haematemesis of two cupfuls of fresh blood. He is intoxicated and is pale, anxious and there is blood-staining around his mouth. His colleagues tell you that they were at a social event together at a local buffet restaurant and that he usually never gets drunk but had been drinking heavily on this occasion.

73 A 54-year-old man is brought in to A&E by ambulance after collapsing at his home 10 minutes away from the hospital. On arrival, he looks pale and there is blood staining down his shirt, trousers and around his mouth. His past medical history includes a previous open AAA repair, asthma and hypertension.

74 A 43-year-old woman is 3 days post-laparoscopic gastric bypass for morbid obesity. The nurses call you early in the morning as she started to bring up dark red blood with intermittent bouts of vomiting. A sample of the vomitus has been kept and you notice a characteristic heavily dark brown appearance to the blood consistent with coffee ground vomiting. Her drug prescription chart reveals once daily aspirin for previous MI, diclofenac (a non-steroidal anti-inflammatory drug [NSAID]) for knee arthritis and paracetamol.

75 A 58-year-old Korean man presents to his GP with a 6-week history of feeling tired at work. He has a microcytic anaemia on routine blood work, in addition to weight loss. He asks whether he will still be able to donate blood on a regular basis as he is blood group A and has been asked regularly for donations.

Specific pneumonias

a. Pneumococcal
b. Staphylococcal
c. *Klebsiella*
d. *Pseudomonas*
e. *Mycoplasma*
f. *Legionella*
g. *Chlamydia*
h. *Streptococcus*

The following patients have all presented with pneumonia. Please choose the most correct pathogen from the above list. Each option may be used once, more than once, or not at all.

76 An 80-year old woman with a history of COPD and heart failure ☐ has a 2-day history of cough and fever. Her chest X-ray shows a right lower lobe pneumonia. Which is the most likely pathogen?

77 A 30-year-old man with a history of cystic fibrosis presents with ☐ a 5-day history of worsening productive cough and fever. Which of the pathogens is likely to be the cause of his pneumonia?

78 A 24-year-old man complains of myalgia, headaches and ☐ malaise. He has a productive cough and some mild shortness of breath although, clinically, his chest is clear to auscultation.

79 A 34-year-old street dweller presents with a productive cough ☐ and fever. He has needle marks on his forearms, and chest X-ray confirms a mid-zone consolidation. What is the likely cause?

80 A 45-year-old man, who has recently returned from a business ☐ trip to Europe, presents with a 3-day history of a dry cough and associated chest pain and diarrhoea. On attendance he has a fever of 40°C with bibasal inspiratory crepitations.

Investigation of renal disease

a. Renal biopsy
b. Autoantibody screen
c. Renal tract ultrasound
d. 24-hour protein collection
e. Daily urea and creatinine
f. Bence–Jones protein
g. IVU
h. Renal artery Doppler scans
i. CT scan of abdomen

The following patients have all presented with renal disease. Please choose the key diagnostic investigation from the list above. Each option can be used once, more than once, or not at all.

81 A 34-year-old man complains of arthralgia, abdominal pain and vomiting, a facial rash that is worse in the summer and haematuria. His urea and creatinine are slightly elevated, with urinalysis demonstrating red cell casts. Past medical history is remarkable for childhood eczema.

82 A 42-year-old woman with a past medical history of left hemispheric stroke presents to hospital with signs and symptoms of renal failure. She has been seen by her GP for hypertension and abdominal pain with outpatient investigations pending.

83 A 78-year-old woman is brought to hospital complaining of abdominal pain and is referred to the surgeons. She has been saying that her mother is due to visit her today and that somebody must have broken her lower back as she is in agony. Her blood results show creatinine 295 μmol/L and calcium 3.03 mmol/L.

84 A 32-year-old man presents with shortness of breath and swollen legs and face. He describes feeling progressively more unwell in the weeks preceding admission. On examination, there are signs of renal failure. He is admitted to hospital and rapidly deteriorates over a matter of weeks, requiring emergency renal replacement therapy.

85 A 72-year-old man is admitted to the ward with chest pain and managed on the acute coronary syndrome protocol. He is started on a beta-blocker, 3-hydroxymethylglutaryl coenzyme A (HMG-CoA) reductase inhibitor (statin) and an angiotensin-converting enzyme (ACE) inhibitor. Shortly after the nurse administers the medications, he desaturates and become acutely short of breath.

Peripheral nerve lesions

a. Common peroneal nerve
b. Median nerve
c. Tibial nerve
d. Radial nerve
e. Obturator nerve
f. Lateral cutaneous nerve of the thigh
g. Ulnar nerve
h. Axillary nerve

Which nerve from the above list is likely to account for the symptoms in the cases below? Each option can be used once, more than once, or not at all.

86 A 27-year-old man has been admitted to hospital following a football injury. He remembers that during the match, another player went for the ball but hit his leg over the fibular head. His leg was immediately painful but he also noticed that he was experiencing difficulty in lifting his foot up towards him and also everting his foot.

87 A 43-year-old man has suffered an anterior dislocation of his humerus following trauma. He describes weakness in shoulder elevation and abduction, with numbness and altered sensation over the lateral aspect of the arm.

88 A 49-year-old secretary visits her GP with numbness and tingling in both of her hands. She mentions that it affects the lateral $3^{1}/_{2}$ fingers and it often wakes her at night.

89 A 76-year-old woman suffered a fall that resulted in a fracture of her proximal ulna bone. Following the initial injury she notes pain over her elbow and weakness in her same hand. She complains of numbness and tingling in her ring and little fingers.

90 A 55-year-old man has noticed a burning and stinging sensation antero-lateral aspect of his thigh. It is aggravated by walking or standing and relieved by lying down with the hip flexed.

PART 2

Answers to Practice Papers

PAPER 1

Answers

Single Best Answer Questions

1 a. Approximately 45% of breast cancers occur in the upper outer quadrant of the breast. A quarter of cancers occur in the retro-areolar region, with the lower inner quadrant being the least common site of tumours.

2 d. An echocardiogram is the most important next step in the management of this man. This will aid in the decision about anticoagulation. If an echocardiogram shows a structurally normal heart, then the risk of thrombus formation is small and warfarinization would be unnecessary. While atrial fibrillation can commonly be managed in the community, it is appropriate to refer for an echocardiogram. Rate control is unnecessary in this scenario as its upper limit is 90 bpm. There are many known risk factors for atrial fibrillation, including body mass index (BMI) >30, alcohol consumption >42 units per week, chronic respiratory disease, hyperthyroidism and any underlying cardiac problem.

3 e. The majority of breast cancers are hormone sensitive. They are classified as oestrogen receptor positive. For cancers that are hormone sensitive, treatment may be commenced with medications such as tamoxifen, which is an oestrogen receptor antagonist. With this in mind, risk factors for breast cancer can be thought of as those that increase the duration that the body is producing hormones, for example those with an early menarche and late menopause are more at risk. There is some controversy surrounding dairy produce in diet and whether there is any association with the development of breast cancer; however, there is, at present, no firm evidence to suggest that there is an association. Other risk factors for breast cancer include past history,

EMQs and SBAs for Medical Finals, Second Edition. Jonathan Bath, Rebecca Morgan and Mehool Patel.
© 2011 John Wiley & Sons, Ltd. Published 2011 by John Wiley & Sons, Ltd.

use of oral contraceptives, never having breastfed and a family history.

4 d. This man can be safely discharged without follow-up. Troponin is a contractile protein that is not normally found in serum. It is released from necrotic myocardial tissue. In this case, the troponin results represent a 12-hour test by which time if there was cardiac damage the levels would be elevated. This, combined with the fact that there are no ischaemic changes on the ECG, make the risk of a cardiac event minimal. Having ruled out a cardiac cause for his chest pain, a gastrointestinal cause is most likely, given the associated nausea. There is no indication to start this man on aspirin; in fact, it could exacerbate any gastroenterological symptoms.

5 a. Dermatitis (eczema) is a common problem that often affects individuals whose work involves immersion in irritant substances such as bleach, shampoo, chemicals, washing-up liquids, etc. One can therefore predict with some accuracy a period of resolution from the dermatological problem when the person is away from the workplace irritant, for example during holiday periods. This type of dermatitis is sometimes referred to as extrinsic eczema, to differentiate it from intrinsic or atopic eczema.

Lichen planus is typically associated with characteristic fine white lines that lie over the papules (Wickham's striae) and may affect the wrist. A chemical burn is a possibility; however, this does not usually present with an itchy rash. Porphyria cutanea tarda is a rare form of porphyria that manifests as cutaneous photosensitivity. Psoriasis typically favours the extensor surfaces and usually presents as a non-itchy silver scale on an erythematous base.

6 d. Investigation of breast lumps involves triple assessment. The gold standard for this varies in accordance with the age of the patient. All patients require:
- clinical assessment,
- imaging (either mammogram or ultrasound),
- cytology/histology.

The imaging is dependent on the patient's age. For patients <35 years old an ultrasound is the most appropriate form of imaging due to the ductal and dense nature of the breast tissue. After the age of 35 years, breast tissue becomes increasingly fatty and is better imaged with mammography. In patients with breast implants, it may be necessary to consider CT scanning.

7 c. This clinical picture is typical of diabetic ketoacidosis occurring secondarily to a preceding infection. In times of stress, such as postoperatively, or after an infection or inflammation or event such as an MI, blood glucose levels may rise owing to an increase in the stress response and release of gluconeogenic hormones. Insulin requirements may increase remarkably during these periods and it is important to establish close blood glucose control.

Education of patients with type I diabetes mellitus is key to preventing diabetic ketoacidosis; these patients should be taught to increase the frequency of their blood glucose monitoring and increase insulin appropriately in line with any increase in blood glucose. Failure to do this will result in glucose levels rising but the lack of insulin leads to increased production of glucagon, resulting in increased amounts of gluconeogenesis, glycogenolysis and lipolysis. A combination of osmotic diuresis leads to dehydration and tissue hypoxia (leading to lactic acid production through anaerobic metabolism) and lipolysis (leading to increased production of ketone bodies, which are inherently acidic). This results in a florid metabolic acidosis, which may be severe enough to be life threatening.

Treatment involves replacing any fluid losses with 0.9% normal saline (up to 6 L may be required in a 24-hour period) and commencement on a constant infusion of insulin at, for example, 6 units/hour in order to suppress ongoing ketogenesis, which will occur for some hours after blood glucose has been controlled. Monitoring of blood glucose and urinalysis for ketones is imperative to guide management. When blood glucose drops to <15 mmol/L then the infusion can be halved to 3 units/hour and 5% dextrose solution written up instead of saline as fluid replacement. Once the blood glucose is under adequate control, the urine is free from ketones and the patient is eating and drinking normally, then consideration of normal insulin regimen is appropriate. If the patient is not yet fully established on eating and drinking, then conversion to an insulin sliding scale may be a step-down until oral intake is established. Potassium replacement should also be considered, as although levels may appear normal acutely, when the insulin infusion is started and resolution of acid–base deficits occurs then potassium will inevitably fall and must be replaced accordingly.

8 b. Rectal examination is avoided in neutropenic patients as trauma to the ano-rectum is easily manifested and may provide an easy access route to the bloodstream for gastrointestinal flora. Where possible, these patients should be nursed in isolation in a side-room with full barrier nursing precautions. These patients should be subjected to the minimal number of examinations and procedures and clinical staff should also be restricted to essential members only.

9 e. Measuring digoxin levels in this woman will detect any potential toxicity that would account for her symptoms. In this case, blood tests confirmed digoxin toxicity and a binding agent was administered. There is no indication to insert a pacing wire in this woman, as her heart rate is being maintained at 40 bpm although there is complete heart block. Having stopped this woman's digoxin, her heart rate increased to approximately 120 bpm and ultimately she had a permanent pacemaker inserted. Amiodarone is indicated in refractory tachycardias. Indications for temporary pacing include symptomatic bradycardia and second- or third-degree heart block with associated haemodynamic compromise, among others.

10 a. Hypothyroidism may manifest with a plethora of features, including constipation, bradycardia, hypothermia and confusion. Thyroid function tests should always be taken when investigating the cause of confusion in an elderly patient not otherwise known to be confused, as extremes of both hyper- and hypofunction may lead to confusion. General reduction in mobility may be the root cause of falling in patients with hypothyroidism and should prompt investigation of thyroid dysfunction before more specialized investigation is performed.

ECG may reveal a sinus bradycardia, which along with an element of postural hypotension may well contribute to falling; however, the cause of bradycardia should be investigated. Echocardiography may be useful in detecting any clinically significant valvular disease, of which the most relevant to falls is aortic stenosis. The triad of symptoms typically associated with aortic stenosis (syncope, angina and dyspnoea) is often subtle in the elderly and often the only sign of severity is a fall leading to admission.

CT scan of the head is part of the screen for confusion and reversible causes of dementia but it may also reveal a subdural haematoma that may be contributing to, or be a result of, head injury sustained during a fall. In the presence of such florid clinical indices of thyroid dysfunction, this should be considered only after blood tests have returned normal and the cause of confusion is still undiagnosed.

Addison's disease (primary adrenocortical failure) may present in many different ways; however, the classical presentation is of hypotension, hyperkalaemia, hyponatraemia with nausea and vomiting. The short synacthen test is a specific test for Addison's disease and involves measurement of the cortisol level at baseline before and 30 minutes after injection of *syn*thetic adrenocorticotropic hormone (*ACTH*) (hence the name). Treatment is of the underlying cause and replacement of steroids with prednisolone or hydrocortisone if oral intake is compromised.

11 **c.** Dermatitis herpetiformis forms crops of itchy blisters that are commonly found on elbows, knees and scalp. The itch can drive people to suicide and can be usually very effectively, and with much gratitude, relieved by oral dapsone. Dermatitis herpetiformis is associated with coeliac disease and as the risk of lymphoma is greatly increased by having both conditions, regular surveillance is recommended. Psoriasis does commonly affect the elbows but usually does not present with itch and eczema may present in such sites and with pruritus, but is not strongly associated with coeliac disease. Scabies should always be kept in mind when considering itch, usually in children in the web spaces of the hands and feet. Track marks from the burrowing *Sarcoptes scabiei* mite can often be seen and harvested for microscopic diagnosis.

12 **a.** Ventricular septal rupture is a rare but serious complication of MI. The event occurs 2–8 days after an infarction and often precipitates cardiogenic shock. Dressler's syndrome is a pericarditis and is more likely to present 2 weeks after MI. Other complications can include arrhythmias, bradycardias, pulmonary oedema and depression, which occurs in around 20% of patients.

13 **c.** There is radiological evidence of an abscess that will require drainage. In the first instance, a needle aspiration under local anaesthetic is the most appropriate treatment. In the event that this is unsuccessful due to the pus being too thick or not achieving symptomatic relief, an incision and drainage should be considered. This treatment should always be followed up with a course of antibiotics, usually flucloxacillin or erythromycin if penicillin allergic. Patients should be advised to continue to breastfeed. Although this may provide discomfort, it will aid the healing process and in addition it is safe to do so while on antibiotics. In all cases, pus should be sent off for examination to exclude an inflammatory carcinoma.

14 **e.** Cushing's disease is associated with hyperglycaemia due to the glucocorticoid effect of cortisol and associated steroids. **141**

Cushing's disease describes a specific disease of hypercortiso-laemia owing to excess ACTH from a pituitary tumour. It is a subdivision of Cushing's syndrome, which describes gluco-corticoid excess, usually due to excess ACTH (90% of cases) of which the majority are due to ACTH-producing pituitary tumours.

Other causes of excess ACTH leading to Cushing's syndrome include ectopic production from certain lung and carcinoid tu-mours and, rarely, over-administration of ACTH. Primary causes of Cushing's syndrome include steroid use, adrenal tumours and alcohol abuse. Addison's disease can be thought of simplistically as the opposite of Cushing's syndrome, as primary adrenal fail-ure leads to low levels of circulating corticosteroids. Thus hypo-glycaemia, hypotension and hyperkalaemia and hyponatraemia occur. Liver failure tends to present with hypoglycaemia due to impaired liver function leading to poor glycogen production (resulting in low 'glucose' stores during periods of fasting) and impaired fatty acid metabolism.

Insulinomas are classically associated with severe hypogly-caemia due to excess production of insulin and may be bio-chemically tested for by assay of c-peptide levels (which are cleaved from insulin pre-cursors to release physiologically ac-tive insulin). In cases where exogenous insulin may be abused thus mimicking the effects of an insulinoma, c-peptide levels can be taken; they will be high in cases of insulinoma and within normal limits or low in exogenous insulin administration (as c-peptide is not present in synthetic insulin).

Gliclazide is a sulphonylurea that is similar in structure to sul-pha antibiotics. The mechanism of action as a hypoglycaemic agent was discovered when malnourished and starved patients were given sulpha antibiotics leading to hypoglycaemic attacks and acts by increasing endogenous insulin production (*sulphony-lureas squeeze* the pancreas). Sulphonylureas should be used with caution in the elderly because of the decreased awareness for hypoglycaemic attacks and thus inability to counteract the ef-fects (e.g. by taking sweet foods/drinks). The duration of action of the sulphonylureas is long and therefore any diabetic pre-senting to hospital with hypoglycaemia on sulphonylurea tablets must be either admitted for blood glucose observation for a 24-hour period until the effect has worn off or in exceptional cir-cumstances where they themselves or those around them are able to measure the blood glucose and know how to counteract any hypoglycaemia, may be allowed to return home but with a low threshold to return to hospital if there is any doubt about the effectiveness of treatment.

15 a. This woman has no history of alcoholism (her profession was specifically selected to hint at this). She has no signs of outflow tract obstruction. The most likely cause of her dilated cardiomyopathy is viral. The commonest viruses implicated in this condition include coxsackie A and B, influenza A and B, adenovirus and echovirus.

16 a. Hodgkin's lymphoma typically presents with a picture of painless localized lymphadenopathy with systemic features associated with malignancy such as weight loss, fevers, night sweats and lethargy. It is often seen in young men around the age of 20 years and there is a second peak in middle age. Almost pathognomonic of Hodgkin's lymphoma is the interesting association of pain upon drinking alcohol and this may sometimes be the primary complaint of those presenting with the disease. The pathological hallmark of Hodgkin's lymphoma is the Reed–Sternberg cell, sometimes referred to as owl's eyes.

Infectious mononucleosis is caused by the Epstein–Barr virus and commonly presents insidiously with fatigue and malaise, with a sore throat being the second most common symptom. Penicillin derivatives, such as amoxicillin, should be avoided in the treatment of infectious mononucleosis as they may cause a maculopapular rash.

Non-Hodgkin's lymphoma is typically classified into low-grade, intermediate-grade and high-grade, depending on the clinical behaviour of the tumour. Presenting most often with peripheral lymphadenopathy, there may be involvement of bone marrow causing abnormal blood counts and constitutional features of cancer are common reported symptoms.

Polycythaemia rubra vera is a disorder affecting the totipotent haematopoietic stem cells and causes a varying degree of overproduction of erythrocytes, leucocytes and platelets. Often causing vascular thromboses, patients may present with stroke, MI, deep vein thromboses or pulmonary emboli. Interestingly, arterial thromboses are seen three times more commonly than venous thromboses.

Myelodysplastic syndrome actually describes a group of haematopoietic disorders that many authors group as a form of premalignancy. Characterized by either a hypercellular or hypocellular bone marrow with abnormal forms seen on peripheral blood smear, this disorder is probably underestimated in the population over 70 years and may be increasing in incidence due to the relative increase in blood tests taken on arrival to hospital as compared with years ago. Clinically, the symptoms of anaemia or thrombocytopenia may be the only clues to an abnormal bone marrow and are often the mode of diagnosis in the majority of elderly patients presenting to hospital with nebulous constitutional upset.

17 d. The question asks for the most *diagnostic* investigation. While measuring the blood pressure in all limbs raises the suspicion of aortic dissection, the most diagnostic investigation is a chest CT scan. Other diagnostic investigations include an MRI and a transoesophageal echocardiogram. This case is suggesting a diagnosis of dissecting aortic aneurysm and there are no typical diagnostic ECG changes seen. LFTs are of no use in confirming the diagnosis.

18 c. Molluscum contagiosum is caused by a poxvirus and is most commonly seen in children. Lesions are typical in appearance and present as discrete papules sometimes with a surrounding area of mild erythema due to an eczematous process. A distinctive feature of molluscum contagiosum is the presence of a central core of keratin, which can be expressed from the lesions. They are treated conservatively and will resolve on their own or can be squeezed between two fingernails to express the central keratin plug.

VZV does give a similar picture, however, the absence of significant itch, blistering vesicles and distribution in a particular dermatome makes the diagnosis unlikely. HSV is found in two subtypes: HSV 1 affecting the oral and buccal mucosa causing 'cold sores' and HSV 2 affecting primarily the genital tract (although both types can be found almost anywhere in the body). The lesions are transmissible through direct contact e.g. kissing and may be painful and ulcerated with small eruptive vesicles. The lesions will settle spontaneously although in the immuno-compromised or elderly a prolonged course may occur.

Eczema presents as an itchy rash with typical erythema and excoriation of the skin from scratching. Lesions are neither papular nor discrete entities and characteristically affect flexor surfaces.

Pityriasis versicolor is a skin condition affecting primarily young adults and is due to *Malassezia* yeasts, a normal skin commensal. Areas of macular hypopigmentation are seen in persons of dark skin colour with a faint brownish colour in persons of light skin colour. Microscopic examination of skin scrapings reveals the yeasts clumped in short balls and longer hyphae.

19 e. While all of the options are correct, the most important is to complete a primary survey (*a*irway, *b*reathing, *c*irculation, *d*isability, *e*xposure). Once this has been done, the full extent of the situation will become clear and it will then be more appropriate to ask for help and order further investigations. There may be scenarios where it is clear that you may need more assistance, for example cardiac arrest; however, it is really important to maintain a structured approach to these situations to ensure the best outcome for the patient.

20 a. The most likely diagnosis in this case is a fibroadenoma of the breast. It is most commonly seen in women aged between 15 and 40 years old. Characteristically, fibroadenomas are smooth, firm and well circumscribed lumps. They may vary in size from 1 to 5 cm and are often very mobile. Along with all other breast lumps, these should be investigated using the triple approach and, if small, their management should include reassurance. For larger fibroadenomas, management may include excision to restore symmetry to the breasts. Approximately 30% of fibroadenomas shrink and disappear completely. There is no association between fibroadenomas and breast cancer.

21 b. This question is difficult only because it requires a knowledge of the genetic translocation associated with the more familiar *bcr-abl* fusion gene (Philadelphia chromosome). Genetic translocations are responsible for a large number of genetic predispositions to cancer. Another commonly seen translocation associated with cancer is the t(8;14) *c-myc* activation leading to an increased risk of developing Burkitt's lymphoma. A handy way to remember the chromosomes involved in the Philadelphia chromosome is as follows. Philadelphia chromosome – the 'P' of Philadelphia is located at the ninth position and there are 22 letters in the two words put together (hence 9;22). The t(11;22) translocation is commonly associated with a rare bone tumour seen almost exclusively in children and young adults. It is a highly malignant tumour that has a high mortality rate in those who are afflicted.

Robertsonian translocations are a type of genetic transfer of chromosomal material that occurs in association with a number of disorders, most commonly with Down syndrome. Robertsonian translocations can be one of two types: (i) balanced – where there is no loss or addition of chromosomal material and the person with that karyotype will be a carrier of Down syndrome and not be afflicted; or (ii) unbalanced – resulting in trisomy or monosomy (the latter of which is lethal) and will exhibit the Down syndrome. Down syndrome involves trisomy of chromosome 21 and may involve a combination of nearby chromosomes. The translocation t(14;21) is relatively frequently identified as the cause of this disease.

22 e. Erythema nodosum is often indicative of an underlying infectious disease but a cause is not always found. It has no association with infective endocarditis. Causes for erythema nodosum include sarcoidosis, tuberculosis and mycoplasma pneumonia. Retinal haemorrhages are seen in the form of Roth spots. Vasculitis accounts for Osler's nodes, splinter haemorrhages, Roth spots and Janeway lesions.

23 c. The T4 level is elevated in the face of a high TSH, which in the absence of a secondary cause for hyperthyroidism (e.g. hypothalamic or pituitary disease producing high TSH) is discordant with the clinical state. The most likely explanation is chronic undertreatment of hypothyroidism leading to a raised TSH as the pituitary tries to compensate for low levels of T4 followed by over-replacement prior to the clinic appointment in order to try to give the biochemical appearance of compliance. Subclinical hypothyroidism presents with a T4 that is in the normal range but at the low end of the spectrum with a raised TSH. Treatment of subclinical hypothyroidism depends on the clinical state and often these patients are followed up with regular-interval blood tests to assess the need for thyroxine replacement.

Sick euthyroid syndrome is often seen biochemically as a low TSH and low T4 (and T3) and occurs in the absence of any pre-existing thyroid or hypothalamo-pituitary disease. It can occur for a number of reasons, including gastrointestinal and cardiovascular disease, and is defined from intrinsic thyroid dysfunction by the resolution of abnormal thyroid tests with resolution of the underlying non-thyroid illness. Inadequate replacement with thyroxine would lead to a low T4 and a high TSH (simply slightly 'milder' biochemical indices of hypothyroidism than frank untreated hypothyroidism) and the opposite would lead to high T4 associated with a depressed TSH (by the negative feedback mechanism).

24 b. Furosemide is a loop diuretic. When given intravenously, furosemide can reduce arteriolar vasodilatation, which is a beneficial action independent to its diuretic effect. ACE inhibitors have an adjunctive effect when used in combination with diuretics but in this situation optimization of the diuretic therapy is the first step in management of this patient. While bumetanide is a useful drug it is a loop diuretic and there is limited benefit of adding this in to his current treatment regime.

Metolazone is an example of a thiazide diuretic and is known to cause a profound diuresis. It has a role in severe heart failure resistant to large doses of loop diuretics.

25 b. Cocaine is known to cause spasm of coronary arteries and its abuse should always be suspected in cardiac sounding chest pain in a young person. Amphetamines are also known to cause cardiac arrhythmias, and 'crystal meth', an amphetamine that is slowly rising in popularity, has led to cardiac events in some documented cases.

26 d. Arthropathy is a condition that is usually associated with psoriasis and may in fact sometimes be the first presentation of psoriasis in a patient with no obvious skin lesions. The arthropathy can mimic many other rheumatological conditions, including rheumatoid arthritis and osteoarthritis; however, usually presents in one of four patterns:
- distal interphalangeal joint involvement,
- rheumatoid-like joint changes,
- large joint involvement,
- seronegative type joint changes.

Up to 10% of psoriatics will suffer with some kind of joint change associated with skin disease. Eczema can be broadly classified into exogenous, i.e. usually due to an allergic or irritant stimulus and endogenous, i.e. no identifiable precipitant. The latter classification further subdivides into: atopic eczema, eczema associated with venous insufficiency, eczema affecting the sebaceous glands, discoid eczema and asteatotic eczema, which tends to affect the elderly, especially those who are subject to hospital and nursing home washing and bathing.

Eczema responds to emollients to keep the skin from drying and atopic eczema usually benefits from topical steroid cream. Secondary bacterial infection can manifest in broken eczematous skin and a topical steroid and antibacterial combination therapy or even systemic antibiotics may be employed to both eradicate the infection and return the skin to a more balanced level of hydration.

27 d. This case describes Marfan's syndrome. The description given highlights the main phenotypic picture. Marfan's is associated with mitral valve prolapse and a dilated aortic root. The prolapse gives a mid-systolic click, followed by a systolic murmur heard at the apex. Associations of Marfan's syndrome also include lens detachment and a marfarnoid habitus, where arm span is characteristically longer than body height.

28 b. Serum potassium is important to monitor in patients on digoxin as hypokalaemia can potentiate the effects of digoxin leading to toxicity.

29 e. Dapsone is a sulpha-derivative drug that is employed in the effective treatment of dermatitis herpetiformis. Treatment modalities used in the management of psoriasis include agents to keep the skin hydrated, such as moisturizers and emollients, cold tar, topical steroids, vitamin D analogues and vitamin A analogues such as tazarotene. Erythrodermic or acute generalized pustular psoriasis is one of the few true dermatological emergencies and should be initially managed with topical treatments and immunosuppressants such as methotrexate and cyclosporine. Cold tar has anti-inflammatory properties that make this most effective in treating chronic plaque psoriasis; however, patient concordance with treatment is poor. Systemic treatments are also employed to managed chronic stable psoriasis and guttate psoriasis and may consist of ultraviolet light therapy or photochemotherapy such as PUVA, which can be effective in almost all kinds of psoriasis.

30 b. In this man with a history of peripheral vascular disease an ETT would provide inadequate information. A thallium cardiac scan can assess the heart without putting pressure on the peripheral vasculature. The results of an ETT can be influenced by pain from intermittent claudication and therefore the thallium scan is the obvious choice for risk stratification in this patient.

31 d. Amiodarone is a drug notorious for its detrimental effect on the lungs, thyroid and liver and is best remembered for these derangements by the mnemonic pulmonary function tests (*PFTs*), *LFTs* and thyroid function tests (*TFTs*). Amiodarone can cause a picture of hyperthyroidism as it is structurally similar to thyroxine and thus thyroid function tests must be monitored on a regular basis with a low threshold to stop or reduce dosing if thyroid derangement is detected. Pulmonary fibrosis and skin manifestations such as photosensitivity reactions have also been reported.

Atorvastatin has been linked to myositis (like all statin drugs) and attention to the development of muscle pain and weakness should prompt assessment of dosing and/or consideration of changing to another statin or other class of lipid-regulating drug. Statins must be used with caution in hypothyroidism due to the increased risk of myositis with untreated hypothyroidism and correction of thyroid dysfunction may itself lead to an amelioration of lipid profile.

Amlodipine is associated with many diffuse symptoms, including gastrointestinal upset, but the main problem with use is the development of ankle swelling, which may only partially respond to diuresis. Atenolol and other beta-blocking medication may exacerbate asthma and other bronchospastic diseases; however, this effect may be minimized by the use of cardioselective beta-blockers such as bisoprolol.

Acarbose is an inhibitor of intestinal glucosidases (acting at the brush border) and may cause diarrhoea and loose stools due to the osmotic effect of a higher glucose load in the stool. Flatulence is also a side-effect reported by those taking acarbose owing to the amount of glucose present in the colon available for metabolism by lower gastrointestinal organisms.

32 b. The most likely cause for this man's gynaecomastia is liver failure. The history states that he has suffered with pancreatitis and acute liver failure in the past, which suggest that this is likely to be due to hepatobiliary failure. Although it is a physiological change seen in the elderly, this man's condition is most likely to be secondary to further liver problems. There is no evidence that he is suffering with thyroid dysfunction and the history does not state that he is on any medications that are known to cause this condition, including digoxin, steroids, methyl-dopa and anti-androgens.

33 a. Both verapamil and diltiazem are calcium-channel blockers. They block calcium entry into the cell and its utilization within the cell. They relax the coronary arteries and reduce the force of left ventricular contraction, which in turn reduces oxygen demand. Diltiazem has a negative chronotropic effect, which helps alleviate the symptoms of angina as will regular long-acting nitrates.

34 b. Eyelid retraction is a sign of sympathetic overactivity and can be seen in normal individuals who ingest large amounts of thyroxine with normal thyroid function. It can be used as a fairly reliable measure of the degree of treatment with thyroid-blocking medication. Hyperthyroidism is assessed clinically and confirmed biochemically with high levels of thyroid hormones (T4 and T3) and low levels of TSH due to negative feedback.

The normal thyroid produces T4 and T3 as driven by TSH from the pituitary, which in turn is driven by hypothalamic thyroid-releasing hormone (TRH). T4 is produced in abundance relative to T3; however, T3 is four times more metabolically active than T4 and is converted from T4 in peripheral tissues.

Symptomatic control of hyperthyroidism is achieved acutely with beta-blockade such as propranolol until thyroid-blocking agents such as propylthiouracil or carbimazole have taken effect. This usually occurs over a period of weeks and therapy must be monitored in this period with regular tests of thyroid activity until a stable dosage regime has been established. Beta-blockade is not usually required as long-term therapy if control of over-activity can be managed medically or surgically with subtotal or total thyroidectomy (if refractory to medical treatment).

35 b. Warfarin is not indicated in the immediate management of MI. The antiplatelet effect of aspirin and clopidogrel has been shown to be beneficial in the treatment of MI.

36 a. The presentation is strongly suspicious for scabies, which in this age group should be high on the differential diagnosis of an itchy rash. Scabies is caused by the *Sarcoptes scabiei* mite, which has a predilection for the epidermis. Typical features of scabies are an intensely itchy rash, which is caused by a delayed-type hypersensitivity reaction to the mite itself, with characteristic inflammatory papules and almost pathognomonic burrows or tracts. Areas commonly affected include the hands and feet with fingers, wrists and web spaces the most often afflicted.

Treatment modalities include one or two applications of malathion or permethrin cream, which are left on the skin for a period of 24 or 12 hours. Aqueous cream is used in the treatment of eczema and while it may give some mild symptomatic relief, it is not effective in treating scabies. Flucloxacillin 500 mg tds is usually given in conjunction with another penicillin derivative for cellulitic infections. If a viral infection was suspected in a young child it may be appropriate to adopt a conservative management policy; however, this will not lead to adequate symptom control and resolution in scabies. Cold tar is a very effective but messy treatment option in the management of psoriasis and acts as an anti-inflammatory agent when applied topically to psoriatic areas.

37 e. New-onset atrial fibrillation should ideally be converted to sinus rhythm by DC cardioversion. DC cardioversion may precipitate systemic emboli from intracardiac thrombus. To avoid

thromboembolic events, formal anticoagulation is required for 1 month before and after the cardioversion, unless:
- the arrhythmia is of less than 72 hours' standing, or
- no intracardiac thrombus is apparent on transoesophageal echocardiography.

Co-ordinated atrial activity may not resume for 2 weeks following cardioversion even if sinus rhythm is apparent on the ECG. For this reason, anticoagulation should continue for 1 month usually in the form of warfarin. In this case it is inappropriate to start conservative medical management since the atrial fibrillation is of new onset and the patient is compromised.

In those patients with a new diagnosis of atrial fibrillation, management can be challenging, particularly if it is not clear of the duration of the arrhythmia. In stable patients, most commonly management with medications including beta-blockers is appropriate. There has been a move away from rhythm control with digoxin in the past few years and rate control with beta-blockade is now favoured.

38 c. PTCA is the most appropriate management option for this man. PTCA restores artery patency in more than 90% of patients. PTCA has fewer bleeding complications and recurrent ischaemia when compared to thrombolysis. However, a major drawback of PTCA is the need for 24-hour availability of an angioplasty suite and staff. The time for treatment is longer for patients receiving primary PTCA as compared with those receiving thrombolysis; however, if the facilities are available, it is the preferred treatment option. None of the other options listed is appropriate in the management of this case.

39 c. Pituitary adenoma accounts for over 95% of all causes of acromegaly and results in a plethora of clinical features, often noticed by those around the patient rather than the patient themselves. Headache and visual disturbance are common complaints due to the enlarging adenoma causing compression of the neighbouring optic chiasm, usually in the central portion, leading to the classical pattern of visual loss and bitemporal hemianopia (tunnel vision). Adenomas are almost always benign and can be classified as secretory or non-secretory (null-cell tumours). In total, 25% of the secretory adenomas produce prolactin, 20% produce growth hormone and 10% produce ACTH, accounting for the endocrine disturbance in addition to the mass effect of the adenoma.

Craniopharyngioma is a squamous, calcified cystic tumour arising from the remnant of the craniopharyngeal duct or **151**

Rathke's pouch and manifests with similar signs and symptoms as acromegaly. Headache due to mass effect is a predominant complaint but over 50% present with signs of endocrinopathy such as hypothyroidism, adrenal failure or diabetes insipidus and around 75% may present with visual disturbance. Craniopharyngioma exhibits a bimodal distribution in children aged around 6–10 years and then again in adults in their mid- to late 50s.

Hypothalamic glioma is typically a disease of children and young adults and tends to be aggressive in nature. Subtle endocrine disturbance may occur related to the area of hypothalamus affected and range from disturbance in temperature regulation and appetite to SIADH and cranial diabetes insipidus.

Parasella meningioma usually causes local compression effects and causes a local osteoblastic reaction to the surrounding bone that is usually depicted on plain radiographs and CT scan. MRI is the definitive imaging modality and may help to assess surgical resectability by defining involvement of the cavernous sinus and carotid artery.

Metastases can also be seen to the pituitary and are usually clinically silent unless large in size. Lymphoma, breast and bone marrow tumours are the most commonly seen metastases at this rare site and most diagnoses of pituitary metastases are made only at autopsy. Diabetes insipidus may sometimes be a consequence of large secondary deposits.

40 b. Macule is a descriptive term for a flat but well-defined area of skin change. Papule refers to a raised macule that is <0.5 cm in diameter, i.e. a circumscribed area of skin that is elevated. A nodule is the counterpart to a papule that is >0.5 cm in diameter. Plaques refer to more discoid elevations of the skin that are small <2 cm in diameter or large when >2 cm. A vesicle describes a localized collection of fluid <0.5 cm in diameter, such as found typically in herpes zoster. A bulla describes the counterpart that is >0.5 cm in diameter. A pustule is simply a collection of pus in the skin. A weal is usually associated with allergic reactions such as seen in urticarial disorders and represents a localized area of oedema within the skin.

41 b. Contraindications to thrombolysis include:
- known active bleeding source, e.g. peptic ulcer, active dyspepsia,
- active menstruation,
- cerebrovascular accident within 3 months,
- surgery or head injury within last 3 months,

- severe hypertension:
  - systolic >200 mmHg or diastolic >100 mmHg,
  - must be sustained, e.g. not responding to IV nitrates,
- hypotension:
  - systolic <90 mmHg and not corrected by atropine (if brady-cardia) or other rhythm correction,
- chest trauma due to prolonged cardiac massage – if cardiopul-monary resuscitation more than 5 minutes, assess risks with senior staff,
- on warfarin,
- known or suspected aortic aneurysm,
- known sensitivity to streptokinase or prior administration within last 24 months (for streptokinase administration only).

42 a. DCIS is a premalignant condition. Approximately 40% of DCIS lesions will progress to become invasive breast cancers. As carcinomas *in situ*, they are unable to metastasize. They present in the same way as invasive breast cancers but are more readily picked up on mammography – they account for approximately 25% of all cancers picked up in that way. Management nor-mally involves a wide local excision with possible radiotherapy, depending on the clinical decision made at the time of surgery. If the lesion is large, axillary node clearance may also be required.

43 b. If the causative organism is not known, empirical therapy is as follows:
- IV benzylpenicillin and gentamycin unless staphylococcal in-fection is suspected, when vancomycin is substituted for peni-cillin,
- if patient is allergic to penicillin, use vancomycin and gen-tamycin.

44 e. Cullen's sign is peri-umbilical bruising or yellow blue discol-oration. Originally, it was described in ruptured ectopic preg-nancy but it is more commonly associated with severe, acute pancreatitis. The cause of the discoloration is pancreatic en-zymes tracking along the falciform ligament and digesting sub-cutaneous tissues around the umbilicus. Aortic regurgitation is associated with De Musset's sign (head-bobbing) and Quincke's sign (visible nail bed pulsations). Kussmaul's sign is a rising JVP on inspiration associated with a diagnosis of constrictive pericarditis and cardiac tamponade. Corrigan's sign is associated with aortic valve incompetence.

45 e. Long-term use of steroids (>2 weeks) with abrupt withdrawal causes the clinical state of hypoadrenalism similar to Addison's **153**

disease due to exogenous suppression of the endogenous production of corticosteroids. Patients who are on steroid medications should carry a 'steroid card' with information regarding
dosing and length of dosing and side-effects of abrupt cessation
of steroids. High-dose regimens for acute flares of autoimmune
diseases are usually tapered over a matter of weeks, usually with
fixed-increment reduction in dose (e.g. 5 mg/week) to prevent a
hypoadrenal crisis by slow regaining of endogenous adrenal axis
function.

Intravascular depletion is often a cause of hypotension in the
elderly and is usually seen in the context of an infective process, such as a urinary tract infection or pneumonia with good
response to IV fluids. In this case, there were abnormal requirements for parenteral fluids to maintain a barely adequate blood
pressure, indicating an underlying process more complex than
intravascular depletion.

Septic shock (especially with Gram-negative organisms) can
cause a profound hypotension that is refractory to fluid resuscitation and may in fact lead to fluid overload and pulmonary
oedema. The pathophysiology is one of a decreased systemic
vascular resistance due to bacterial endotoxins and intravascular
depletion and hypotension. Inotropic support in a critical care
setting with an agent such as noradrenaline may be required.

Haemorrhagic stroke usually presents acutely with neurological signs and symptoms and hypertension due to a reflex response to cerebral injury and loss of autoregulation in order to
ensure adequate cerebral perfusion pressure (CPP). As cerebral
perfusion is a function of mean arterial pressure (MAP) minus
the intracerebral pressure (ICP), in the face of increased ICP, for
example cerebral insult, adequate CPP is achieved by an increase
in the MAP manifest as hypertension. It is vital not to treat this
primary hypertension acutely. Vasovagal syncope is unlikely to
cause such a long-lasting hypotension and would be responsive
to fluid resuscitation.

46 a. The scenario describes a classic history of pericarditis. This
is often associated with a history of a recent upper respiratory
tract infection. The history of chest pain that is exacerbated by
lying flat and inspiration is characteristic of pericarditis. Classical ECG findings are described, including concave upwards ST
segment elevation (saddle-shaped). Management of pericarditis
includes NSAIDs for pain control and rest. A&E referral would
be appropriate management if there was uncertainty about the
diagnosis. No further useful information would be gleaned from
a chest X-ray or an echocardiogram.

47 d. Indications for performing a mastectomy *in lieu* of any other procedure include:

- a lump of 4 cm or greater,
- a multifocal cancer,
- a centrally located cancer,
- patient choice (in the presence of a breast lump).

fibroadenomas are often managed conservatively and one third regress and disappear in their own time. If they cause significant discomfort or are >4 cm, they may be considered for removal.

48 a. Identification of cardiac tamponade relies upon Beck's triad: hypotension, jugular vein distention and muffled heart sounds, resulting from fluid accumulation in the pericardial sac, which dampens the transmission of sounds through the chest wall. Identification of the quiet heart sounds can be difficult using a stethoscope, which is why a hospital setting is useful for further investigations. Bradycardia is not associated with cardiac tamponade; in fact, tachycardia is often seen as there is reduced filling time in the cardiac cycle due to reduced capacity of the chambers.

49 b. A PDA is a defect between the pulmonary artery and the aorta. The ductus arteriosus normally closes within the first 48 hours of life. In premature babies, it may remain open for longer, sometimes up to 3 months. If it remains patent longer than this it is unlikely to close spontaneously. A persistently patent ductus is a common congenital heart lesion, occurring either singly or in combination with other defects. Girls are more likely to be affected by PDA. Also those affected by congenital rubella syndrome are more likely to suffer a PDA.

All other options are correct.

50 c. Phentolamine and phenoxybenzamine are the agents of choice in the rapid treatment of hypertension caused by phaeochromocytoma. Beta-blockade can be added to control dangerously high blood pressure but only after institution of an alpha-blocker, otherwise there is a significant risk of exacerbating hypertension. Surgical intervention in patients with phaeochromocytoma must only be performed once the patient has been medically treated and blocked from the effects of excess circulating catecholamines. Catecholamine-induced cardiomyopathy and life-threatening hypertensive crisis due to uncontrolled release of catecholamines intraoperatively are a significant cause of mortality and morbidity.

Imaging modalities, such as a CT scan of the abdomen and renal artery Doppler scans, are useful studies in the investigation of any patient with uncontrolled newly diagnosed hypertension. However, these are not urgent and CT scan would be contraindicated in an unstable patient (the 'doughnut of death'). Renal artery ultrasonography is used commonly to detect clinically significant arterial stenosis, which can lead to hypertension and flash pulmonary oedema.

Surgical management of phaeochromocytoma is usually performed transabdominally with identification and ligation of the adrenal veins to isolate the tumour from releasing a surge of catecholamine into the systemic circulation. Laparoscopic approaches have been favoured recently but prove more difficult to assess for extra-adrenal sites of catecholamine production, for example elsewhere in the sympathetic chain.

51 d. Hypothyroidism is associated with bradycardia. It often has an insidious onset with symptoms such as fatigue, weight gain and cold intolerance. Cardiovascular symptoms include angina, cardiac failure, pericardial and pleural effusions. Ehlers–Danlos syndrome is associated with joint laxity and hypermobility and mitral valve prolapse. While superficially Turner's syndrome is associated with a webbed neck, cardiovascular complications can include coarctation of the aorta, which can be how the syndrome is discovered in young girls. Cardiovascular lesions in Noonan's syndrome affect the right side of the heart, for example pulmonary valve stenosis.

52 b. Hypertrophic cardiomyopathy is defined as the unexplained, asymmetrical or concentric hypertrophy of the undilated left ventricle. There is also hypertrophy of the right ventricle. It may be inherited as an autosomal dominant condition, but at least half of cases may be the result of sporadic mutation and therefore the patient may be unaware of the condition.

Symptoms may include:
- angina,
- dyspnoea,
- palpitations,
- syncope,
- sudden death.

Clinical signs include:
- jerky pulse,
- JVP: large 'a' waves, indicating right ventricular flow obstruction,
- double impulse at apex,

- loud fourth heart sound due to the left ventricular hypertrophy,
- third heart sound,
- late systolic murmur.

It is unlikely that this episode has been caused by a pulmonary embolus as she is a fit and well woman with no obvious risk factors. A pneumonia or pneumothorax would have caused some symptoms but would have been unlikely to have resulted in a cardiac arrest.

53 d. Seborrhoeic keratoses are encountered universally in medicine in whichever specialty one trains as they are frequently an incidental finding in the elderly population. Most often found on the back and chest, the lesions may take on an oily appearance due to the sebaceous nature of the growth and resemble segmented discrete flat brown abnormalities that arise from the skin surface.

Malignant melanoma may be suspected in seborrhoeic keratoses that have a darker, more atypical appearance; however, malignant melanomas occur in a younger population than other skin cancers and are predisposed by frequent sun exposure, typically in a pale-skinned patient with a history of repeated sun-burning episodes. Malignant melanomas are aggressive once spread past the superficial layers of the skin has occurred and must be caught early if effective curative resection is to be achieved.

Keratoacanthoma is often classified as a benign tumour, although histologically it closely resembles a squamous cell carcinoma. However, excision and further histological analysis is usually recommended if the diagnosis is not clear. It often presents as a round discrete nodule with a central darker area filled with keratin.

Campbell de Morgan spots are again often seen in the elderly population and are essentially abnormal vascular regions developing within the deeper layers of the skin. They present as cherry red round lesions in the skin and are harmless.

Basal cell carcinoma is the commonest malignant skin tumour seen in dermatological practice and is locally invasive, with metastasis being extremely rare. It is classically described as having a pearly appearance with areas of superficial telangiectasia and a rolled edge surrounding a sunken central area. Treatment is with excision and biopsy, with or without radiotherapy.

54 c. Warfarin acts as a vitamin K antagonist and so affects the synthesis of active factors II, VII, IX, X and protein C. The therapeutic goal is to cause a partial inhibition of clotting factor synthesis, to prolong prothrombin time two- to four-fold. Once administered, warfarin does not exert its effect for 2–3 days and therefore during this lag period alternative anticoagulation should be used. This anticoagulation is usually in the form of a low molecular weight heparin; its anticoagulation action is via factor Xa and is much more rapid in its onset.

55 c. All of the signs are suggestive of a locally invasive breast cancer. A growing mass with overlying skin ulceration is highly suggestive of malignancy. Other signs to look out for include *peau d'orange* skin changes and axillary lymphadenopathy, which are not mentioned in the case. A breast abscess or mastitis are unlikely to be the case in this woman, as she reports no pain from the lump and is not strictly in the right age range for those conditions. Although DCIS may present in a similar manner to an invasive breast lump, the extent of the spread of this lump suggests that a more sinister cause is responsible.

56 a. Inhibition of HMG CoA in the liver, which is the rate-limiting step in cholesterol synthesis, is the mechanism of action of statins. They are appropriately prescribed in the evening, since the synthesis of cholesterol appears most active overnight.

The cytochrome p450 is a group of enzymes that control concentrations of drugs and endogenous substances. Succinate co-A is involved in the Krebs cycle.

57 c. Adenosine is a naturally occurring purine nucleoside with a pharmacological half-life of less than 2 seconds. Its principal role is in the diagnosis and management of paroxysmal supraventricular tachycardia. Cautions include atrial fibrillation or flutter caused by accessory pathways and contraindications include second- or third-degree heart block and sick sinus syndrome. Before administering adenosine to a patient, it is important to tell them that they may experience a strange sensation, which may make them feel as if they are about to die. This sensation may last for a few seconds.

Atenolol is a beta-blocker and has limited use in an acute setting, while atorvastatin has a role in reduction of cholesterol in a chronic capacity. Amlodipine is a calcium-channel blocker and amiodarone has a role in refractory ventricular fibrillation or atrial flutter.

58 e. Pyoderma gangrenosum is associated with inflammatory bowel disease such as ulcerative colitis and Crohn's disease. It presents as wet sloughy ulcers with heaped edges and scattered areas of black necrotic tissue. Pyoderma gangrenosum may also be associated with haematological malignancy and rheumatoid arthritis.

The cutaneous manifestations of diabetes mellitus are legion and range from diabetic foot ulcers to atrophy of the fat layers in the skin, causing thinning and an abnormal appearance to the area (lipoatrophy). Necrobiosis lipoidica diabeticorum is usually found on the shins and presents as shiny, yellow-brown heterogeneous areas of skin discoloration with associated skin thinning and predisposition to breakdown. Xanthoma and xanthelasma are seen in condition of hypercholesterolaemia and are not discrete to diabetes; however, endocrine disturbance, as seen in diabetes mellitus, is frequently associated with derangement in other biochemical profiles such as lipid homeostasis.

Acanthosis nigricans (the presenting complaint of this man) manifests as a result of insulin resistance, although it may be seen in association with gastrointestinal malignancy.

Granuloma annulare often presents in association with diabetes when generalized rather than discrete and is characteristically described as crops of hard raised areas of skin in a ring-like arrangement occurring on the back of the hands and soles of the feet. A conservative approach is adopted in most cases as spontaneous resolution tends to be the rule.

59 b. Simvastatin has been linked to inflammation of muscle tissue (myositis), causing a rise in CK associated with muscle aches, malaise and abdominal pain. Also reported is a derangement of liver enzymes, especially of aspartate transaminase (AST) and alanine transaminase (ALT).

A rare but serious side-effect of simvastatin in particular is the development of rhabdomyolysis, leading to acute renal damage. Diclofenac may be associated with abdominal pain but the mechanism of pain is usually due to gastric ulceration caused by the inhibition of protective prostaglandins in the gastric mucosa.

Metformin is a diabetic medication that, unlike the sulphonylureas, does not cause hypoglycaemia due to a mechanism of action that increases insulin sensitivity in tissues rather than increases insulin levels. Metformin can cause a metabolic acidosis and renal impairment when given in conjunction with contrast agents, such as those used in radiographic investigations. It should be stopped on the day of the investigation and the patient should be encouraged to drink fluids for the 24–48 hours post-contrast.

60 b. Ventricular fibrillation is uncoordinated ventricular activity that can be corrected by unsynchronized DC shock. Pulseless ventricular tachycardia can also be managed by unsynchronized DC shock. Atrial fibrillation, provided it is new in origin, can be managed by electrical current but this requires synchronized current. Asystole and pulseless electrical activity do not benefit from treatment with electrical current.

Extended Matching Questions

61 d. *Cryptosporidium parvum* is a protozoal infection that can cause a severe diarrhoea in immunocompromised individuals. Protozoal cysts adhere to the gut wall and cause a florid secretory diarrhoea that requires large volume fluid resuscitation. The organism can be found in cattle and can cause self-limiting diarrhoea in immunocompetent individuals. Treatment is mainly supportive, as antibiotic therapy has not been proven to be effective.

62 e. *Cryptococcus neoformans* is a fungal infection usually associated with meningitis in HIV. The clinical signs may be masked by the damped immune response seen in immunocompromised individuals and thus the fever, neck stiffness and photophobia associated with inflammation of the meninges may be impaired or even lacking. *Cryptococcus* may be diagnosed by India ink staining of a sample of cerebrospinal fluid (CSF) at lumbar puncture and carries a 20% mortality even with treatment.

63 b. Candidiasis is often seen in diabetics, those on immunosuppressive therapy and those with immunodeficiency. The most common manifestation is oral candidiasis with white plaques in the mouth and oropharynx. Oesophageal candidiasis presents with odynophagia (pain on swallowing – usually retrosternal) and dysphagia due to the pain. Treatment is usually with fluconazole or another associated 'azole' by mouth for a couple of weeks. Severe cases may merit using amphotericin with caution ('*amphoterrible*' – coined because of severe nephrotoxic side-effects).

64 c. Infection with the protozoan *Toxoplasma gondii* can cause encephalitis and cerebral abscesses, of which the latter may catastrophically be misdiagnosed as primary cerebral tumour or stroke. The symptoms are those of a space-occupying lesion and may cause fitting, focal neurological deficit, confusion, personality change and may be difficult to distinguish from a cerebrovascular event. magnetic resonance imaging (MRI) is the investigation of choice in imaging suspected *Toxoplasma* infection and can prove to be spectacularly superior to CT scanning in defining numbers and character of lesions with ring-enhancing lesions classically described. Treatment with pyrimethamine in combination with sulfadiazine and folinic acid for at least 6 weeks can produce remarkable reversal of the clinical state.

65 a. *Pneumocystis jiroveci* pneumonia (formally called *Pneumocystis carinii* pneumonia) is one of the most common life-threatening infections in HIV/AIDS. It can act as a benchmark for the severity of immunosuppression as it is rarely seen with CD4 counts >200/mm^3. Prophylaxis is given when CD4 counts drop <200/mm^3 and co-trimoxazole (trimethoprim and sulfamethoxazole) is the agent of choice. Chest signs may be clinically absent but the usual scenario is an HIV-positive individual who is in frank respiratory compromise with hypoxia, tachypnoea and tachycardia with fine crepitations throughout the chest. Treatment is with high-dose co-trimoxazole for up to 3 weeks, with systemic corticosteroids for severe disease (defined as a PaO2 <9.5 kPa).

66 b. This woman is suffering from a pneumonia, which can be associated with chest pain. Risk factors for her developing chest infections include the fact that she has a history of lung disease and that she resides in a nursing home. Sedentary lifestyles are often associated with acquiring infections, particularly in institutionalized patients.

67 e. Bornholm disease is a post-viral illness that is associated with costochondritis. Patients describe a chest pain that can be recreated by sternal pressure – similar to Tietze's syndrome or idiopathic costochondritis but on further questioning its incidence closely follows a viral illness.

68 g. The clue in this scenario is the recent addition of diclofenac into his medication list. The man's history suggests a diagnosis of gastro-oesophageal reflux disease. Exacerbation of his symptoms on lying flat suggests a gastric association and deficiency in the distal oesophageal sphincter. The nausea associated with this pain could be associated with cardiac pain but in the context of this history we can be reassured that the likely cause of this gentleman's pain is gastrointestinal in origin.

69 h. Acute-onset chest pain that is described as radiating to the back is characteristic of aortic dissection. Aortic dissection is defined as separation of the layers within the aortic wall. Tears in the intimal layer result in the propagation of dissection (proximally or distally) secondary to blood entering the intima–media space. Aortic dissection is more common in males than in females, with a male to female ratio of 2:1. The condition commonly occurs in persons in the sixth and seventh decades of life. Patients with Marfan's syndrome present earlier, usually in the third and fourth decades of life.

DeBakey classified aortic dissection into three types:
- type I: the intimal tear occurs in the ascending aorta, but the descending aorta is also involved,
- type II: only the ascending aorta is involved,
- type III: only the descending aorta is involved:
  ○ type IIIA: involves the descending aorta that originates distal to the left subclavian artery and extends as far as the diaphragm,
  ○ type IIIB: involves the descending aorta below the diaphragm.

The pain of aortic dissection may be distinguished from the pain of acute MI by its abrupt onset, although the presentations of the two conditions overlap to some degree. Aortic dissection should be strongly considered in patients with symptoms and signs suggestive of MI but without classic ECG findings.

70 c. Risk factors for pulmonary embolus include: immobility, malignancy, postoperative period for abdominal or pelvic surgery, lower limb fractures, previous thromboembolic disease, pregnancy and hip or knee replacements. In addition to these there are further minor risk factors, including long-distance travel, use of the combined oral contraceptive pill or hormone replacement therapy. In the case in question, this woman is 1 week into the postoperative period from having a knee replacement. In this case, right calf swelling that progresses to chest pain exacerbated by inspiration is a classical description of a pulmonary embolus.

A ventilation/perfusion scan or a CT pulmonary angiogram should be organized to confirm the diagnosis and treatment-dose anticoagulation should be commenced as soon as the diagnosis is suspected and, if confirmed, this should be replaced with warfarin.

71 f. Bacterial vaginosis, although a cause of vaginal discharge, is not usually classified as a sexually transmitted infection as it can present unrelated to sexual intercourse. The terminology 'vaginosis' is used as there is usually no inflammation of the vagina, separating this condition from diseases causing vaginitis. A change in the normal pH of the vagina is thought to play a role in the alteration of the normal flora and encourages overgrowth of bacteria such as *Gardnerella vaginalis*, *Mycoplasma hominis*, *Mobiluncus* spp. and anaerobes such as *Bacteroides*. Microscopy of vaginal epithelial cells reveals the presence of 'clue cells', which are squamous vaginal cells on which the causative bacteria are attached.

72 g. Gonorrhoea typically presents in men with a yellow purulent discharge from the urethra with associated dysuria and irritation. However, *Neisseria gonorrhoeae* has a predilection for epithelium of the cervix, rectum, conjunctiva and pharynx, depending upon exposure to such sites. In women, the presentation is much more subtle and insidious. Up to 50% of women may be asymptomatic and may eventually present with altered vaginal discharge, dysuria and intermenstrual bleeding with fertility problems as *Neisseria gonorrhoeae* a long-term consequence of severe untreated infection. *Neisseria gonorrhoeae* are Gram-negative intracellular diplococci and are easily recognizable on microscopy. Treatment involves using fluoroquinolones such as ciprofloxacin or ofloxacin for uncomplicated disease, amoxicillin (sometimes with probenecid) in penicillin-sensitive areas or ceftriaxone in areas of high penicillin resistance.

73 a. *Candida albicans* is an extremely common non-sexually transmitted infection of females and males. In females, it can cause a very itchy vulvovaginal rash (pruritus vulvae) with a creamy white, curd-like discharge from the vagina. In men, infection with *Candida albicans* may occasionally arise due to cross-infection from a partner but more usually is the manifestation of an underlying disorder, such as immunosuppression, diabetes or overuse of broad-spectrum antibiotics. In this case, the patient was a known diabetic and some would argue that the routine work-up of male patients presenting with balanitis (infection of the head of the penis) should include investigation of undiagnosed diabetes. Treatment can be obtained over the counter, as either a topical antifungal pessary, cream or oral tablet.

74 c. *Chlamydia trachomatis* is a common sexually transmitted infection with up to 5% of the UK population of sexually active women infected. It is often clinically silent until the long-term consequences are discovered and a retrospective diagnosis is offered. Some authorities report figures as high as 80% for asymptomatic infection in women with approximately half of all infected males demonstrating no clinical symptoms. Well-recognized sequelae of infection with *Chlamydia trachomatis* are infertility (due to salpingitis and pelvic inflammatory disease) and Reiter's syndrome – a triad of conjunctivitis, arthritis and urethritis. Diagnosis of *Chlamydia trachomatis* is complicated by the fact that it is an obligate intracellular bacterium and thus complex cell culture, direct fluorescent antibody and DNA testing form the mainstay of diagnostic techniques.

75 b. *Trichomonas vaginalis* is a sexually transmitted infection that causes inflammation of the vagina (vaginitis) and can often be confused with bacterial vaginosis, a non-sexually transmitted infection that does not affect the vagina itself. The discharge is classically described as a *champagne* discharge as it is green-yellow and frothy and may accompany a *strawberry* cervix – so called as the cervix if often dotted with small haemorrhagic areas. Diagnosis is with dark-ground microscopy on a wet preparation and treatment involves metronidazole 400 mg bd for 1 week.

76 a. The mechanism of action of atropine is via blockage of the vagus nerve and subsequently enhances sinus node automaticity and atrioventricular conduction:
- atropine causes blockade of parasympathetic activity at both the sinoatrial (SA) node and the atrioventricular (AV) node; it may increase sinus automaticity and facilitate AV node conduction,
- dosages of atropine for adults in asystole, or pulseless electrical activity with a rate < 60 bpm, is 3 mg IV.

Atropine may increase myocardial oxygen demand and unmask sympathetic overactivity.

77 e. The dose of magnesium sulphate is 8 mmol (4 mL of a 50% solution) for refractory ventricular fibrillation if there is any suspicion of hypomagnesaemia, especially if the patient is on potassium-losing diuretics.

Other indications for the use of magnesium sulphate are:
- ventricular tachyarrhythmias in the presence of possible hypomagnesaemia,
- torsades de pointes,
- digoxin toxicity.

78 c. The use of amiodarone in shock-refractory ventricular fibrillation is believed to improve survival. Experts believe that there is a role for amiodarone in ventricular fibrillation or pulseless ventricular tachycardia resistant to three shocks. Initially, 300 mg IV should be given before continuing with shocks. The UK Resuscitation Council suggests that a further dose of 150 mg may be given for recurrent or refractory ventricular fibrillation/ventricular tachycardia followed by an infusion of 900 mg over the next 24 hours.

79 f. Adenosine slows conduction across the AV node but has limited effect on myocardial cells. This makes it very effective for terminating paroxysmal supraventricular tachycardias associated with re-entrant circuits. Adenosine has a short duration of action and therefore the affect of the drug may be short lived. Induction of AV nodal block can reveal underlying atrial rhythms and in those patients presenting with narrow complex tachycardias, it slows down the ventricular response. Side-effects of administration of adenosine include episodes of severe bradycardia.

80 h. Flecainide is a potent sodium-channel blocker and therefore slows conduction. The effect of flecainide can be seen on the ECG as lengthening of the PR interval and widening of the QRS complex.

Flecainide is known to be negatively inotropic and may result in bradycardia and hypotension. Other side-effects documented include blurring of vision and oral paraesthesiae.

81 e. A diagnostic coronary angiogram is indicated in this case. The mildly positive troponin and associated ECG changes increase the likelihood that this woman is suffering from cardiac chest pain. While she has no cardiovascular history, it is not inconceivable that this could be the first presentation of underlying problems. Information could be gleaned from an echocardiogram but the most appropriate diagnostic investigation is a coronary angiogram.

Risk factors for cardiovascular disease include:

- male sex,
- hypertension,
- hypercholesterolaemia,
- diabetes,
- smoking,
- family history,
- homocysteine levels.

82 b. An ECG is the most sensible place to start in investigation of this woman's symptoms. The most likely cause for her symptoms is either sinus pauses or arrhythmias. If she had been taking a lot of medication this would have been a sensible place to start. If an ECG does not yield a diagnosis it may then be sensible to proceed on to a 24-hour tape to hunt for further answers.

83 c. An echocardiogram would provide useful information about the necessity for anticoagulation in this case. In cardiovascular disease, anticoagulation may be divided into two levels, warfarinization or antiplatelet therapy. Antiplatelet therapy includes both aspirin and clopidogrel. In the absence of a dilated left atrium, warfarinization is unnecessary as the likelihood of a thrombus forming in a normal atrium is slim. Should an echocardiogram reveal a dilated left atrium, warfarinization should be discussed with the patient, since there are serious indications to warfarin, particularly in elderly patients.

84 d. An ETT is the next logical step in risk stratification of this patient. He has ECG changes, a history of chest pain but negative troponin. Any changes on ETT will help to identify risk of this patient developing cardiovascular disease or symptoms. Depending on the findings, it may be necessary to proceed on to a coronary angiogram.

85 f. These findings are suggestive of some form of arrhythmia. With rate variations such as this, in excess of 40 bpm, a cause should be sought. A 24-hour tape should provide adequate information about the cause of these rate variations. Based on this information, treatment may be commenced. An ECG alone is unlikely to show any cause for this rate variation as it only captures a period of 6 seconds.

86 a. Cushing's syndrome manifests clinically with a plethora of clinical signs due to excess amounts of corticosteroid. The typical clinical picture is of an obese patient who exhibits a moon-face appearance, abnormal fatty pads over the neck and upper back leading to the classical buffalo hump, with easily bruised and paper thin skin. Hypertension and diabetes mellitus are commonly found due to both the mineralocorticoid and glucocorticoid effects of excess corticosteroid and a picture of hypernatraemia and hypokalaemia provides a clue to the pathology in the face of a strong clinical suspicion.

Cushing's syndrome can be as a result of Cushing's disease, which describes the above clinical findings as a consequence of a primary pituitary neoplasm (usually adenoma). Other ACTH-dependent causes may be due to an ectopic focus of ACTH secretion, such as a small-cell carcinoma of the lung. ACTH-independent causes include a primary adrenocortical tumour such as an adenoma or, commonly, exogenous steroid use such as that seen often in those requiring steroid immunosuppression for transplants or autoimmune disease.

87 g. Hypothyroidism may present in the elderly with very non-specific signs and should be considered in the differential of anyone presenting with confusion (so-called part of the 'dementia' screen) and general deterioration with no readily identifiable cause. One of the most common endocrine disturbances alongside diabetes mellitus, it should not be missed as a cause of symptoms ranging from neurological signs, typically bradykinesia, reduced deep tendon reflexes and paraesthesia from nerve entrapment (especially carpal tunnel syndrome) to abdominal pain from chronic constipation to mental disturbance manifest as confusion and apparent memory impairment. Other subtle signs of hypothyroidism include loss of the outer one third of the eyebrows with male-pattern frontal balding, hypothermia (leading to the aptly named 'granny's tartan' – erythema ab igne from sitting close to or being in close contact with a source of heat such as a fire, electric heater or hot-water bottle), bradycardia and dry, coarse skin. Thyroid function tests are usually diagnostic and demonstrate a low free T4 with a compensatory high TSH in primary hypothyroidism. Very occasionally, a low TSH and a low free T4 may be seen in the context of panhypopituitarism and assay of levels of sex hormones, ACTH and other pituitary hormones will confirm the diagnosis.

88 c. Diabetes mellitus can often present in a similar fashion to other endocrine diseases and thus it is important that investigations be interpreted in the correct fashion. Loss of weight, fatigue, polydipsia and polyuria are features of not only diabetes mellitus but also of diabetes insipidus (loss of free water due to an inability to secrete or respond to vasopressin and thus concentrate urine). Occasionally, hysterical polydipsia manifests with the above clinical features and can be difficult to clinically distinguish from diabetes insipidus. In this case, performing urine electrolyte and osmolality studies can differentiate between these two very different conditions; in diabetes insipidus there is secretion of free water and thus urine osmolality is very low. However, in hysterical polydipsia urine osmolality is normal as intake is matched by output, keeping an overall isotonic balance to osmolality. Clues in the above case to a diagnosis of diabetes mellitus are the concurrent infection (which raises stress hormone levels, e.g. cortisol, causing an increase in blood glucose levels), the high urine osmolality (due to high glucose load as the renal tubular threshold for glucose absorption has been exceeded) and the very high plasma osmolality. This can be approximated thus:

$$P_{osm} \sim 2(Na^+) + K^+ + urea + glucose \qquad (units = mOsm/L)$$

Plugging in the values for sodium, potassium and urea leaves the remaining component (glucose) at 20.1. This high glucose in the absence of any previous history of diabetes mellitus suggests a type II manifestation of high blood sugar, i.e. a hyperosmolar hyperglycaemic state. Urine dipstick will confirm the presence of heavy ketonuria (suggestive of diabetic ketoacidosis or an element of hyperosmolar hyperglycaemic state/diabetic ketoacidosis overlap) and an ABG would demonstrate the pH. As a general rule, any event such as surgery, illness or even MI can manifest clinically in addition to the primary event with features of high blood glucose control, which may then progress to hyperosmolar hyperglycaemic state or diabetic ketoacidosis.

89 b. The diagnosis of acromegaly can often be very subtle, with those closest to the patient often bringing the changes to attention. It is often helpful to look at old photographs if there is a suspicion of acromegaly as coarsening of features, protrusion of the jaw (prognathism) and change in clothing or shoe size may all point to a retrospective diagnosis. Most often due to a pituitary adenoma (80% macroadenoma, 20% microadenoma), visual symptoms may be a complaint alongside headache and even bedside visual field testing may reveal a defect, commonly a bitemporal hemianopia (tunnel vision). Sausage fingers (leading to an inability to wear rings), greasy coarse skin and a thickening of the forehead are all signs of the growth hormone excess that characterizes acromegaly. Trans-sphenoidal hypophysectomy is usually employed as a treatment modality, sometimes in conjunction with medical therapy to reduce the size of a very large macroadenoma or surgically incompletely resected tumour.

90 e. Phaechromocytoma is a rare tumour of the sympathetic nervous system, notable for the production of catecholamines. Tumours may be adrenal or extra-adrenal and occur in both children and adults. The *Rule of 10* mnemonic is a helpful way of remembering that phaeochromocytomas are *10%* ectopic, *10%*

malignant, *10%* multiple and *10%* extra-adrenal. Symptoms may often be mistaken for anxiety attacks or cardiac symptoms, as palpitations, tremors, severe anxiety with no basis and chest pain may all be manifestations of the tumour. Severe hypertension is commonly associated and this may prompt more serious investigation of otherwise subtle symptomatology.

Plasma metanephrines (metabolic products of catecholamine pathways) is the most sensitive investigation but a useful screening tool is the 24-hour urine collection for metanephrines and catecholamines. Imaging modalities should be used only on the basis of a strong clinical suspicion and/or biochemical evidence of a catecholamine disturbance as the incidence of adrenal mass (so-called incidentaloma) found on imaging has been estimated to be around 7% in the elderly population. MRI scanning of the abdomen is the preferred and most sensitive and specific modality and should be employed after positive biochemical tests have been confirmed.

Answers

Single Best Answer Questions

1 d. Polycythaemia is commonly found in COPD patients and in other respiratory diseases where gas transfer is reduced. Chronic hypoxia stimulates the production of erythropoietin from the kidneys, which acts on the bone marrow to augment the oxygen-carrying capacity of the blood. Usually this is the most important derangement that is found in the full blood count in the absence of an exacerbation.

2 c. This case presents a difficult ethical dilemma that is not infrequently encountered and can require extremely sensitive handling of the situation. An adult that is unconscious or otherwise incompetent to make a decision with respect to understanding, weighing up the options and retaining information in order to make an informed decision about their medical care presents difficulty in deciding what is in the patient's best interest. A discussion with family members may sometimes help inform the decision; however, there is no legal requirement (for an otherwise competent adult) for assent from the family or close relatives before making decisions about medical care in situations where that adult cannot consent to treatment.

Refusing to perform surgery without blood is indeed a surgeon's prerogative as a splenectomy following trauma may be dangerous without the back-up of blood products and may ultimately cause more harm than good. However, this is not the right course of action, as without surgery the prognosis is poor. Using crystalloid replacement is similarly not correct for the reasons above.

The brief clinical indicators point to a ruptured spleen in a hypotensive road traffic accident victim in whom delaying surgery any longer than is necessary would be seriously detrimental to

EMQs and SBAs for Medical Finals, Second Edition. Jonathan Bath, Rebecca Morgan and Mehool Patel.

the prognosis and would be labelled as medically unsafe. Awaiting a court order in an emergency situation would take too long and would not allow the appropriate timely intervention (emergency surgery) to occur, thus this should not be considered.

As the child is 14 years old and a legal minor, the parents have a legal right to dictate what medical treatment is appropriate for their child. However, in the case of emergency or life-threatening situations this may be overcome by the need to do what is in the patient's best interest. The four pillars of ethics – beneficence, nonmaleficence, autonomy and justice – should always be borne in mind when addressing ethical situations. Applied to this case, the surgeon would be covered from a legal and ethical standpoint to act in the patient's best interest and take the child to surgery, even if this is against the religious view of the parents.

Further justification is that religious values of parents are not intrinsically inherent to children and should not be assumed to represent the true wishes of the child in a situation such as this. A sensible strategy would be to take the onus from the parents by stating that clinical need dictates this course of action and if there was any other way to proceed without transfusion, it would have been explored. Often this abdicates the feeling of blame and responsibility that comes with making an active decision by taking the decision out of their hands.

3 e. There is no evidence that cannabis abuse is linked with epistaxis. One of the most common causes is trauma to the nose. In the anterior portion of the nose, 'Little's area' represents the anastomosis of the sphenopalatine artery, superior labial artery and the anterior ethmoid artery. This area is prone to bleeding following direct trauma and is the commonest site of bleeding from the anterior part of the nose. Other causes of bleeding include medications, for example warfarin and aspirin, blood disorders and granulomatous diseases including sarcoidosis. Other more unusual causes include hereditary haemorrhagic telangiectasia, which can occur in other parts of the body including the bowel resulting in a rectal bleed.

4 c. INR is derived from the prothrombin time, which is then normalized against a laboratory standard to give values that are interpretable and standardized wherever the tests are taken. The INR is a very specific and sensitive indicator of liver damage and is the investigation of choice when assessing liver function (although many laboratories persist with using the incorrect liver function test [LFT] terminology when assaying

levels of liver transaminases). Albumin is also a product of liver synthesis and can be expected to fall with chronic liver diseases. Glycaemic control is also regulated in a large part by the liver and hypoglycaemia due to impaired gluconeogenesis and glycogen storage is often a complication of patients with advanced liver impairment. AST and ALT are useful markers of acute liver insult such as hepatitis; however, they are not well correlated with the degree of liver failure. Alkaline phosphatase and bilirubin are often associated with obstruction of the biliary system and will often rise in obstructive jaundice preferentially to the transaminases. Fibrinogen is a useful indicator of consumption and turnover of clotting products and can be low in disseminated intravascular coagulation and venous thromboembolism.

5 d. This woman is suffering an allergic reaction to the antibiotics. Despite having had five previous doses and no known drug allergies, these symptoms of facial flushing and tingling in her hands are characteristic of an allergic reaction. More severe cases of allergy/anaphylaxis may result in shortness of breath and chest pain. Although this was not the case here, these should always be noted as important negatives in the patient's notes. It is important to stop all antibiotics in this case to assess the response to steroids and antihistamines, as there may be another underlying cause for these symptoms.

6 b. This woman has developed *Clostridium difficile* diarrhoea, which is associated with pseudomembranous colitis. It is particularly a complication of clindamycin use but few antibiotics are completely free of this side-effect. Treatment is with either metronidazole or vancomycin for more seriously ill patients. Her blood results can be explained by dehydration due to fluid and electrolyte loss from the gastrointestinal tract. IV potassium replacement is rarely indicated in patients with hypokalaemia and in fact in inexperienced hands may be extremely dangerous due to cardiac arrhythmias. Diuresis is not indicated as this woman is in negative fluid balance and the addition of amoxicillin is not effective at treating *C. difficile* diarrhoea. Blood is not needed in this case for fluid replacement; 0.9% normal saline is adequate.

7 e. Acute glaucoma, one of the most important ophthalmological emergencies, presents with a fixed dilated and often oval-shaped pupil.

Features of ophthalmological disease are as follows:

- *Acute glaucoma* – entire eye is red, both conjunctiva and ciliary vessels are injected. Pupil is fixed, dilated and oval in shape and the intraocular pressure is high.
- *Iritis* – redness is most marked around the cornea and does NOT blanch on pressure. Pupil is small and fixed.
- *Conjunctivitis* – conjunctival vessels injected, blanch on pressure. Pupil is normal and reactive.
- *Subconjunctival haemorrhage* – bright red sclera with rim around limbus. Pupil is normal.

8 a. Endogenous depression, i.e. depression that occurs without an easily identifiable precipitant, is typically more difficult to treat than exogenous (reactive) depression. Depression can be subclassified according to severity and the components required to fulfil the diagnostic criteria for a major depressive episode are at least five of the following, during the same 2-week period, representing a change from previous functioning; these must include either (a) or (b):

a. depressed mood,

b. diminished interest or pleasure (anhedonia),

c. significant change in weight,

d. insomnia or excessive sleepiness,

e. psychomotor agitation or retardation,

f. suicidal ideation or planned suicide,

g. fatigue or loss of energy,

h. feelings of worthlessness,

i. reduced ability to concentrate.

The above symptoms must also not be associated with signs of mania or excessive elevation of mood (leading more towards a diagnosis of bipolar affective disorder). They must cause clinically significant distress or impairment of functioning and organic causes for symptomatology must be ruled out. Symptoms must also not be associated with a grief response or bereavement. Females have been shown to be more prone to medication overdose and deliberate self-harm behaviour, with males favouring more violent modes of suicide.

A lack of a confiding relationship has previously been described as a vulnerability factor for depression along with early maternal loss, more than three children under 14 years at home and unemployment. These features are part of the Brown and Harris model of depression and have been postulated to be associated strongly with the development of depression.

Organic causes of depression or any change in mood or mental status *must* be ruled out prior to a diagnosis of psychiatric disease. This may include CT scan of the head and should include as routine blood glucose evaluation, thyroid hormones, vitamin B12 and folate levels, infection screen (including syphilis and, if indicated, HIV) and electrolyte and full blood count. Thyroid disease is the second most common endocrine disorder (after diabetes) and can present insidiously in the elderly population with features of depression or mood alteration.

9 **d.** Autoimmune hepatitis tends to affect young to middle-aged women and may present either acutely with features of hepatitis, or more insidiously with features of chronic liver disease. Extrahepatic involvement is common, with rash, arthralgia and arthritis accompanying more constitutional features of hepatitis such as nausea, malaise, vomiting, loss of appetite and weight loss. An interesting finding is that many women experience amenorrhoea and the clinical picture of a young woman of childbearing age with vomiting, loss of appetite and some abdominal pain can easily lead to misdiagnosis if an accurate history is not taken. Antibody screens are useful in making the diagnosis and a dichotomy is classically described between those individuals with type I and type II autoimmune hepatitis:
   - type I – involvement of antinuclear antibodies with or without anti-smooth muscle antibodies,
   - type II – mainly children involved and with liver/kidney microsomal type I antibodies (LKM1).

   Budd–Chiari syndrome presents with acute epigastric pain and shock and is due to occlusion of the hepatic vein. It presents rapidly and would not fit the clinical picture in this case. Viral hepatitis is an option to be considered in any young person with a tender right upper quadrant especially in the face of mild jaundice and hepatomegaly and risk assessment should be carried out for blood-borne viruses and possibly hepatitis serology. McArdle's syndrome is a glycogen storage disease (type V) and presents with muscular pain after exercise due to deficiency in myophosphorylase. A muscle biopsy is diagnostic. A useful mnemonic for remembering the rare disorders of glycogen storage is *V*ery *P*oor *C*arbohydrate *M*etabolism standing for Von Gierke's disease, Pompé's disease, Cori's disease and McArdle's disease.

10 **b.** Hypertension is a common cause of retinopathy and the history alone may aid in making a diagnosis, which is further confirmed on fundoscopy. Classification schemes for hypertensive

retinopathy wax and wane in popularity and may exist in the normal population as well as overlap with other syndromes, such as diabetic retinopathy. The Scheie classification provides a simplified format from which to work:

- grade 0 – hypertensive but no visible retinal abnormalities,
- grade I – arteriolar narrowing,
- grade II – arteriolar narrowing with focal constriction,
- grade III – diffuse narrowing with retinal haemorrhage,
- grade IV – papilloedema and hard exudates.

The changes seen in diabetic retinopathy are often classified by the degree of retinopathy seen; however, this system is more useful clinically as local treatment, for example laser photocoagulation, may be influenced by the degree of retinopathy. The following classification represents a simplified format as schemes are in constant flux:

- background DR – microaneurysms (dot), microhaemorrhages (blot) and hard exudates,
- preproliferative DR – cotton-wool spots and extensive blot haemorrhages,
- proliferative DR – neovascularization,
- macular disease – hard exudates encroaching on fovea or macular oedema.

Age-related macular degeneration (ARMD) can occur as 'dry' or 'wet' degeneration, with the defining feature being the presence of choroidal neovascularization (leading to 'wet' ARMD). Although dry ARMD is by far the more commonly encountered type, wet ARMD is the more rapidly progressive and requires attention due to the accompanying visual deterioration that is seen. CMV retinitis usually occurs in the immunosuppressed and is sometimes seen in AIDS patients. It manifests as cotton-wool spots with flame haemorrhages, often given the name pizza-pie fundus because of this appearance. Ankylosing spondylitis usually presents with uveitis (inflammation of the components of the uveal tract; namely the iris, ciliary body and choroid) and is thought to occur in autoimmune disorders due to immune complex deposition in the uveal tract.

11 **a.** This woman needs to continue rehabilitation before being discharged home. Being a recurrent attender should pose the question of whether there is an underlying social issue. Although medically fit, she would not benefit from being immediately discharged under GP care, as this option has been available to her but she has repeatedly chosen to call an ambulance. Remaining in hospital until she feels ready to leave would lead to a

number of problems, both financially and physically in terms of acquiring hospital infections and taking up an acute bed. Being assessed by social services is a realistic option, although in reality this takes time and means an extended stay in hospital while the process is completed. Placement in a short-term rehabilitation facility is a good compromise; it allows continued rehabilitation with physiotherapists while she is less at risk of developing further infections.

12 **a.** Pharyngeal pouches (Zenker's diverticulum) occur more commonly in women and in the elderly. The features described are classically associated with the presence of a pharyngeal pouch. There have been instances of rupture of the pouch, most usually at OGD, if there has not been a significant suspicion of pouch disease. However, most cases are diagnosed early and are surgically amenable to excision and repair. The pouch forms at an anatomical weakness between the inferior pharyngeal muscle complex and the cricopharyngeus posteriorly, known as Killian's dehiscence. Diagnostically is it best seen on contrast swallow where the pouch is clearly delineated.

Plummer–Vinson syndrome describes iron-deficiency anaemia and dysphagia caused by the formation of a keratinized web. Features associated with iron deficiency, such as koilonychia (spoon-shaped nails) and atrophic glossitis, may be rarely seen. The post-cricoid web is a direct but very rare consequence of severe iron-deficiency anaemia.

Chagas' disease was described by a Brazilian physician who described the characteristic symptoms of achalasia (failure of the oesophageal cardia to relax) in the South American population in association with *Trypanosoma cruzi* infection. Contrast swallow shows the level of obstruction often with hugely dilated and poorly functioning proximal oesophagus. A failure of neuromuscular co-ordination is thought to be the pathogenesis behind the disease.

Mallory–Weiss tear often follows a large meal and binge-drinking leading to a small linear tear in the oesophageal mucosa. Oesophageal carcinoma presents with progressive dysphagia for solids then liquids, often with florid constitutional signs of cancer.

13 **c.** Marfan's syndrome is an inherited connective tissue disorder that affects the expression of the fibrillin gene, leading to defects in the connective tissue of the ocular, skeletal and cardiovascular system. Mitral valve prolapse, tall, spindly stature, ectopia lentis (lens dislocation), as well as aortic involvement such as

aortic-root dilatation, aortic regurgitation and aortic dissection, are associated with the syndrome.

William's syndrome is a neurodevelopmental disorder with cardiovascular abnormalities and typical facial appearances. Hypercalcaemia is also commonly seen. Most importantly in this syndrome is the association of supravalvular aortic outflow obstruction, which may be severe enough to cause sudden death.

Down syndrome is a disorder of mental development and behaviour and is associated with characteristic features, including a single palmar crease, upslanting palpebral fissure and a flat nasal bridge. Ocular involvement is legion, ranging from refractive errors, the most common, to congenital cataracts. However, lens dislocation is a relatively rare event.

Turner's syndrome is a disease affecting females and presents with short stature and signs of ovarian dysfunction. Widely spaced nipples and a webbed neck are often quoted features of this disease and genetic analysis reveals a 45 X0 karyotype.

Reiter's syndrome is a rheumatological manifestation of the triad of conjunctivitis, urethritis and arthritis and classically occurs following a sexually transmitted infection, although it can also be seen after a bout of infectious diarrhoea. It is a seronegative arthropathy, so-called because rheumatoid factor is negative, and is grouped with reactive arthropathy, enteropathy-associated arthropathy and ankylosing spondylitis.

14 d. The scenario is describing a case of acute epiglottitis. The commonest cause of epiglottitis is a viral infection with *Haemophilus influenzae*. This is a respiratory emergency and without prompt action may result in death. There are obvious signs of respiratory distress that alert us to a serious condition, including the use of accessory muscles.

The other diagnoses in the question are unlikely to be correct. Although tonsillitis can be a serious condition and may present acutely, it is unlikely to present with use of accessory muscles. A chest infection or an acute exacerbation of asthma are most likely to present with either inspiratory or expiratory wheeze, but not both. This clinical picture could represent an allergic reaction but the history of a gradual fever and general unwell feeling rule out this diagnosis.

15 b. ERCP would be the next most appropriate investigation as this man has symptoms and blood tests most likely to be primary sclerosing cholangitis (PSC). The association between ulcerative colitis and PSC is well recognized and up to 75% of patients with PSC may have inflammatory bowel disease.

Liver biopsy is a useful investigation to confirm the diagnosis in cases with equivocal or borderline investigative results and shows a characteristic 'onion-skin' appearance to the intrahepatic biliary system. ERCP in most cases will make the diagnosis with a 'beaded' appearance due to alternating section of dilatation and stricture of the bile ducts.

CT scan may detect areas of liver damage due to chronic back pressure from strictured bile ducts but is far less superior at imaging the biliary tree than magnetic resonance cholangiopancreatography.

Colonoscopy is useful for detecting inflammatory bowel conditions in patients who present with abdominal pain and change of bowel habit but may have additional benefit in screening for colorectal cancer, which is increased in risk by PSC. Plain abdominal radiography is only of benefit in the diagnosis of complications of inflammatory bowel conditions such as bile duct fistula (aerobilia) and bowel obstruction due to stricture.

16 **c.** Section 4 refers to a provision by the Mental Health Act for detention of an individual against their own wishes for assessment of a mental health condition and is valid for 72 hours. It requires only one responsible medical officer and should only be used in the very acute situation when obtaining a Section 2 would not be easily achieved (a similar order that is backed by two medical recommendations and is valid for up to 28 days for assessment of a presumed psychiatric condition). A Section 4 may be converted into a Section 2 by the addition of a second medical recommendation during the period of validity.

It would not be an appropriate course of action to allow this man to be discharged, either against medical advice or with follow-up with a community psychiatrist, as he is likely to be a danger to himself or others and has already exhibited behaviour that would merit at least a brief period of assessment, if not psychiatric treatment as an inpatient.

A Section 3 order refers to a detention order for a period of up to 6 months per Section 3 (i.e. it can be renewed) for treatment of a psychiatric condition. It is typically a conversion from a Section 2 when the assessment has been made and the decision to start treatment has been deemed appropriate. It again requires two medical recommendations to be held valid.

Cuff and restraint under common law is not an appropriate modality to use in this case, where a psychiatric diagnosis is suspected, and would have to be justified on a case by case basis under the direct decision by a consultant physician.

17 c. The clinical picture is one of carcinoid syndrome secondary to a carcinoid tumour. The syndrome of facial flushing, watery diarrhoea, abdominal pain and cardiac abnormalities implies hepatic metastases of a carcinoid tumour. Common sites in the bowel are terminal ileum, rectum and appendix (25% of all tumours); however, involvement of other organs, such as ovaries or testes, have been reported.

Diagnosis is elegantly made from the clinical picture and 24-hour collection of urine for levels of 5-HIAA, a metabolite of 5-HT (serotonin) that is postulated to be responsible for the cardiac manifestations of the disease and profuse watery diarrhoea. Twenty-four-hour urine collection for protein is useful in cases of renal disease where the amount of proteinuria can be quantified.

Urine and plasma osmolalities are usually taken together in the diagnosis of disorders of free water clearance such as the syndrome of inappropriate antidiuretic hormone (SIADH). A low plasma sodium is seen in the face of inappropriately high urine osmolality, indicating free water retention. Fluid restriction may be used to bring the level of sodium up slowly. Too rapid correction of plasma sodium is associated with the development of central pontine myelinolysis – a catastrophic shrinking in the size of brain cells due to rapid osmolarity shifts and may be fatal.

Twenty-four-hour urine collection for the presence of VMA (metabolites of catecholamines) may be helpful in making the diagnosis of phaeochromocytoma, a rare catecholamine-producing tumour; 90% of tumours are in the adrenal medulla, 90% are benign and 90% of these unilateral.

18 e. Panic disorders are seen two to three times more commonly in females than males and are diagnosed according to strict criteria involving sensations of choking, tingling or numbness, chest tightness and shortness of breath, fear of losing control and a variety of other perceived symptoms. In addition to the presence of these symptoms, a diagnosis of panic disorder is only valid if there is an additional persistent worry for a period greater than 1 month about recurrence of attacks, the consequences of having another attack and a significant behavioural modification as a result of a panic attack, for example avoiding public places. Panic disorders exhibit a bimodal distribution in prevalence with peaks seen in late adolescence and then again in the mid-thirties.

There have been a wide variety of medical comorbidities associated with panic disorders, for example irritable bowel syndrome, COPD, cardiomyopathy, hypertension, migraine

headache, mitral valve prolapse to name a few of the more stud-
ied examples. Agoraphobia is often seen with panic disorder and
is estimated to be present in between 30 and 50% of cases of diagnosed panic disorder.

Treatment for panic disorder includes cognitive behavioural
therapy involving exposure and subsequent desensitization to
panic-inducing stimuli, respiratory training to help break the
cycle of reinforcement of panic-induced hyperventilation and
medical therapy, usually in the form of antidepressant medication with selective serotonin reuptake inhibitors (SSRIs) as first-
line, followed by tricyclic antidepressants (TCAs) as a second-
line modality.

19 d. Sjögren's syndrome (keratoconjunctivitis sicca) manifests as
dryness of the mucous membranes, leading to dry eyes, dry
mouth (xerostomia) and occasionally dryness of the tracheo-
bronchial tree. Investigations include the Schirmer test, which
assesses the amount of tear production from the eye with a reduction to less than 5 mm of tearing after 5 minutes on a strip of
filter paper suggestive of the condition. ESR and autoantibodies;
especially anti-Ro and anti-La (SS-A and SS-B), are frequently
raised in Sjögren's syndrome.

Anterior uveitis is associated with the seronegative arthro-
pathies, a group of arthritic conditions so-called because they
do not exhibit a positive rheumatoid factor. Classified into
enteropathy-associated arthritis, reactive arthritis (including
Reiter's syndrome), psoriatic arthritis and ankylosing spondylitis, they are commonly associated with extra-articular features
such as inflammation of the (anterior) uveal tract comprising
iris, ciliary body and choroid. Symptoms of anterior uveitis include pain in the affected eye, tear production, blurred vision
and occasionally photophobia.

Acute glaucoma can present in a similar fashion to anterior
uveitis and must be differentiated if appropriate treatment can
be instituted. One of the true ocular emergencies, it presents
with an acutely painful, red eye with both conjunctival and
ciliary vessel injection. The pupil is fixed, dilated and oval in
shape and the intraocular pressure is high. Beta-blockade, acetazolamide and topical steroids form the mainstay of treatment.

Subconjunctival haemorrhage presents with an acute red eye
consisting of bright red sclera with a rim around the limbus.
The pupil is normal, which allows differentiation from the other
causes of red eye. Retinal vein occlusion commonly occurs in
elderly hypertensive patients and presents with an acute deterioration in visual acuity. It can be detected on fundoscopy as

either a wedge deficit on the retina (due to a branch retinal vein occlusion) or, when central, presents with dot and blot haemorrhages or florid retinal haemorrhages leading to the description of the appearance as a 'stormy sunset'. Photocoagulation is the treatment of choice in preventing the neovascular complications of retinal vein occlusion; however, no medical therapy has been demonstrated to be curative once the event has occurred.

20 d. *Bacillus cereus* is often associated with refried rice and is the culprit behind diarrhoea and vomiting that occurs soon after ingestion of food colonized by the bacterium. A mnemonic to help remember the association between *Bacillus cereus* and rice is '*Eat refried rice? Be Serious!*' The onset of symptoms can be very rapid, anywhere between 1 and 5 hours from ingestion.

Clostridium botulinum can be found in many processed foods and has been associated with 'floppy baby syndrome'. This is due to the release of botulinum toxin, usually associated with babies who have been fed honey and subsequently suffer vomiting and even paralysis.

Rotavirus is another important cause of diarrhoea in children and is often responsible for outbreaks of playground diarrhoea. It is self-limiting and will resolve with adequate fluid rehydration and rest.

Cryptosporidium parvum is a fungal infection commonly associated with HIV infection and usually resolves unless the patient is severely immunocompromised, i.e. CD4 count <200 cells/µL. Treatment is supportive, as there are no effective antimicrobial agents of proven value.

Escherichia coli is possibly one of the more notorious causes of infective diarrhoea and has many subtypes. Enterotoxic *E. coli* is frequently associated with travel to different climates and cultures and has been aptly named 'traveller's diarrhoea'. As with almost all the types of diarrhoea, the treatment is fluid rehydration. Antibiotics are not used unless there are signs of systemic compromise.

21 e. Budd–Chiari syndrome is due to obstruction of the hepatic vein causing back pressure and eventual damage to the liver. Approximately one third of cases have no identifiable cause; however, associations between hypercoagulable states have been well described in the literature. The oral contraceptive pill, polycythaemia rubra vera and haematological and intra-abdominal malignancy may all predispose to this catastrophic syndrome. Diagnosis is usually by venous phase CT scan, which delineates the filling defect in the hepatic vein, and even inferior vena cava ultrasound of the liver may be a useful non-invasive bedside investigation to demonstrate retrograde flow in the portal system due to outflow obstruction and hence strengthen the diagnosis.

Viral hepatitis may present similarly but usually with jaundice and right upper quadrant pain, with or without a palpable liver. Gross ascites and signs of portal hypertension are not usually manifest without chronic liver disease and this goes against an acute infectious cause.

Epstein–Barr virus infection can cause hepatomegaly and may occur post infectious mononucleosis but, as with viral hepatitis, does not usually cause a picture of chronic liver disease. Wilson's disease is a rare inherited disorder of copper metabolism causing hepatolenticular degeneration and deposition of copper in the liver and basal ganglia. It causes movement disorders and liver failure in those not identified and treated early. Deposition of copper in Descemet's membrane in the eye causing Kayser-Fleischer rings is pathognomonic of this disease.

α1-Antitrypsin deficiency affects both lungs and liver, causing emphysema and chronic liver disease. α1-Antitrypsin is a protease involved in damping down inflammatory cascades and plays an especially important role in the protection of alveoli from protease damage in the lungs. It is associated with chronic liver disease and hepatocellular carcinoma in adults in approximately one quarter of all α1-antitrypsin-deficient patients.

22 d. The protein content of the fluid aspirated from the pleural effusion is consistent with a transudate. Causes of transudates can be grouped together as "failures", for example cardiac failure, liver failure (cirrhosis), renal failure (nephrotic syndrome) and thyroid failure (hypothyroidism). Exudates are defined by a protein content >30 g/L and caused by infections such as pneumonia, inflammations or malignancies, for example bronchial carcinoma.

23 c. This man is suffering from Crohn's disease. The combination of clinical pattern and colonoscopic appearance make the diagnosis unlikely to be ulcerative or other types of colitis. Aphthous ulceration is often one of the earliest signs on colonoscopy and occurs anywhere from mouth to anus, thus differentiating Crohn's disease from ulcerative colitis, which occurs proximally from the rectum, occasionally involving the terminal ileum (backwash ileitis). Crohn's disease can be thought of as a transmural inflammatory process with multiple skip lesions associated with a cobblestone pattern. The mnemonic 'a thick *old Crone skipping down a cobblestone pavement'* neatly sums up the histological and colonoscopic appearance of Crohn's disease. Anal and perianal disease are also a hallmark of Crohn's disease. Barium follow-through is an extremely useful investigation in eliciting small-bowel involvement and the pathological hallmark of small bowel Crohn's disease, rose-thorn type ulceration, may be seen.

24 **c.** The sudden onset of the symptoms suggests an acute pathology. The two likeliest diagnoses include a foreign body in the auditory canal or a perforation of the ear drum. Foreign bodies in the ear canal tend to be seen in children rather than adults. Any infection in the ear would typically result in pain in the ear or peri-aural region. Difficulty in hearing both high and low pitch sounds suggests a perforation of the drum. Causes of a perforated ear drum include infection, barotrauma, direct injury, sudden loud noises or postsurgical procedures, for example grommet insertion in children. Most tympanic perforations heal without intervention over the course of 6–8 weeks.

25 **h.** Acute glaucoma is a common condition affecting the elderly and one of the few true ocular emergencies that presents acutely. Classified as acute angle-closure and open-angle glaucoma, pain is typically unilateral and may be associated with headache. Blurred vision and visual distortion are symptoms experienced frequently and may be severe enough to reduce acuity to recognition of hand movements only. Dim light, anticholinergic drugs and intrinsic anatomical predisposition such as a shallow anterior chamber all predispose to acute angle-closure glaucoma and may be relieved by drugs reducing aqueous humour production, such as beta-blockers and acetazolamide. A few doses of a topical steroid preparation may aid in dampening the inflammatory response that accompanies glaucoma.

Endophthalmitis describes an intraocular inflammation usually caused by infection affecting the aqueous or vitreous humour and may occur as a result of direct inoculation of infectious agent to the eye, for example foreign body penetration or endogenously via spread from a pre-existing primary focus. Systemic antibiotics are usually indicated for infectious causes and may be treated adjuvantly by administration of antibiotic and steroid directly into the eye. Involvement of an ophthalmologist is always indicated and should be performed immediately once the diagnosis is suspected.

Retinitis pigmentosa is a complex inherited disorder of the retinal photoreceptors and pigment epithelium. There is a slight male predominance due to the more frequent X-linked varieties. Loss of night vision and peripheral vision are the most common complaints in those affected. Treatment modalities have been shown to have modest benefit and are mainly involved in symptom control. These include massive vitamin A dosing, the use of acetazolamide along with experimental procedures such as retinal prosthesis or transplantation.

Retinal detachment may occur as a result of traction from retinal neovascularisation with attachment to the vitreous humour, a tear in the surface with mechanical detachment by subretinal vitreous humour invasion or as a result of vascular changes in the retina e.g. hypertension or vasculitis. The sensation of flashing lights and floaters associated with patches of lost vision (scotomata) is the most commonly described phenomenon.

Retinal artery occlusion usually presents with painless sudden loss of vision in one eye and is caused by an embolus. The pathophysiology is similar to that of cerebral stroke. There may be a role for thrombolysis if an embolus is detected within the first 4-6 hours but the mainstay of treatment is expectant management with investigation of the underlying cause.

26 b. A typical regimen for the management of diabetic ketoacidosis is outlined below:

- Start an infusion of 50 units of short-acting insulin in 50 mL of 0.9% sodium chloride at a high rate (e.g. 6 units/hour) with 5 L fluid replacement with 0.9% sodium chloride.
- Once blood glucose levels are below 15 mmol/L, convert to 5% dextrose fluid replacement and halve infusion rate (e.g. 3 units/hour).
- Monitor urine for ketones and once ketones are negative or very low and the patient is eating and drinking normally, stop the insulin infusion.
- If the patient is not eating normally, convert insulin infusion to sliding scale with hourly blood glucose measurement.
- Potassium is driven into cells by insulin and will thus appear initially high due to lack of insulin but will rapidly drop with sliding scale. Titrate up to 40 mmol/hour against the serum potassium.

The rationale for large volume fluid rehydration is that high levels of blood glucose cause a massive osmotic diuresis and may be associated with vomiting. Fluid losses through the kidneys and gastrointestinal tract lead to serious dehydration. High levels of insulin infusion are used to suppress ongoing ketogenesis, which will happen hours after the blood glucose levels have been brought down and thus urinary monitoring of ketones is vital to guide requirements to sliding scale. Metabolic acidosis will respond to fluid rehydration and will correct with the breakdown of ketone bodies, a by-product of free fatty acid metabolism. Type I diabetics eating and drinking normally should be given subcutaneous insulin 30 minutes preprandially with insulin infusion stopped 1 hour after the meal to ensure adequate insulin cover during the transition. Basal bolus insulin or intermediate-acting insulin will not be adequate to suppress ketogenesis, which is key in correcting the metabolic acidosis and thus should not be used in the acute management of diabetic ketoacidosis.

27 **c.** Post-traumatic stress disorder is defined as a pathological anxiety reaction that develops following an extreme traumatic stressor (often an act of physical violence) witnessed or experienced by an individual. Features manifest as mood disturbance, a re-experiencing of the event, hypervigilance (exaggerated startle reaction) and avoidance of stimuli (e.g. location) associated with the event. It is differentiated from the very similar condition of acute stress disorder by the duration of symptoms. Post-traumatic stress disorder symptoms usually occur a few months from the sentinel event and can last for anywhere between <3 months to >6 months. Acute stress disorders typically occur within 1 month of a traumatic event and last for less than 1 month from onset.

Depressive symptoms make a diagnosis of depression a differential to consider; however, there are only a few of the symptoms of a depressive episode listed in the clinical vignette and the addition of nightmares associated with a history of a traumatic event alongside the features of a pathologically heightened sense of awareness (hypervigilance and exaggerated startle response) make this diagnosis unlikely.

Schizoid personality disorders present with typical behavioural manifestations such as detaching from close relationships, being aloof and exhibiting signs of anhedonia (inability to enjoy oneself). Rarely seen in the clinical setting, this diagnosis forms part of the cluster A (odd, eccentric) classification of personality disorders along with schizotypal and paranoid personality disorders.

Generalized anxiety disorder describes a chronic anxiety state characterized by disproportional worry about a wide range of life events that cause impairment to normal social functioning. The pertinent features associated with generalized anxiety disorder are of anxiety that occurs for most days for more than 6 months and manifests with greater than three somatic symptoms, such as sleep disturbance, poor concentration and mood disturbance.

28 **a.** This woman is exhibiting the symptoms and signs of diverticulitis. Left iliac fossa pain associated with a high white cell count, raised inflammatory markers and constitutional upset makes the diagnosis likely. Faecal peritonitis can be deadly and an operation is warranted as an emergency.

A tender palpable mass in the abdomen is occasionally found on clinical examination but is not an indication for surgery as many can be managed conservatively with antibiotics such as cefuroxime and metronidazole. If an abscess is suspected that is resilient to medical therapy, CT-guided percutaneous drainage is a relatively safe and feasible option. CT scanning of the abdomen is a very useful imaging modality that carries none of the complications, for example perforation, that direct visualization of the bowel does.

Colovesical fistula can be managed in an elective fashion by allowing the inflammation to settle before operating. Recent trials of risk factors for diverticular perforation have identified a possible role for opioid and NSAID analgesia in the development of such complications. Long-term use of opioid analgesia has been shown to increase intracolonic pressure and hence possibly increase the risk of mechanical perforation of diverticulae. NSAIDs have been linked to an alteration in mucosal blood flow via prostaglandin inhibition leading to a consistently identified risk of perforation in up to 20% of diverticular complications. This should, however, not preclude the use of NSAIDs but guide sensible prescribing of this often-feared analgesic agent.

29 **c.** Vomiting in meningitis is due to raised intracranial pressure and is central or neurogenic in origin. Patients may offer this clue to the cause of their vomiting by stating that the episode of vomiting came as a surprise to them and was not preceded by a period of nausea. Other causes of neurogenic vomiting are centrally acting drugs and any other cause of raised intracranial pressure, such as space-occupying lesion. The other options, while feasible, are less likely to be the cause of vomiting in an otherwise healthy young man. NSAID-associated gastritis would be more likely to occur in an elderly patient but more often presents insidiously as an iron-deficient anaemia or occasionally as melaena.

30 **d.** Normal portal venous pressure is between 8 and 15 cmH$_2$O. Portal hypertension occurs when there is outflow obstruction to

the portal system and can be evidenced by clinical manifestations and ultrasonographically, with reversal of flow along the portal vein. Obstruction can be classified as: (i) prehepatic, for example portal vein thrombosis secondary to neonatal umbilical infection; (ii) hepatic, for example cirrhosis; or (iii) posthepatic, for example tumour compression. As there is a rich collateral supply to the abdominal viscera, a substantial rise in portal pressure will cause the formation of porto-systemic anastomoses. The most clinically significant of these are oesophageal varices, which can present with life-threatening gastrointestinal bleeding. Splenomegaly can occur secondary to back pressure through the splenic vein and may cause leucopenia, thrombocytopenia and anaemia. Diaphragmatic varices can complicate surgery at the time of liver transplantation and may cause subphrenic haematomas that may become secondarily infected and form abscesses.

31 **e.** Hyperglycaemia and diabetes have been linked to the development of posterior subcapsular cataract by a mechanism thought to be due to chronic osmotic changes, modification of lens protein and oxidative damage in the lens. A distortion in vision can often be experienced with accumulation of high blood glucose levels and is often complained of in patients who present with hyperosmolar hyperglycaemic and diabetic ketoacidotic states and who experience large and often rapid shifts in the osmotic content of the lens while on treatment.

Steroids, hypertriglyceridaemia, obesity and hypertension have all been demonstrated to be associated with this type of senile cataract at a young age. Posterior subcapsular cataracts tend to present with more florid and disabling visual disturbance than cortical, nuclear or mixed cataracts (the other subclassifications of senile cataracts). Glare, especially in sunlight or with bright headlights at night, causes reduction in visual acuity and sometimes a reduction in accommodation.

Treatment is primarily surgical with lens extraction and replacement providing great improvement in vision. Cataract operations have become almost standard procedures in day surgery units and can be performed with complete removal of the lens (intracapsular cataract extraction) or with removal of the lens nucleus only with retention of the posterior capsule (extracapsular cataract extraction). Extracapsular cataract extraction is the currently preferred method of extraction; however, the choice of procedure depends on the surgeon, patient and the type of cataract present.

32 a. CEA may be raised in gastrointestinal cancers, especially colorectal carcinoma. As with all tumour markers it can be raised in a variety of cases, notably pancreatitis, cirrhosis and smoking, and must be interpreted within the clinical context. Tumour markers should never be used as a diagnostic tool; the use of markers is to add weight to an already strong clinical index of suspicion and to help guide investigation of possibly sites of neoplasm.

CA19-9 is often raised in pancreatic cancer, but can be elevated in benign biliary obstruction. AFP is most specific for hepatocellular carcinoma but also may rise in germ cell tumours as well as other liver disorders. NSE is specific for small-cell carcinoma of the lung and hCG is raised in pregnancy as well as with germ cell tumours. CA 15-3 is raised most commonly in breast disorders, including cancer and benign breast disease.

33 a. An ultrasound of the right upper quadrant is an easy, non-invasive evaluation of the biliary tree and can detect postoperative fluid collections. It should be the first-line investigation of any patient with right upper quadrant pain.

HIDA scan is a nuclear medicine scan involving intravenous injection of a ^{99m}technetium-labelled derivative of iminodiacetic acid. It can be helpful in the investigation of bile duct leakage postoperatively. The radionuclide is excreted by the liver into the biliary system and through into the duodenum. Imaging is taken serially after injection and will define the gallbladder to duodenum. Identification of leaks is evident as a nuclear signal in areas external to the biliary system. HIDA scan has an additional purpose in the identification of acute cholecystitis and has a sensitivity of around 96% and a specificity of around 94%. The easily performed and non-invasive ultrasound examination of the gallbladder has, however, rendered HIDA obsolete as a first-line investigation for the diagnosis of cholecystitis.

Plain abdominal radiograph will not detect a bile leak; however, it may be useful in showing air in the biliary tree as may occur with conditions such as choledochal fistula seen in gallstone ileus and with gas-forming organism infection of the biliary tree. CT scan of the abdomen will detect hepatic abnormalities such as cysts, tumours and collections but is poor at visualizing the biliary system and will not demonstrate bile leak. ERCP is both a diagnostic and therapeutic tool for imaging the biliary and pancreatic tree; however, is not as sensitive as HIDA for demonstrating bile leak.

34 e. Charcot's triad describes the clinical findings of right upper quadrant pain, jaundice and fever/chills. It is associated with acute (ascending) cholangitis most often due to Gram-negative bacterial infection such as *Escherichia coli, Enterobacter* and *Pseudomonas*. Reynold's pentad simply adds features of shock and altered mental state to Charcot's triad and occurs in acute cholangitis. Fitz–Hugh–Curtis syndrome occurs in young women who have been exposed to chlamydia and manifests as perihepatic adhesions involving the diaphragm and nearby structures. The pain experienced may mimic that of biliary obstruction and may spread transcoelomically to involve other abdominal viscera, causing generalized peritonitis.

Leriche's syndrome is found in arteriopathic patients who exhibit absent femoral pulses with buttock pain and claudication and impotence. The syndrome occurs because of occlusion of the aortic bifurcation by atherosclerosis or thromboembolism. Wernicke–Korsakoff syndrome is comprised of the triad of Wernicke's encephalopathy; nystagmus, ophthalmoplegia and ataxia and Korsakoff's psychosis, which is manifest as the inability to acquire new memories with confabulation of missing information. The latter is irreversible but may be prevented by parenteral administration of thiamine.

35 c. The biggest clue to this question is in the patient's age, as is true of many examination questions and real life. The symptoms are not unlike those experienced by patients with colon cancer but the infrequency of cancer in this age group makes this one of the most unlikely possibilities. Ulcerative colitis is bimodally distributed, peaking between the ages of 15 and 30 years and then again in later life. The patient's ethnic background is also suggestive of the diagnosis as there is a slightly increased prevalence among the Jewish population. Pseudomembranous colitis is typically due to antibiotic-associated overgrowth of *Clostridium difficile* and both angiodysplasia and haemorrhoids usually present with fresh rectal bleeding in the absence of abdominal symptoms.

36 d. The clinical picture shows many of the characteristic hallmarks of hereditary haemochromatosis. This autosomal recessive disease is common in older males of northern European descent and has been genetically linked to the C282Y mutation on the short arm of chromosome 6. Abnormal iron metabolism leads to deposition of iron and haemosiderin in liver, heart, pancreas, pituitary, joints, adrenals, testes and kidneys. This in turn leads to a spectrum of cirrhosis, pancreatic dysfunction and diabetes mellitus, skin pigmentation, cardiac dysfunction and dilated cardiomyopathy and hypogonadism.

Diagnostic investigations include radiography of joints for chondrocalcinosis, fasting transferrin saturation (a level >45% is very sensitive for hereditary haemochromatosis), liver biopsy to assay the degree of hepatic iron loading, MRI scan if liver biopsy is contraindicated, and genetic mutational analysis. Management of hereditary haemochromatosis is by twice weekly venesection to render the patient mildly iron deficient then maintenance venesection every 2 months. The iron-chelating agent, desferrioxamine, has some clinical benefit in reducing iron levels.

37 d. This woman most likely has Wilson's disease (hepatolenticular degeneration), a rare inborn error of metabolism that leads to a failure to excrete copper. The build-up of copper can sometimes be seen as a green-brown pigmented ring at the junction of cornea and sclera known as a Kayser–Fleischer ring. Four-vessel neck angiography would be a useful discriminative test in cases of suspected arteriovenous malformations or vessel occlusion. Hyperthyroidism can lead to a slender frame and an anxious disposition but this is not the clinical picture of thyroid dysfunction. Serum bilirubin and liver enzymes would be a useful test to do if there were any clinical signs of jaundice or any liver disease, which is associated with Wilson's disease; however, it would not be the most discriminative test. Peripheral blood films and vitamin B12 levels are useful in cases of suspected subacute combined degeneration of the spinal cord secondary to vitamin B12 deficiency.

38 a. Haloperidol is an extremely useful medication for the acute management of a confused patient with agitation and behavioural symptoms. An alternative agent used to manage behavioural effects of dementia is risperidone, which shares a similar incidence of parkinsonism side-effects but is more expensive than haloperidol. Given orally, intramuscularly or intravenously these are effective first-line medications for the treatment of acute behavioural crises.

Benzodiazepines should be avoided in demented patients due to the paradoxical exacerbation of behaviour and sedation that occurs. In the acute setting a demented patient should never be assumed to suffer from intrinsic dementia until all organic and reversible causes have been ruled out. A nice mnemonic for tying in the causes of dementia is *DEMENTIAS* – standing for *d*egenerative diseases (Parkinson's disease, Huntingdon's disease, Alzheimer's disease), endocrine disorders, metabolic derangement, exogenous factors (heavy metals, drugs, medications), neoplasia, trauma (e.g. subdural haematoma), infection, affective disorders (e.g. pseudodementia) and vascular (vascular dementia, ischaemic stroke, vasculitis).

Memantine is an N-methyl-D-aspartic acid (NMDA) antagonist used in the treatment of cognitive symptoms of Alzheimer's disease. It may be most effective when used in conjunction with cholinesterase inhibitors, such as galantamine and rivastigmine. These medications act to increase acetylcholine levels, thought to be the biological correlate responsible for memory and concentration. There is evidence that the cholinesterase inhibitors may ameliorate the so-called secondary (behavioural) component to Alzheimer's disease; however, they are not appropriate for use acutely in the demented patient.

Olanzapine and the other atypical antipsychotic agents are effective agents when used as maintenance of behavioural disturbance; however, they are not as predictable in effect when used acutely and thus tend to accede to the 'older' neuroleptic medications such as haloperidol and risperidone.

Sertraline is an SSRI and is a useful adjunct in the treatment of depressive symptoms associated with dementia. It has a good side-effect to the treatment profile and may have some benefit for psychotic disturbance as well as mood disturbance.

39 c. The patient is showing a response to a placebo. Normal saline is not known to have any pain-reducing qualities and this amount of normal saline is unlikely to alter any electrolyte abnormality this man may have. His pain could be psychogenic in origin; however, further work-up for organic pathology in necessary before assigning this diagnosis. There is no evidence in the question that he is suffering from a personality disorder. His pain may be somatic in origin but this is unlikely to be directly affected by a bolus dose of normal saline and is likely to improve with rest and conservative measures.

40 a. Proliferation of new blood vessels on the retina is associated with the development of vitreous haemorrhage and retinal detachment (usually by attachment of new vessels into the vitreous humour with traction detachment of the retina) as the most clinically significant sequelae of retinal neovascularization (new blood vessel formation). Treatment modalities include laser photocoagulation of peripheral parts of the retina with theoretical reduction of retinal oxygen requirements. Another rationale for laser therapy is that photocoagulation is thought to supplement the oxygenation of the retina by increasing the supply from the choroid layer and thus reducing the ischaemic burden shouldered by the retinal vessels.

Aqueous haemorrhages are not seen due to the lens capsule separating the posterior (vitreous) compartment of the eye from the anterior (aqueous compartment). The pathogenesis of retinal neovascularization is thought to be a direct consequence of retinal ischaemia with resultant compensation in blood flow through the rapid formation of new but friable blood vessels. Rupture and haemorrhage of these delicate vessels can cause acute changes in vision due to clouding of the vitreous humour with blood and patients may experience floaters and progressive deterioration in visual acuity.

Optic neuritis most often occurs in association with demyelinating conditions such as multiple sclerosis and is due to inflammation of the optic nerve. Typically presenting as pain on eye movement with distortion of central vision, it may be associated with a relative pupillary afferent defect detectable upon examination of pupillary reflexes to light.

A bitemporal hemianopia is sometimes referred to colloquially as 'tunnel vision' and is seen in conditions of central compression of the optic chiasm, such as an enlarging pituitary tumour. Often a focused history will lead to a diagnosis of pituitary disease such as acromegaly, presenting with symptoms of coarse skin, thick heavy-set features and other manifestations of soft tissue overgrowth.

41 **c.** Antihypertensive medications are known to cause a depressed mood in susceptible individuals. Other drugs that are strongly associated with depression are steroids and hypnotic medications. Digoxin, calcium supplements and oral hypoglycaemics are not usually associated with depression.

42 **e.** An increase in adipose tissue in the elderly resulting in a reduction in number of insulin receptors available for glucose leads to a mild glucose intolerance. Bone changes and degenerative arthritis are responsible for an increase in alkaline phosphatase, while creatinine clearance reduces with age owing to a reduction in glomerular filtration rate. With age and reduction in the level of testosterone, stimulation of erythropoietin falls, resulting in a mild anaemia in the elderly.

43 **a.** Digoxin is the first-line agent in treating atrial fibrillation with fast ventricular rate (note the concept of 'fast' atrial fibrillation is a misnomer as atrial fibrillation is, by definition, fast – it is the

rate of conduction to the ventricles that should be described). Loading is given as 500 μg oral (there is no evidence that IV digoxin works better) once every 12 hours for two doses, then conversion to digoxin maintenance, usually at a dose of 62.5 μg. Patients should be placed on a cardiac monitor in a ward setting where this can be adequately observed. Digoxin will act over a 24–48-hour period and care must be taken not to over digitalize patients, leading to bradycardia. If the rate is not adequately controlled with digoxin in the first instance, then beta-blockade may be added if left ventricular function is adequate.

Finally, although still somewhat controversial, anticoagulation should be considered in patients with persistent atrial fibrillation. If there is documented evidence of either known atrial fibrillation or structural heart disease, the evidence weighs heavily in favour of long-term anticoagulation with an agent such as warfarin. In cases where patients are younger than 65 years, with echocardiographically normal hearts and a potentially reversible reason for atrial fibrillation, then the decision to anticoagulate over the long term becomes more subjective.

44 c. There are few clues to the diagnosis in the question; however, the clinical picture suggests an episode of acute pancreatitis with classical radiological features. The best discriminatory investigation is serum amylase, which, if raised four-fold above the upper limit of normal (90 IU/dL), is highly suggestive of pancreatitis. Diabetic ketoacidosis should also be ruled out and a simple bedside blood glucose and urine dipstick is a quick and easy screen while serum levels are awaited. A pleural tap is unlikely to be useful in the diagnosis of this patient's abdominal pain and transoesophageal echocardiography is usually employed in the visualization of the heart and cardiac function. Endoscopy is a useful option if amylase levels are normal and an upper gastrointestinal cause of pain is suggested.

45 a. *Candida albicans* is a fungal infection responsible for causing thrush in women and balanitis in males. Although it is common in normal healthy women it is relatively uncommon in males and thus any male presenting with signs of candidal infection should have blood glucose levels checked. Diabetes mellitus predisposes to infection and the clinical history of polyuria, polydipsia and a candidal infection in the absence of genitourinary tract infection in a young male is almost enough to make the diagnosis itself.

Full blood count might be useful if a sexually transmitted infection with systemic involvement was suspected. ESR is a **193** non-specific index of disease, for example inflammatory conditions, disseminated malignancy and infection, but would not be beneficial in this case. ESR rises with age and anaemia and an easy guide to interpreting ESR with respect to age is by using the Westergren formula:

Males − (Age in years)/2   Females − (Age in years + 10)/2

HTLV-1 and -2 are oncogenic retroviruses that are of the same family as HIV. HTLV-1 has been linked to the development of T-cell leukaemia and lymphoma and neurological diseases such as tropical spastic paraparesis and Brown–Séquard syndrome. Urine analysis would be useful in determining the clinical probability of urinary tract infection and on the basis of dipstick positive findings would be evidence enough to start empirical antibiotics. Urine specimen for microscopy, culture and sensitivities should be considered if there is a negative urine dipstick or suspicion of a more resistant or atypical organism.

46 b. The tricyclic antidepressants have a recognizable pattern of toxicity that occurs in overdose, which can be summed up: *Tri-C's of toxicity – convulsions, coma, cardiac arrhythmias.* Patients may present asymptomatically, having been found by someone close to them, or they may sometime self-refer to hospital feeling remorseful of their actions; however, serious side-effects may be delayed for between 2 and 6 hours post-ingestion and careful monitoring should be undertaken of anyone suspected of having an overdose. Cardiac monitoring is essential due to the inhibition of normal cardiac conduction (due to inhibition of the fast sodium channel) leading especially to a prolonged QT interval. Anticholinergic effects are also seen commonly with overdose of the tricyclics due to their potent competitive antagonism at central and peripheral muscarinic acetylcholine receptors.

Monoamine oxidase inhibitors (MAOIs) such as tranylcypromine, when taken in overdose, usually manifest with symptoms of catecholamine excess such as sweating, tachycardia, hypertension, tremors and seizures but arrhythmias are typically uncommon in the setting of pure MAOI ingestion. A well-recognized phenomenon occurring in individuals who are prescribed MAOIs is a hyperadrenergic state resulting from the ingestion of foods containing tyramine, such as cheese, red wine and some meats. Tyramine is not broken down normally, due to enzyme inhibition by MAOIs, and therefore acts as a sympathomimetic.

A similar phenomenon, known as a serotonin syndrome, may occur in individuals coprescribed MAOIs and SSRIs or even those who overdose with SSRIs (e.g. sertraline), with symptoms of flushing, a change in mental status, sweating and hyperthermia as well as neuromuscular agitation.

Beta-blockade usually causes symptoms of bradycardia and hypotension, which may be life threatening. Other effects less commonly seen are bronchospasm in sensitive individuals and hypoglycaemia in diabetics. The agent of choice to reverse beta-blocker overdose is glucagon, which seems to act independently of the beta-receptor to increase heart rate and myocardial contractility.

Digoxin toxicity is manifest by a yellow-green colour disturbance to normal vision, confusion and/or agitation in addition to the distinctive *reverse tick sign* on electrocardiography. Premature ventricular contractions, bigeminy and trigeminy are often encountered signs of digoxin toxicity. Hypokalaemia, hypomagnesaemia and hypernatraemia can all potentiate digoxin toxicity, even at normal therapeutic doses, and should be considered as a cause of toxicity. Reversal is by use of digibind (a digoxin-binding antibody).

47 b. Benign oesophageal strictures are associated with gastro-oesophageal reflux disease (GORD) and are caused by backwash of acid through an incompetent lower oesophageal sphincter with resultant scarring, fibrosis and stenosis of the lower oesophagus. The history of taking antacid remedies points the clinician to a diagnosis by proxy of GORD and the patient's body habitus makes acid reflux a likely problem. GORD can be treated medically with antacids, proton-pump inhibition or H_2 antagonism and surgical therapy (Nissen fundoplication) may be necessary for those refractory to medical treatment.

Systemic sclerosis would likely manifest with clinically obvious features, such as periorbital or digital skin changes or lung, cardiac or renal involvement. Autoantibody screen, especially for Scl-70 and RNA polymerases, will aid in diagnosis if any doubt is present. Oesophageal carcinoma is very unlikely given the patients age; however, if there were any sinister features to the history or examination, an outpatient barium swallow study would aid in making the diagnosis.

The typical radiological finding suggestive of oesophageal carcinoma is of an apple-core appearance as the tumour encircles a portion of oesophageal lumen, causing dilatation of the proximal segment. Oesophageal candidiasis would again be unlikely in an immunocompetent individual but if retrosternal pain on swallowing persists in the face of effective proton-pump or H_2-receptor inhibition for GORD, then further investigation may be warranted. There is no history of radiotherapy to the chest or mediastinum that may raise the suspicion of a radiation stricture.

48 c. Drug therapy is one of the causes of gynaecomastia but must not attributed as a cause without exclusion of the aggressive male breast cancer. Spironolactone, digoxin, cimetidine, alcohol and ketoconazole have been linked to the development of gynaecomastia and the mnemonic '*S*ome *D*rugs *C*ause *A*wesome *K*nockers' aids in remembering these. Other causes of bilateral benign breast swellings include liver cirrhosis, testicular and adrenal tumours, hypogonadism and renal failure with the pathogenetic link being an abnormality in the normal ratio of oestrogens to androgens (either due to failure of production in liver cirrhosis, testicular and adrenal tumours or a failure to clear hormones from the body as in renal failure).

49 c. Retinoblastoma is the most common ocular malignancy of childhood and exhibits a peak in incidence between 10 and 20 months. There is no significant difference in sex and both unilateral and bilateral disease has been described with bilateral disease presenting an average of 7 months before unilateral disease. The aetiology of retinoblastoma has been linked to a mutation in the retinoblastoma gene located on the long arm of chromosome 13. A deletion or non-functional mutation causes inactivation of this gene, which actually suppresses the formation of retinoblastoma, and when both loci are inactivated the tumour occurs. Treatment is directed at preservation of as much visual function as possible and can be delivered through external beam radiotherapy (however, with a very unfavourable side-effect of facial hypoplasia due to cessation of bony growth with radiotherapy), chemotherapy to achieve local control, or radionuclide plaque treatment. However, surgical treatment still remains the most definitive option in retinoblastoma and involves enucleation for very poor prognosis tumours with photocoagulation and cryotherapy additional options in very selected cases.

Endophthalmitis is inflammation of the internal cavities of the eye and can occur after trauma to the eye with inoculation of bacteria, after retained lens material during cataract operations, or by metastatic spread to the eye from a distant focus. It presents with pain in the eye, redness, swelling and a decrease in visual acuity. Antibiotic therapy, both systemic and occasionally into the ocular cavities, is merited and the choice of antibiotic will depend upon the putative organism responsible, for example skin flora inoculation during eye surgery, and on any possible patient allergy to antibiotic therapy.

Congenital cataract presents with opacity of the lens, which may be very subtle, and irregularity of the red reflex. If the cataract is in the visual axis then reduction in vision may occur and this must be corrected as soon as possible to minimize long-term deficits in vision. Congenital cataract may be associated with infection, genetic diseases such as Down syndrome, and prematurity. Retinopathy of prematurity is a disease that is related to the degree of prematurity of a newborn and is a serious disorder of vascular proliferation due to underlying retinal ischaemia from untimely birth. Laser therapy, cryotherapy and even ablative therapy are the main modes of treatment.

50 e. Rectal bleeding is a distressing symptom and every effort should be taken to reassure the patient. An accurate history can be more useful than investigation and should always be undertaken, as the difficulty in finding an occult source of bleeding should never be underestimated. Classifying rectal bleeding into fresh red and altered dark bleeding can help to differentiate between upper and lower gastrointestinal causes. The presence of melaena, i.e. altered changed blood, almost exclusively locates the source of bleeding to the upper gastrointestinal tract as blood is altered by digestive enzymes and acid found in the stomach and proximal small intestine. Fresh red blood suggests lower tract bleeding. Further classifying lower tract bleeding into painful versus painless helps to exclude conditions such as anal fissure, which causes excruciating pain on passing stool.

Angiodysplasia is a cause of fresh rectal bleeding from an arteriovenous malformation, often seen in the elderly. It can be seen at colonoscopy as a luminal vascular abnormality that may bleed on pressure over it. Rectosigmoid carcinoma typically presents with anaemia or obstruction and may only bleed when advanced. Inflammatory bowel disorders tend to present with altered bowel habit and bloody diarrhoea mixed in with mucus rather than bright red blood.

51 b. Schizotypal personality disorders form part of Cluster A of the *Diagnostic and Statistical Manual of Mental Disorders* (*DSM-IV*), which groups personality disorders by similarly matched characteristics. The definition of a personality disorder is an enduring pattern of inner experience and behaviour that differs markedly from the expectations of the individual's culture, is pervasive and inflexible, has an onset in adolescence or early adulthood, is stable over time, and leads to distress or impairment.

Schizotypal personality disorders manifest with behaviour or thinking that is odd, often associated with excessive social anxiety, an inability to form close, confiding relationships with other individuals, and often paranoid ideation. It can be difficult to distinguish from schizoid personality disorders, which typically exhibit an emotionally flat affect with a lack of enjoyment for activities, close relationships and sexual activity.

Antisocial personality disorders are usually found in those over 18 years but many have evidence of early conduct disorder in early adolescence. A lack of respect for authority and lawmaking characterizes this disorder, which is one of the few psychiatric conditions that one may be put in prison for. A lack of remorse for aggressive and often dangerous behaviour is a common feature.

Dependent personality disorders refer to a cluster of character traits that include dependence on other individuals, an inability to be alone or not in a close relationship and making excessive demands on those around them for support and reassurance. They are similarly clustered with the avoidant personality disorder, which differs slightly in a lack of a close relationship unless acceptance is guaranteed. Avoidant personalities tend to shun social situations and activities that bring attention to themselves for fear of criticism and they exhibit anxiety in social contexts.

52 a. Microcytic anaemia with weight loss in an elderly patient is colorectal carcinoma until proven otherwise. Right-sided tumours, for example caecum and ascending colon, tend to cause occult bleeding and a microcytic anaemia, while left-sided tumours, for example rectosigmoid, tend to cause obstruction and sometimes fresh red rectal bleeding. The derangement of liver enzymes is a sinister sign of potential hepatic metastases and a coagulation profile should be requested in case of liver dysfunction.

In the first instance, an OGD and colonoscopy (top and tail) should be performed as this will both identify any suspicious masses and allow tissue harvest for histological analysis. A staging CT scan of the chest, abdomen and pelvis should then be performed if endoscopy results demonstrate a lesion. The images and case details should ideally be discussed in a multidisciplinary meeting involving surgeons, oncologists, palliative care physicians and radiologists, so active decisions regarding management can be made. A simple chest radiograph is a useful screening tool if a colorectal cancer is suspected and will be done more quickly than a staging CT. Liver biopsy is rarely necessary unless disseminated malignancy is found with no apparent primary focus and histological diagnosis will influence management strategy.

53 c. Upper gastrointestinal bleeds manifest themselves both as haematemesis, typically with coffee ground vomiting from the alteration of blood by digestive enzymes and stomach acid, or with the presence of melaena (dark, offensive, altered blood per rectum). Evidence of an actively bleeding source in the upper gastrointestinal tract can often be difficult to assess objectively as the subjective description of passing melaena stools may vary greatly. Clinical and laboratory indices of bleeding are often relied upon as a proxy measure and include:

- pulse rate,
- lying versus standing (or sitting if patients are not able to stand) blood pressures looking for significant postural hypotension (arbitrarily described as a drop in systolic of greater than 20 mmHg,
- a systolic pressure lower than 90 mmHg,
- a drop in haemoglobin (which will only occur after a period of bleeding lasting longer than about 24 hours due to the acute effect of haemoconcentration during an acute bleed leading a falsely normal haemoglobin reading), and
- a rise in urea due to breakdown of blood into nitrogenous products.

Once the diagnosis of upper gastrointestinal bleeding has been made, patients should be commenced on proton pump inhibitors and any non-steroidal drugs should be stopped, as these increase the risk of gastrointestinal bleeds by inhibiting the protective effect of prostaglandins in the gastrointestinal tract.

Decisions as to the urgency of endoscopy should then be made. Indications for urgent endoscopy depend on the clinical risk prediction for active bleeding and in this case are fulfilled. A postural drop and tachycardia approximates at least a 20% blood loss and with biochemical evidence of a clinically significant bleed, endoscopy may identify and treat any actively bleeding source. Surgical referral is not merited at this time as the patient may be adequately and safely treated endoscopically. Persistent bleeding in an unstable patient who may not be treatable endoscopically and in whom urgent control of bleeding is required are candidates for laparotomy and direct surgical intervention, although the mortality is high in cases of emergency surgery for upper gastrointestinal bleeding.

Coeliac arteriography is an option to consider in a patient in whom no readily identifiable lesion has been demonstrated but who continues to bleed and a small bowel source of bleeding is suspected. Colonoscopy is only useful for assessing sources of bleeding in the lower gastrointestinal tract and is most often applied in the investigation of colonic malignancy.

54 b. Meigs' syndrome describes the association of an ovarian thecoma or fibroma with ascites and pleural effusion. Usually occurring to women of child-bearing age, the benign ovarian thecoma is one of the commonest sex-cord stromal tumours. The Jarisch–Herxheimer reaction occurs secondary to penicillin use in syphilis and is caused by a release of tumour necrosis factor α (TNF-α), interleukin (IL)-6 and IL-8. As it is not a dose-related phenomenon, penicillin should not be withheld or reduced in dose.

Fitz–Hugh–Curtis syndrome is seen in chlamydial infection of young women leading to perihepatic adhesions through transcoelomic spread of chlamydia from the genitourinary tract. Peyronie's disease is seen in males leading to angulation of the penis due to fibrosis of soft tissue. It is associated with Dupuytren's contracture and atheroma. Raynaud's syndrome describes intermittent digital ischaemia with colour changes in the hands, often precipitated by cold weather or emotion. It has been linked with the use of vibrating machinery, CREST syndrome (*c*alcinosis, *R*aynaud's phenomenon, *o*esophageal dysmotility, *s*clerodactyly and *t*elangiectasia) and smoking.

55 c. The presentation of abdominal pain and new-onset neuropsychiatric symptoms in a young woman should always alert the clinician to the possibility of acute intermittent porphyria as the diagnosis. The porphyrias are a set of genetic disorders of haem biosynthesis resulting in increased levels of porphyrin precursors, such as porphobilinogen and 5-δ-aminolaevulinic acid. Skin involvement is a feature of some varieties of porphyria and may be the presenting feature. Other clinical features can be summed up by the four *Hs, Ps and Ss*:

*H*ypotonia, *h*ypotension, *h*yponatraemia and *h*ypokalaemia
*P*roteinuria, *p*sychosis, *p*aralysis and *p*eripheral neuritis
*S*eizures, *s*hock, *s*ensory impairment and visual abnormalities

The urine may appear dark or deep red especially on standing and testing for urinary porphobilinogen and 5-δ-aminolaevulinic acid levels aids in diagnosis. TFTs may be helpful in patients with features of thyroid dysfunction and confusion or psychiatric symptoms; however, the clinical picture is not typical for thyroid dysfunction. Phaeochromocytoma may cause symptoms of anxiety, depression and a sense of impending doom. Levels of adrenaline metabolites can be assayed in a 24-hour urine collection; however, a phaeochromocytoma crisis manifests with sympathetic overactivity, which can help to differentiate organic from functional causes of psychosis. CT scan of the abdomen is a reasonable line of investigation to proceed with once simple causes of abdominal pain and psychiatric disturbance have been ruled out as malignancy, and especially hormone-secreting tumours, may cause the above picture.

56 **a.** A fluctuating level of consciousness suggests a diagnosis of delirium rather than dementia. Dementia can be defined as the deterioration of cognitive functions, such as memory, concentration and judgment, and personality and behavioural changes resulting most commonly from an intrinsic disorder of the brain but infrequently from a reversible organic cause. Dementia typically presents with features of cognitive impairment manifesting as forgetfulness, inability to recognize familiar objects, persons and places, and behavioural manifestations that may range from wandering behaviours to aggression or emotional lability and inappropriateness. Dementia encompasses a wide range of disease pathologies, such as vascular dementia, neurodegenerative aetiologies such as Pick's disease and Alzheimer's disease, infectious processes and metabolic, endocrine and traumatic derangements, some of which may ameliorate with correction of the abnormality.

Sundowning is a phenomenon that is common to both dementia and delirium and describes the worsening of symptoms that occurs towards the end of the day. It has been postulated that the reduction in ambient light levels and external cues causes an increase in disorientation and this forms the basis of simple nursing strategies for orientating demented patients. Strict adherence to routines, such as medication timing, bright lighting and set sleep–wake patterns, and reinforcement of external cues such as the time, date and place are important nursing tasks that can make a significant difference in the care for this often difficult but vulnerable population.

57 **a.** Faecal impaction with overflow diarrhoea is a common cause of spurious diarrhoea in an elderly poorly mobile patient. Radiological and clinical features show a ground-glass appearance throughout the gastrointestinal tract with hard faecal matter per rectum and a lumpy abdomen. Treatment involves the use of phosphate enemas once obstruction has been ruled out, or aperients such as senna, lactulose or sodium docusate. Faecal stool softeners such as glycerine suppositories can

additionally be used if constipation is not relieved by the above measures.

Sigmoid volvulus is a cause of large bowel obstruction and a surgical emergency if absolute constipation (obstipation) has set in. It is commoner in men than women and presents acutely with sudden-onset colicky abdominal pain with radiographic appearance of a 'bent inner tube' if the two segments of sigmoid lie adjacent to each other.

Cholesterol embolus can occur from the mobilization of cholesterol atheromatous plaques from the aorta or renal arteries causing back and abdominal pain with evidence of end-artery ischaemia, for example in retina/digits. Usually occurring after arterial catheterization, especially renal artery angioplasty, it may lead to gastrointestinal bleeding, purpura, progressive renal failure and a net-like rash (livedo reticularis).

Cauda equina syndrome is a neurosurgical emergency due to compression of the spinal cord at the level of the cauda equina. It manifests typically with perineal numbness (saddle anaesthesia), loss of anal sphincter tone, incontinence and paraparesis of both legs.

Clostridium difficile infection is usually associated with the use of antibiotics, in particular clindamycin and the cephalosporins. Diarrhoea is profuse, watery and offensive and direct imaging of the colon demonstrates a pseudomembranous colitis appearance. Oral metronidazole and fluid rehydration is the first line in treatment along with stopping other antibiotic therapy.

58 e. Extraocular muscles are supplied by three main cranial nerves; the oculomotor (III), trochlear nerve (IV) and abducens nerve (VI). The abducens nerve supplies motor innervation to the lateral rectus muscle, the trochlear nerve supplies motor innervation to the superior oblique muscle and medial rectus, inferior oblique, superior and inferior rectus are all motor innervated by the oculomotor (III) nerve. A useful way of remembering this information is the 'chemical formula' – $LR_6SO_4AL_3$ *(Lateral Rectus 6, Superior Oblique 4, All the rest 3).*

The innervation to levator palpebrae superioris (the muscle responsible for eyelid opening) is dual, involving both the sympathetic nervous system and the third cranial nerve (oculomotor nerve). This dual supply is evident from the degree of ptosis (drooping of the eyelid) seen in oculomotor palsy and in conditions affecting the sympathetic supply to the head and neck, for example Horner's syndrome. Partial ptosis is seen in Horner's syndrome due to sparing of the oculomotor innervation to levator palpebrae superioris, while complete ptosis occurs in oculomotor palsies due to loss of both oculomotor *and* sympathetic tone (as sympathetic fibres run along the course of the oculomotor nerve). Supply to the lacrimal glands is from the parasympathetic nervous system and is delivered via the greater petrosal nerve, the deep petrosal nerve and zygomatic and lacrimal nerves.

59 b. TPN has been linked with derangement of liver enzymes, sepsis, thrombosis and hyponatraemia. Cholestasis has been shown to occur after commencement of TPN and frank liver damage can occur. It is extremely common for patients to exhibit a rise in liver enzymes after starting TPN and these must be monitored three times weekly for acute rises. Enteral nutrition is the preferred route of administration of nutrition even in the face of gastrointestinal disease and recent advances in the management of pancreatitis aim to re-establish enteral feeding slowly once vomiting and abdominal pain allow.

Blood transfusion reactions are usually acute events occurring within minutes to an hour of the transfusion with pyrexia, flushing and in severe cases anaphylaxis. Biliary leak usually occurs after hepatobiliary surgery and manifests in the days postoperatively with pain, peritonitis and a rise in liver enzymes. Hepatitis in a very rare complication of blood transfusion and, although a theoretical risk, nowadays would be low down on the differential diagnosis of a rise in liver enzymes in this case.

Sedation on the Intensive Care Unit (ICU) is usually maintained with infusion of benzodiazepine and opioids such as midazolam and morphine. Neither agents have been linked with hepatic damage in doses used for sedation, although use in pre-existing severe hepatic dysfunction may prolong the sedative effects and is recommended with caution.

60 a. This man has a ventricular septal defect, which is an unusual but serious complication of MI. It is confirmed by echocardiography and requires surgery to close the defect. On auscultation, a pansystolic murmur is heard, which should raise suspicion. The shortness of breath without radiological changes is caused by increased release of atrial natriuretic peptide caused by increased pressure in the right atrium.

Aortic regurgitation would give a diastolic murmur and heart failure would produce characteristic changes on the chest X-ray. Dressler's syndrome is a late complication, occurring weeks to months after the initial insult and presents with recurrent pericarditis and pleural effusions associated with fever, which does not fit this clinical presentation.

Extended Matching Questions

61 i. Haemophilia A and B and von Willebrand's disease may manifest as bleeding from the gastrointestinal tract and mucous membranes into joints and from any wounds (including surgical wounds). von Willebrand's disease is the most common inherited coagulopathy and results from either a reduction or lack of von Willebrand factor (vWF) or abnormally functioning vWF. vWF is involved in platelet function thus manifests in laboratory studies as an increase in bleeding time, high APTT with a normal INR. Haemophiliacs are much more likely to exhibit major bleeding than von Willebrand's disease sufferers and bleeding into joints after trauma or exercise and into muscle after intramuscular injections are more commonly seen. The haemophilias are caused by a deficiency of factor VIII (haemophilia A) and factor IX (Christmas disease, haemophilia B) and behave clinically similarly. It should always be borne in mind when considering the differential diagnosis of any cause of bleeding that general bleeding diatheses may be responsible.

62 d. Internal haemorrhoids (or piles) are congested vascular cushions that aid the anal sphincter mechanism in maintaining continence. It is postulated that poor dietary fibre and straining at stool may contribute to the increase in rectal venous pressure that may precipitate haemorrhoid formation but mechanical factors, such as rectal carcinoma, pelvic tumours and pregnancy, all predispose to haemorrhoids. Typically, bleeding is bright red and painless, unless a prolapsed haemorrhoid becomes trapped in the sphincter or thrombosed. Sometimes patients have a sensation that something is descending in the rectum and may actually be able to feel prolapsed haemorrhoids. These are termed second-degree when they reduce spontaneously (first-degree haemorrhoids do not prolapse) and third-degree when they remain prolapsed. Sclerotherapy, banding or surgical removal form the mainstay of treatment measures.

63 a. Angiodysplasia may be clinically asymptomatic or present with rectal bleeding, either occult in nature or associated with life-threatening haemorrhage. Owing to their frequency in the elderly as opposed to the young population, the diagnosis is often only made at colonoscopy or mesenteric angiography. Angiodysplasia refers to vascular abnormalities, usually of veins, and are most commonly found in the caecum or ascending colon. Treatment is restricted to hemicolectomy if bleeding is severe or recurrent. If lesions are small or solitary, then a trial of electrocoagulation during colonoscopy may be of benefit.

64 b. Osler–Weber–Rendu syndrome (hereditary haemorrhagic telangiectasia) is an autosomal-dominant disease involving dilation of small arterioles and capillaries causing an increased tendency to bleed. Anticoagulation and antiplatelet agents should be avoided if the syndrome is diagnosed. At one end of the spectrum, small red blanching lesions are found on skin, mucous membranes and the gastrointestinal tract but at the other end the syndrome has been associated with the development of hepatic and pulmonary arteriovenous fistulas leading to high-output heart failure, cerebral embolism and cerebral abscesses. Recurrent epistaxis and gastrointestinal bleeds are the most common presentation of Osler–Weber–Rendu syndrome, although stroke and cerebral abscess in young patients should always alert the clinician to the possibility of this disease.

65 f. Mesenteric embolus is a difficult diagnosis to make due to the myriad of insidious causes of rectal bleeding. The presentation of shock may be a feature of both hypovolaemia and infarction of bowel, leading rapidly to faecal peritonitis and overwhelming sepsis if not caught early. Atrial fibrillation, bruit or other risk factors for thromboembolism may aid in pointing the surgeon to the right diagnosis. A careful history may reveal preceding symptoms of intermittent pain on eating and resultant weight loss due to reduction in blood flow through the mesenteric system; however, this is often uncommon in acute-on-chronic cases with the development of good collateral supply in the gastrointestinal tract even in the face of marked blockage. Resection of the necrotic bowel with either primary anastomosis or secondary closure of colostomy depending on site, age and comorbidities is often the only treatment available at emergency presentation.

66 c. Gardeners expose themselves to many organisms if durable gloves are not worn and infections of the nail bed and surrounding area are common. These conditions are occasionally confused with fungal infections of the nail bed and scrapings for mycology can be taken if there is any doubt. Another common infection spread characteristically following rose-thorn pricks is with *Sporothrix* spp. This usually presents with characteristic tracks that spread distal to proximal.

67 i. Glomus tumour typically presents as a mass under the nail with severe pain as the most common feature. The bluish hue is another feature of this rare tumour that can resemble a subungal melanoma. Looking for other signs of melanoma can often be useful in differentiating between these two conditions.

68 e. Self-harm injuries commonly occur on the forearms and are more common in the female population. Injury to the radial and median nerves is most common in injuries to the wrist, the median nerve being especially vulnerable to slash injuries due to its relatively superficial course at the carpal tunnel. Radial nerve injury typically presents with an inability to extend the hand leading to wrist drop. The aide memoire *BEST* (*b*rachioradialis, *e*xtensors of the forearm, *s*upinator and *t*riceps) describes the muscle of the forearm supplied by this nerve.

69 h. This injury is one of the most commonly injured bones of the carpal row, thought to be due to the higher stresses imposed on the scaphoid due to its unique position spanning both proximal and distal rows of the carpal bones. Falling on an outstretched hand is the mechanism of injury usually encountered in this type of injury, occasionally complicated by neurovascular compromise as with any fracture. Tenderness in the anatomical snuffbox forms a useful clinical reckoner if scaphoid fracture is suspected.

70 j. Associated with a diverse variety of conditions such as diabetes mellitus, acromegaly, rheumatoid arthritis and pregnancy, carpal tunnel syndrome manifests with tingling and numbness that patients often describe as being relieved by shaking out their hands. Pain is typically complained of at night, and can be exacerbated by tapping over the carpal tunnel with the wrist extended (Tinel's test) or by stressing both wrists together into forced flexion (Phalen's test), forming a useful clinical screen for carpal tunnel syndrome. It is thought to be due to fluid retention in the case of pregnancy, diabetes and acromegaly, although the exact mechanism is not known.

71 i. Lithium carbonate is a frequently used drug for both prophylaxis and treatment of mood disorders and has been termed a 'mood-stabilizer'. Classically used as a first-line agent in the long-term treatment of bipolar disorder (manic depression), it helps maintain euthymia and reduces up- and downswings of mood. Side-effects of lithium can be severe and drug monitoring must be undertaken on a regular basis. Lithium toxicity can be precipitated by electrolyte derangements, most notably hyponatraemia, and may lead to nephrogenic diabetes insipidus characterized by an inability to concentrate water in the kidney, leading to dehydration and polydipsia that is resistant to desmopressin.

72 e. EMDR has been used with some success in those suffering from post-traumatic stress disorder following violent acts, especially sexual abuse and trauma from combat. EMDR usually takes place over multiple sessions and involves the assessment of a patient for EMDR therapy, including whether they are emotionally stable enough to start the process of therapy. Subsequent therapy sessions involve identifying a negative thought or image relating to the trauma and a positive thought or belief. The remainder of the therapy involves uncoupling the negative thought process by typically following the therapist's fingers across the visual field multiple times and to express the thought processes experienced at the time. Other modalities, such as music or other tactile stimuli, can be employed instead of eye movements. The aim of the process is to slowly replace the negative emotion experienced during sessions with the positive belief identified at the beginning of therapy. Closure of sessions involves written reflection of events between sessions and evaluation of the effectiveness of the self-calming measures.

Other modalities used in the treatment of post-traumatic stress disorder involve the use SSRIs and beta-blocking medication to reduce the symptoms of hyperarousal.

73 a. Schneider's first rank symptoms describe the spectrum of symptoms experienced by those with schizophrenia and are as follows:
- auditory hallucinations,
- thought insertion,
- thought withdrawal,
- thought block,
- thought broadcast,
- somatic hallucinations,
- lack of control over bodily function, e.g. controlled by external forces,
- delusions (fixed unshakeable beliefs).

Treatment involves the use of neuroleptics, either the older classes such as haloperidol or risperidone (with their risk of extrapyramidal side-effects, e.g. parkinsonism and sedation profile) or the newer classes of neuroleptics such as olanzapine, clozapine and quetiapine. Haloperidol and risperidone are commonly used in the acute management of psychosis with the newer agents more useful for longer-term management. Clozapine must be monitored frequently for the serious side-effect of agranulocytosis, defined as a white blood cell count $<500/mm^3$.

74 **g.** Anxiety attacks are often associated with situations such as speaking in public or being in a public place and share similar characteristics to the specific phobias. Agoraphobia (the fear of being in a public place) is one of the most commonly associated phobias with anxiety. Generalized anxiety disorders have no readily identifiable precipitant and anxiety attacks can occur daily over long periods of time. In this case, this woman is exhibiting a panic disorder manifest as anxiety when performing in public. There are many modalities used to counteract anxiety such as SSRIs, other classes of antidepressants and benzodiazepines (which should only be used as a last resort in intractable anxiety due to the dependence-forming effects of benzodiazepines). Simple measures, however, are often overlooked and these include breathing exercises, dietary modifications including avoiding all caffeine-containing products and relaxation techniques. These should be at least considered as a first-line before instituting medication, which may eventually become a long-term and unnecessary crutch.

75 **d.** ECT is a highly effective form of treatment for severe depression that is refractive to medical therapy and especially useful in the treatment of depression associated with delusional symptoms. The process involves undergoing a short course of general anaesthesia with a muscle relaxant (to prevent muscle damage and rhabdomyolysis associated with rapid muscular contraction during the procedure) then passing of current via two electrodes across the brain. The effect is similar to a tonic–clonic seizure in both electrical brain activity and clinical effect with postictal amnesia and confusion being infrequent non-anaesthetic related side-effects. The reversal of mood is extremely rapid with the use of ECT and can produce profound effects in a short space of time making it an effective therapy for those at severe risk of self-harm or suicide in which antidepressant medication may take too long to have effect.

76 **b.** Riedel's lobe is a congenital anatomical variant that is benign and often found incidentally on physical examination. It is found as an enlargement of the right lobe of the liver below the costal margin and is usually completely asymptomatic unless it

is hugely enlarged. Patients should be reassured that it is normal and that no further action needs to be taken.

77 h. This woman has the clinical features of reactive systemic amyloidosis (AA amyloid). Amyloidosis can be subdivided into three main categories:

- plasma cell dyscrasia (AL amyloid), associated with abnormal production of amyloidogenic immunoglobulins,
- reactive amyloid (AA amyloid), associated with an increase in the production of an acute phase protein called serum amyloid A and highly associated with chronic inflammatory and infective conditions, and
- familial amyloidosis.

Rheumatoid arthritis is especially linked to the development of AA amyloid due to the chronic nature of the inflammation and may present with multiorgan involvement and even failure. Renal disease is very common in amyloid and manifests as nephrotic syndrome. Hepatomegaly may be found on examination but does not usually present with the acute nature of renal disease. Histological diagnosis (80% pick-up rate from rectal tissue) is preferable with staining either with Congo red or under polarized light, where the fibrillar protein deposits exhibit an apple-green birefringence.

78 e. Colorectal and breast cancer are the two most common metastatic deposits in the liver and a derangement in liver enzymes may be one of the only red-flag signs that an undiagnosed malignancy has disseminated. The liver is richly supplied with venous blood from the gastrointestinal tract via the portal vein and thus is the first organ encountered when haematogenous seeding of primary gastrointestinal malignancy metastasizes. Unlike the other more benign or reversible causes of hepatomegaly, the liver edge is often non-tender, craggy and nodular. Recent advances in hepatobiliary surgery have now allowed restricted case-by-case resection of liver segments in an attempt to provide curative therapy for early metastasized malignancy; however, lesions are usually only considered when single and anatomically accessible. A staging CT scan of the chest, abdomen and pelvis should be performed if there is a high index of suspicion of malignancy with discussion at a multidisciplinary meeting involving oncologists, palliative care clinicians, surgeons, gastroenterologists and radiologists.

79 a. Right heart failure can occur secondary to many causes but in the main is due to pulmonary hypertension and left heart failure leading to the clinical syndrome of congestive cardiac failure. Commonly after large MIs a part of the left ventricular muscle becomes non-functional and reorganizes to become scarred fibrotic tissue, leaving the rest of the viable tissue to take on the burden of systolic output. With time, the remaining left ventricle will start to fail causing back pressure through the pulmonary system and eventual pulmonary vascular changes, which may manifest as pulmonary hypertension. This in turn increases the work of the right heart due to increased afterload and the resultant pressure overload will cause hypertrophy and eventual failure. Functional regurgitation may occur through any of the valves involved in the failing heart and tricuspid regurgitation, although rare, may be a mechanical consequence of changes in the right myocardium. A pulsatile liver is a sign that there is an open communication between the right ventricle and the inferior vena cava (as a patent tricuspid valve will direct pressure waves up through the pulmonary valve during systole). Other causes of tricuspid regurgitation such as endocarditis caused by IV drug use may give the same clinical picture of right-sided heart failure without the coexistent left-sided signs and may aid the diagnosis.

80 **i.** Falls are a common presenting complaint in those who abuse alcohol. Right upper quadrant pain may also be complained of and suggests the development of alcoholic hepatitis. Signs may vary from florid signs of chronic liver disease (e.g. ascites, spider naevi, oesophageal, rectal and umbilical varices) to mild signs such as an unwell patient with a faint jaundice. Typically, there is a tender, smoothly enlarged liver edge; however, if the patient has progressed to alcoholic cirrhosis (with a shrunken impalpable and fibrotic liver) there is an increased risk of the development of hepatocellular carcinoma, which may present with nodular hepatomegaly and raised alpha-fetoprotein. Alcoholic hepatitis is usually treated with adequate pain relief, alcohol withdrawal programmes and IV or high-dose oral vitamins and thiamine to prevent complications such as Wernicke–Korsakoff syndrome and neurological sequelae of vitamin B12 deficiency such as peripheral neuropathy and subacute combined degeneration of the spinal cord.

81 **a.** Cocaine is a presynaptic reuptake inhibitor effectively increasing the synaptic concentrations of dopamine, noradrenaline and serotonin at higher doses. Dopamine is involved in the so-called 'reward' pathways of the brain and hence higher levels lead to the feeling of euphoria and 'high' that is produced by cocaine

use. Cocaine is also a vasoconstricting drug and this action can be seen with disastrous effect in those individuals who swallow packets of cocaine with subsequent eruption of the packets in the gastrointestinal tract. Massive local vasoconstriction can occur, leading to ischaemic segments of bowel as well as systemic absorption, leading to tachycardia (due to increased sympathetic drive), myocardial ischaemia (due to vasoconstriction and tachycardia) that may manifest as angina, and increased risk of stroke due to hypertension and localized ischaemia due to vasoconstriction followed by reperfusion injury.

The local anaesthetic effect of cocaine (it was for many years used as the a topical anaesthetic agent) when applied systemically can cause conduction defects in the myocardium and arrhythmias and these must be borne in mind when treating patients with suspected cocaine overdose. Aspirin must not be used in the acute management of angina-like pain, as the risk of cerebral haemorrhage post-vasoconstriction is high and bleeding can be catastrophic.

82 **i.** Marijuana (cannabis) is the most commonly abused illicit substance in the United States. It has a variety of actions that vary from euphoria, an altered perception of space and time, hallucinations, anxiety and paranoia to drowsiness. With chronic use, an 'amotivational syndrome' develops, characterized by a lack of interest in social and occupational life and a lack of energy. The mechanism of effect of marijuana is still largely unknown, although the putative active agent is δ-1-tetrahydrocannabinol (THC), correlating to large numbers of diverse THC receptors found scattered throughout the brain. Long-term effects include orthostatic hypotension and tachycardia and smoking marijuana has been linked with the development of a lung disease similar to COPD. Effects on the central nervous system are controversial but appear to include a type of atrophy that may be related to long-term use. The injected conjunctiva of marijuana use are frequently seen.

83 **g.** Chronic alcohol use has been linked to various vitamin and essential mineral deficiencies owing to both a lack of dietary intake and secondary to vomiting. Most notable are the effects of a lack of thiamine and vitamin B12, which are involved in the development of Wernicke's encephalopathy and Korsakoff's psychosis and when chronic can lead to subacute degeneration of the spinal cord (vitamin B12). This woman is exhibiting signs and symptoms of Wernicke's encephalopathy – a triad of ataxia,

ophthalmoplegia and confusion, which may progress to the irreversible Korsakoff's psychosis, which manifests as confabulation and memory deficits. ECG changes are most likely due to hypomagnesaemia, occasionally seen in alcoholics, those with malabsorption syndromes and diabetics. The widened QT interval has been linked to a risk of developing torsades de pointes and correction of the electrolyte deficit should be part of the standard of care for the acute management of complications of chronic alcohol abuse.

84 f. Opioids are responsible for a plethora of adverse effects if abused, the most serious of which is respiratory depression. This can often be so severe as to cause a life-threatening depression that may occur while the patient retains a level of consciousness. Miosis, nausea, vomiting, constipation, itch and hypotension are some of the other effects that are suggestive of opioid overdose. Florid respiratory depression may manifest clinically as a very low respiratory rate causing a drop in pH as CO_2 is not cleared and a loss of consciousness (hence the high CO_2 and low pH, suggesting a respiratory acidosis in this scenario). Easily reversed by opioid antagonists such as naloxone and naltrexone the clinician must not be lulled into a false sense of security by the apparent improvement in the patient's clinical state as the effects of some of the longer lasting opioids (such as methadone) and large doses can quickly overcome the effects of such antagonists.

85 d. PCP is a powerful dissociative hallucinogen originally used as an anaesthetic agent until the post-anaesthesia side-effects associated with the drug precluded its use. When abused, it has been associated with psychosis, violence and agitation, tachycardia, high temperature and anxiety. Neurological signs such as vertical or horizontal nystagmus are common, as is hypertension. Tachypnoea and irregular breathing patterns have been described in PCP users and, rarely, muscular rigidity syndromes and dystonias are seen. Treatment modalities aim to reduce absorption via the gastrointestinal tract when ingested and to reduce the agitating effects of the drug. Benzodiazepines are a safe antidote to control the behavioural symptoms associated with use and are preferable to antipsychotic agents, which carry the risk of causing neuroleptic malignant syndrome, seizures and malignant hyperthermia. Rhabdomyolysis is a side-effect of muscular rigidity syndromes and merits testing of creatinine kinase levels and careful monitoring of renal function with aggressive fluid therapy if suspected.

86 d. This woman is suffering at attack of inflammatory bowel disease and has a history consistent with a moderate to severe exacerbation. She should be managed initially medically unless any complications such as perforation, uncontrolled bleeding or toxic megacolon should occur and should be started on oral prednisolone and a 5-aminosalicylate (5-ASA) such as mesalazine for symptom relief initially. The history of conjunctivitis and arthritis in a young person with bloody diarrhoea and mucous in the absence of foreign travel or sexually transmitted infection is likely to be an extra-gastrointestinal manifestation of either Crohn's disease or ulcerative colitis.

87 a. *Clostridium difficile* is the most likely agent to have caused this man's diarrhoea. Treatment with antibiotics has been linked to selection of drug-resistant strains of *C. difficile* with resultant overgrowth and the development of pseudomembranous colitis. Clindamycin is particularly linked with the development of pseudomembranous colitis; however, the cephalosporins have also been demonstrated to cause this and few antibiotics are free from this rare but serious side-effect. The colonoscopic appearance is one of an erythematous colonic mucosa with a faint cream or grey pseudomembrane. A stool sample for parasites, bacterium and *Clostridium difficile* toxin should be taken and it is important that antidiarrhoeal therapy is not instituted unless the sample is clear, for fear of prolonging and exacerbating the infection. Treatment is either with oral metronidazole or oral vancomycin and rationalization of antibiotic therapy.

88 b. This man is showing the clinical signs and symptoms of diabetic ketoacidosis with a low pH and metabolic acidosis, ketonuria and hyperglycaemia. Precipitants of diabetic ketoacidosis can range from infection to MI and typically a history is given of an acute illness with a failure to increase insulin requirements appropriately. Travel and erratic eating pattern can disrupt the normal rhythm of blood glucose regulation and a superimposed infection can quickly cause even the most disease-aware individuals to become unwell. The diarrhoea is due to osmotic sequestration of fluid in the gut due to high glucose and electrolyte levels and will cause massive dehydration of up to 5 L quite easily along with polyuria. The treatment strategy includes fast fluid rehydration and high level of insulin infusion to reduce glucose level and suppress ketogenesis. Conversion to sliding scale of insulin can be undertaken after a few days once the initial hyperglycaemia and ketogenesis (as monitored effectively by simple urine dipsticks) has settled.

89 e. These are the classical signs and symptoms of hyperthyroidism with heat intolerance, diarrhoea, mood changes, especially anxiety and mania, and weight loss. Physical signs include increased sweating, tachycardia that does not abate at night or at rest, proptosis, lid lag and exophthalmos if Graves' disease is causative, and a fine tremor. The exact opposite is true for those suffering from hypothyroidism and represents one of the starkest physiological correlates of biochemical disturbance with neurokinetic manifestations. Treatment is aimed to cure and to palliate symptoms and employs both a beta-blocker such as propranolol (in the absence of contraindication) to control symptoms of tremor, tachycardia and excess sympathetic overactivation and a thioureylene such as carbimazole is used to inhibit the iodination of thyroglobulin thereby reducing the synthesis of the end products T3 and T4. A rare but serious side-effect of carbimazole is the development of agranulocytosis and repeat full blood counts must be undertaken. Patients are told to report immediately to hospital or their GP if they develop symptoms such as a sore throat, as this may signify the development of agranulocytosis.

90 i. Bulimia nervosa can manifest in many different ways but the core symptoms that allow a diagnosis to be made are prevalent in all. Typically, the patient is a young female with characteristic episodes of binge eating, particularly of sugar-rich foods and snacks. The period of overeating is then countered with a period of self-induced vomiting, food avoidance or restriction, or even laxative abuse and may present to hospital with diarrhoea. Patients are often aware that their behaviour is detrimental to their health and may be ashamed and disgusted with it. Rapid weight losses can lead to a cessation of periods (secondary amenorrhoea), which usually occurs when total body weight falls below 45 kg. Biochemical disturbances due to vomiting and diarrhoea are common and low levels of potassium may be seen. Treatment strategies may involve psychiatrists when symptoms are severe, especially in cases of self-harm or suicidal behaviour and is focused on changing the behaviour that drives the impulses behind binge eating.

Answers

Single Best Answer Questions

1 b. Acute exacerbations of asthma can be defined as moderate, severe or life threatening. Criteria for diagnosis are as follows:
- *Severe attack:*
  - unable to complete sentences,
  - respiratory rate of greater than 25 breaths/minute,
  - heart rate >110 bpm,
  - PEFR <50% of predicted.
- *Life threatening:*
  - cyanosis, very poor respiratory effort,
  - silent chest,
  - bradycardia and hypotension,
  - PEFR <33% predicted,
  - arterial blood sampling will show normal or high $PaCO_2$ and PaO_2 <8 kPa.

In any case of asthma exacerbation, a chest X-ray should be ordered to exclude a pneumothorax and to look for a concurrent pneumonia. The principles for management of exacerbations should be along the lines of any other emergency and follow a simple airway–breathing–circulation (ABC) approach.

Medications used in the exacerbations of asthma include oxygen, steroids and bronchodilators, with use of aminophylline in some places depending on the clinical situation. Magnesium sulphate is also being used more commonly for the management of acute asthma. Transfer for ventilatory support should always be considered in those patients who appear to be tiring or in those with a history of brittle disease, as fatalities do occur in young asthmatic patients.

2 b. This boy has a classical history of a testicular torsion. This is usually torsion of the spermatic cord in a structurally abnormal

EMQs and SBAs for Medical Finals, Second Edition. Jonathan Bath, Rebecca Morgan and Mehool Patel.

testis. It is possible for it to occur in a structurally normal testis, although it is less common. This constitutes a surgical/urological emergency. Often there is a history of mild trauma or previous attacks of pain due to the torsion and spontaneous untwisting. The supply of the testis is from T10 sympathetic pathway, which is why abdominal pain occurs. These patients require emergency surgery to correct and stabilize the torsion. On occasions, when the torsion has compromised the testicular blood supply for a long duration of time, ischaemia may result and this is usually treated at the time of surgical exploration by orchiectomy.

3 **a.** In a young fit person the two most sensible treatment options include a surgical repair or an above knee backslab with foot in equinus position. After surgery, the re-rupture rate is 2–5%, while it is 8–10% for those treated conservatively. The commonest site for rupture is 4–8 cm above the point of insertion. Characteristic signs of Achilles tendon rupture include difficulty in walking and standing on tip toes, there may be a visible gap in the tendon and a positive Simmonds' test (no plantarflexion on squeezing the affected calf). If there is any doubt clinically, an ultrasound scan may be used to confirm the diagnosis. Conservative treatment is most appropriate for elderly people, while younger and more active patients are usually managed with surgical repair. Infection is the biggest surgical complication involved with this procedure and since the Achilles tendon is quite superficial, any wound infection may result in disrupting the integrity of the tendon repair.

4 **b.** The growth of male breast tissue, known as gynaecomastia, is a normal finding in the neonate, due to maternal oestrogens, and in the pubertal boy and elderly male due to the changing ratio of testosterone to oestrogens in these age groups. This is not a typical finding that would be consistent with non-accidental injury and therefore a referral to social services would be inappropriate. Referral to a breast surgeon and needle aspiration are also unjustified in this case and may even be deleterious to growing breast tissue. Short-course prednisolone is also unwarranted and is not indicated in cases of gynaecomastia.

5 **a.** Sensitivity is defined as the number of disease and test positive (true positive) divided by the number of all the people with the disease. Represented as a formula this can be expressed as $a/(a+c)$. The table below can be used as reference for the following answers:

| | Disease | |
Test	Positive	Negative
Positive	a	b
Negative	c	d

A test that has a high sensitivity is one that is appropriate to use as a screening test for a population as it will pull up few false negatives (high se*N*sitivity = few false *N*egatives) as most of the people who are disease positive will be 'caught' by the test as positive.

A test that has a high specificity, by comparison, should be used once enough individuals have been screened and will 'catch' those individuals who are disease and test negative (i.e. true negatives). This is good for weeding those people out who tested falsely positive in the screening test but are reassured to find out they are truly negative. It can be expressed as $d/(b+d)$.

Positive predictive value refers to the number of true positives who tested positive for the disease and can be expressed as $a/(a+b)$. As the accuracy of any test will increase with population size, it follows that the positive predictive value of a test will increase the higher the prevalence of disease.

Negative predictive value refers to the number of true negatives who tested negative for the disease and can be expressed as $d/(c+d)$.

There were actually 140 false negatives in this case (box c) as these are defined as the number of people who are disease positive who test negative.

Finally, this test should not be used as a screening test as the sensitivity is only 80.1% $(a/(a+c))$, which is not high enough to justify use as you would 'miss' approximately 20% of those with the disease as the test would not pick these people up.

6 c. Testicular tumours are commonly found incidentally after minor trauma to the scrotum, the mass often mistakenly attributed to the trauma itself. Torsion of the testicular apparatus, such as the hydatid of Morgagni, is often heralded by pain and more rarely a blue spot on examination of the scrotum. Previous surgery for undescended and maldescended testes is associated with the development of testicular tumours, of which seminoma is more commonly found in patients over 30 years of age than teratoma.

7 e. While this woman has a strong history of asthma it is important to exclude other causes of shortness of breath. Anaphylaxis refers to a severe allergic reaction including both dermal and systemic signs and symptoms. The full-blown syndrome includes urticaria with occasional angioedema with hypotension and bronchospasm. Anaphylaxis is mediated by immunoglobulin E (IgE) and signs and symptoms are caused by the rapid onset of increased secretion from mucous membranes, increased bronchial smooth muscle tone, reduced vascular smooth muscle tone and increased capillary permeability occur after exposure to an offending substance.

Pneumothorax is a collection of gas in the pleural space resulting in collapse of the lung on the affected side due to the extrinsic pressure on the lung being greater than the intrinsic pressure produced by the respiratory system. A tension pneumothorax can be a life-threatening condition caused by rapidly accumulating air within the pleural space. This causes displacement of mediastinal structures, which in turn compromises cardiopulmonary function.

Tracheal obstruction or a massive pulmonary embolus will understandably cause acute-onset shortness of breath. Stridor may be a clue in upper airway obstruction and a history of risk factors should be sought in a suspected case of pulmonary embolus. An upper respiratory tract infection should not present acutely.

8 e. Ureteric obstruction is confirmed clinically by an IVU. In up to 90% of cases the causative stone can be seen on X-ray of the kidneys, ureter and bladder and this is recommended prior to undertaking an IVU, as contrast may obliterate from view a small but otherwise radio-opaque stone. Delayed excretion and dilatation of ureter or renal pelvis are useful in making the diagnosis and are frequently seen in this investigation. Reduction in kidney size is not due to obstruction of the outflow tract, with the opposite often the case. Perfusion defects can occur in cases of inflow limitation, such as renal artery stenosis, but will not occur due to outflow obstruction. Bladder residual volumes are rarely seen in cases where a stone has travelled the length of the urinary tract and lodges distal to the neck of the bladder.

9 d. This investigation is useful in the screening for two common urological conditions: prostate cancer and benign prostatic hyperplasia (BPH). Epidemiological evidence suggests BPH is more common in the Afro-Caribbean population and may be linked to higher testosterone levels. Suprapubic catheterization is a useful therapeutic and diagnostic procedure for those where urethral catheterization is contraindicated, such as with urethral stricture or pelvic trauma where there is a risk of urethral rupture. In an elderly man presenting with such symptoms, it is usually advisable to perform a digital rectal examination, a PSA test, renal function test and urinalysis as part of routine management.

10 **b.** Although all the investigations should be considered, depending upon the chronicity of the swelling, the most important is to perform a joint aspiration. It is indefensible to miss a septic arthritis by not performing a diagnostic and simple tap in light of the above clinical signs. Septic arthritis will completely destroy a joint in a short space of time and the patient will head down the path of total joint replacement and potential litigation. Fluid should be sent for microscopy to look for organisms, cells and crystals (gout and pseudogout), culture and sensitivities. Blood cultures are merited, preferably prior to antibiotic therapy in light of the features of systemic infection; however, these should not be done in preference to aspiration. Imaging of the knee joint is useful in due course to see the extent of damage if resolution is not achieved with antibiotic therapy.

11 **e.** Pulmonary embolus and deep vein thrombosis risk should be assessed in all patients who present with pleuritic pain and shortness of breath. Patients post-surgery, especially hip surgery, obese patients, those with malignant disease, immobility and taking the oral contraceptive pill all have an increased likelihood of a venous thromboembolism. Carotid massage would be completely contraindicated in this woman as she is hypotensive. It is useful as a first-line manoeuvre in cases of supraventricular tachycardia once the absence of a carotid bruit has been established. Furosemide is useful in cases of heart failure in the presence of relatively normal renal function. CT with pulmonary angiography is the gold standard for diagnosing, but not treating, pulmonary embolus. This patient is tachycardic and hypotensive, therefore close observation and commencement of treatment would be ideal. While investigations need to be carried out, the patient need to be stable enough for the CT scanner.

12 **a.** The common peroneal nerve consists off branches of L4–S1. Its motor supply is to the anterior compartment of the calf, including tibialis anterior and extensor hallucis longus. The sensory component supplies the 1st web space and the dorsum of the foot and front side of the leg. This nerve winds around the head of the tibia and in certain tibial plateau fractures its

integrity may become compromised, usually due to stretching rather than transaction of the nerve, and as a result function usually returns. Given the nature of the nerve supply, crude testing for function may include dorsiflexion of the ankle and toes.

13 d. Rifampicin is known for causing a reddish/orange discoloration to the urine, among other non-therapeutic effects that include liver enzyme induction and resistance when not used in combination with other antituberculous medications. These effects are helpfully summed up by the *three R's of rifampicin (Revs up liver enzymes, Red/orange discoloration and Resistance when used alone)*.

True causes of haematuria are best described anatomically from the kidney downwards and include glomerulonephritic processes, polycystic kidney disease, trauma and urinary tract stone. Infectious processes include tuberculosis, cystitis of the bladder and schistosomiasis (especially if the patient has a positive travel history) and prostatic carcinoma, urethral trauma, urethritis or neoplasm. General causes of abnormal coagulation must always be excluded in any case of bleeding and inherited bleeding disorders, such as haemophilia, and any derangement in coagulation profile must be excluded.

Malaria can cause haematuria and a full history of recent travel must be elicited. Investigation of this often benign but occasionally life-threatening parasitic disease must be undertaken swiftly but should not delay empirical treatment if laboratory turnaround times of thick and thin films looking for malarial parasites are slow. Treatment of *Plasmodium falciparum* malaria is of vital importance due to the association with cerebral malaria and should depend on local sensitivities to antimalarial drugs; however, a week's course of quinine followed by Fansidar (with glucose-6-phosphatase [G6PD] deficiency investigation) is usually an adequate treatment regime. G6PD deficiency poses a risk of haemolytic anaemia with certain medications, notably antimalarials, and G6PD status is usually taken as soon as possible but should not delay the start of treatment.

14 c. Adhesions post-surgery and strangulated hernias are the most common causes of obstruction of the bowel and therefore are not to be missed when assessing a patient. Classically, small strangulated femoral hernias are missed in obese elderly women. Ulcerative colitis is a disease affecting the colon with the exception of backwash ileitis and would not considered as a cause of small bowel obstruction in this woman. Gastrocolic fistulae can occur in Crohn's disease but more commonly lead to faeculent vomiting than obstruction. Intussusception is a disease typically affecting 5–12-month-old infants. Meckel's diverticulum can lead to small bowel obstruction but this is rare and the most common presentation is one of inflammation.

15 d. Patients have the right to be fully informed about their diagnosis in order that they may make informed decisions about their medical care. In the case of patients who are assessed to be competent, this should always be the principle upon which to act. In very special situations where the release of a diagnosis is very strongly thought to be seriously detrimental to the health of the patient (and advice from psychiatrists and ethics departments and close communication with the family is strongly advised) then a diagnosis may be withheld from a patient, although these cases are few and far between and should only be made by the consultant in charge of that patient's care.

It is required of a doctor who has requested an investigation under implied, verbal or written consent (such as laboratory tests or a chest radiograph, etc.) to disclose the results of that investigation as and when the results become available in a timely manner such that the patient is given adequate time and information to make an informed choice regarding their care. For example, informing a patient 10 minutes before surgery that they are to receive a blood transfusion for anaemia, on the basis of blood results known the day before surgery, is not appropriate.

Leaving the breaking of bad news to other healthcare providers who were not responsible for ordering the diagnostic investigation is also not appropriate; for example, requesting an HIV test on a medical inpatient and asking the GP to break the news of a new diagnosis of HIV.

Although family members may be closely involved in the care of their relatives with the consent of the patient, it should not be left to the family to disclose results of investigations or aspects of medical care with the patient without a doctor discussing these directly with the patient. The responsibility of a doctor caring for a patient does not extend to the family and the relationship should be confidential and exclusive, unless explicitly expressed by the patient themselves. As a useful rule of thumb in the clinical setting, if there is ever any doubt regarding the appropriateness of an interaction, then the patient's right to absolute confidentiality from the treating team(s) directly involved in their care must be preserved and consent to extend that confidentiality to include other members must be authorised by the patient him or herself.

16 b. The history is describing a case of pyelonephritis. The features of the vignette suggesting more than a simple urinary tract infection include the systemic signs of fever, tachypnoea, low saturations and tachycardia. In this case, blood results also showed a raised white cell count with a creatinine level of 468 μmol/L, suggesting an acute renal failure secondary to the pyelonephritis. This woman made a good recovery with a combination of IV fluids and reduced doses of gentamicin and Timentin. Since she is experiencing systemic symptoms, oral antibiotics with community follow-up would be an inadequate management plan. Although catheterization and analgesia are important adjuncts to her therapy, alone they are insufficient.

17 b. Intramuscular (IM) adrenaline injection of 0.5 mL of 1:1000 IM adrenaline is the recommended treatment for suspected anaphylaxis. Note that this dose differs from the 10 mL of 1:10 000 IV injection dose of adrenaline used in cardiac arrest. The clues to a severe allergic reaction are manifold from the history; severe shortness of breath occurs secondary to oedema of the upper airway and larynx and his medications reveal an atopic predisposition. Laryngeal mask airway and endotracheal intubation would be possibilities if adrenaline did not work as a first line or if airway control was an issue. Nebulized salbutamol and IV hydrocortisone would provide some relief for airway oedema but are not as effective as adrenaline in the acute management of anaphylaxis.

18 c. This patient needs to be admitted for an open reduction and internal fixation of the fracture. The key feature in this history is the rotation of the fragment. If the fracture was undisplaced and not rotated this could be managed in a backslab and followed up in fracture clinic. However, since there is associated rotation, the patient requires surgical management to achieve a better functional outcome. On examination of this man's hand, it was noted that he was unable to form a fist due to swelling and pain (not uncommon with unrotated fractures either) but there was obvious rotation of his affected little finger.

19 d. The prevalence of disease is defined as the number of active cases in a defined time, divided by the total population surveyed. The number of people with the disease is 20 000 people in that year, with the total population in the same period being 140 000.

   Incidence is defined as the number of new cases diagnosed in a given time period, divided by the total population in that time period. Thus option b (500/140 000) describes the incidence of the disease.

Option e (250/140 000) describes the mortality rate specific to that disease. A similarly calculated figure is the absolute mortality rate (sometimes referred to as the death rate), which describes the total number of deaths per population.

20 b This patient has two main problems: he has severe facial injuries thus may be at risk of losing his airway and on clinical examination he has evidence of a right-sided tension pneumothorax. However, his airway is intact as evidenced by him telling you his was the driver. Most clinicians would consider needle thoracocentesis to drain a tension pneumothorax before considering intubation in a patient with an intact airway, despite severe facial injuries. In addition, intubation in situations of lung compromise carries significant risk from bag ventilation perhaps exacerbating the situation. A nasopharyngeal airway is contraindicated due to the complex facial fractures as the risk of basal skull fracture is high. An emergency cricothyroidotomy is a last resort to secure an airway and can be avoided by early intubation if airway management is likely to become difficult. Chest drain insertion is not the immediate recommended procedure for releasing a tension pneumothorax.

21 a. This question is a commonly tested trauma principle; however, it requires an understanding of trauma triage by severity of injury. Traumatic aortic injuries portend a grave prognosis if the entire category of aortic injuries is examined as a whole. However, broken down into those patients who survive to hospital with a documented traumatic aortic injury, the prognosis is much better than initial appearances. A total of 50% of all patients with traumatic aortic injuries will die at the scene; however, of those that survive the initial event the aortic injury has been self-selected to be stable but requiring urgent repair. In the presence of other life-threatening injuries, such as a shattered spleen – Grade V injury, these should be taken care of first prior to attempt at repair of a (currently) stable aortic injury. This would be accomplished by an exploratory laparotomy.

Blunt traumatic injury most often occurs just distal to the takeoff of the subclavian artery and would likely be attempted endovascularly rather than through a classic open thoracoabdominal incision if the patient is stable. Immediate angiography is likely to delay critical care of the patient and would be unwise. Immediate intubation in A&E is not recommended in a hypotensive patient who needs an emergency operation unless the airway is unprotected (the patient complains of pain therefore we can surmise still has evidence of a patent airway). Finally, cross-matched blood may take up to 30–45 minutes to become available; this patient requires immediate resuscitation with IV fluids and an operation.

22 a. Complex abdominal trauma requiring emergency surgery may require massive transfusion in the peri-operative period. Packed red cells are the most commonly used blood product for transfusion; however, they do not contain platelets and clotting factors. Transfusion of as little as 4 units can predispose a shocked patient to coagulopathy manifest by oozing from all wound sites and bleeding from mucous membranes that cannot be easily controlled. Replacement of clotting factors and platelets forms the mainstay of therapy acutely. Vitamin K can be a useful agent in cases of warfarin overdose; however, it is not beneficial in this situation.

23 d. In patients with advanced cervical cancer, renal failure can occur secondary to bilateral compression of the ureters as they traverse the cervix in the lower pelvis. The mass effect or direct invasion from the cancer exerts pressure on the urinary system, which causes urinary retention. The treatment options are limited at this stage of cervical cancer; however, renal failure secondary to compression must be relieved promptly. This is most often done by inserting bilateral percutaneous nephrostomy tubes in the interventional radiology suite. Tumour lysis syndrome is seen in conjunction with chemotherapeutic agents, causing release of large amounts of purines from DNA catabolism as tumour cells are broken down. Administration of allopurinol, a xanthine oxidase inhibitor, can be used to mitigate this effect.

24 a. Jaundice is a feature of acute pancreatitis due to inflammation of the pancreatic head obstructing bilious outflow. Pseudocyst formation is a late complication of pancreatitis and usually takes about a week to develop thus is not seen in the acute inflammation. Hypocalcaemia as opposed to hypercalcaemia is often seen and is useful as one of the Glasgow criteria for predicting severity of pancreatitis along with a low albumin. Bowel necrosis is not associated classically with pancreatitis.

25 d. Rheumatological disease exhibits a predilection for the female sex. Ankylosing spondylitis is one of the few conditions that goes against this trend, being approximately six times more common in males than females in early teenage years and twice as common in males by 30 years of age. Typically, the patient is a young male presenting with morning stiffness, reduced back movement with back pain and pain over the sacroiliac joints.

Rheumatoid arthritis is unlikely for reasons of sex and age. Prolapsed intervertebral discs may present with symptoms of back and hip pain but would be again unlikely (but not infeasible) in a healthy 23-year-old man. Facet joint arthritis presents in middle to old age with pain, especially on bending backwards as the facets rub against each other.

26 b. Advanced Parkinson's disease can result in many features including a mask-like facial appearance and difficulty in swallowing. This patient suffered an aspiration pneumonia. The commonest site for an aspiration pneumonia, or indeed inhalation of a foreign body, is the lower lobe of the right lung. This is due to the anatomy of the right main bronchus being more vertical than the left due to the positioning of the heart. Parkinson's disease is not known to be closely associated with heart failure. Atypical pneumonias are usually widespread and provide more generalized signs than those described above.

27 c. Causes of testicular swelling can be divided into the following categories:

Painful	Hard and painless	Soft
Torsion of testis	Tumour	Varicocele
Torsion of hydatid of Morgagni	Syphilis	Epididymal cyst
Epididymitis	Tuberculosis	Hydrocele
Orchitis, viral or bacterial	Haematoma	

Other causes of scrotal swelling include an inguinal hernia, which extends above the scrotum, and sebaceous cysts, which sit superficially on the scrotum.

28 a. These signs are characteristic of arterial occlusion. The '6 Ps': *p*ale, *p*ulseless, *p*aresthesia, *p*ainful, *p*aralysed, *p*erishingly cold. The popliteal artery is the most susceptible artery to acute occlusion, being small in calibre.

Cellulitis would cause pain in the leg, erythema and warmth, which is not seen in this case. Reduced circulating volume would provide more generalized symptoms. Distal pulses may be weakened but will be present, although the limbs may be cold there should be no pain. Venous insufficiency would lead to oedema in the limbs and in the longer term trophic skin changes, including venous eczema and lipodermatosclerosis. Vasculitis would provide a different clinical picture with vasculitic lesions on the skin, presence of pulses and blood tests that typically reveal increased inflammatory markers.

29 **a.** The ABG results provided in this question are all within the normal range. The patient has an adequate PaO_2 without retaining carbon dioxide. These results suggest that 35% of oxygen is adequate for this patient; lower levels may not provide adequate oxygenation and higher levels may lead to CO_2 retention. A baseline ABG will have already been performed on air and therefore this is not necessary to repeat. It is important to repeat a blood gas sample on 28% oxygen as this may also provide suitable results. Having established the most appropriate oxygen concentrations, it is sometimes useful to measure saturations after exercise to ensure that no drop is seen in the level of oxygenation. There are strict criteria for long-term domiciliary oxygen and it is important that patients satisfy these prior to the commencement of therapy.

30 **c.** The investigation most likely to be diagnostic is the MRI of the spine. While the bone scan will be useful if the MRI scan does show metastases (which, in this case it did), alone it will not be diagnostic. While in this case it is important to exclude sinister causes of pain, it is also important to exclude more common causes of lower back pain, including discitis and disc prolapse, all of which can usually be identified on CT scan. This man was found to have metastases in his spine and returned to a tertiary centre to have both chemotherapy and radiotherapy.

31 **d.** Taking the patient to CT scan in the first place was a huge risk – the notoriously named 'doughnut of death' should only be considered in the management of trauma patients when the patient is stabilized. The presence of free fluid in the abdomen or pelvis is a red flag, although in women a tiny amount of free fluid may be physiological. Exsanguination into the abdomen, pelvis, chest or from long-bone fractures can occur rapidly and internal bleeding should be considered in any patient who sustains severe trauma.

Noradrenaline would indeed be the inotrope of choice for maintaining blood pressure but is only used in a critical care setting and never to correct a surgical cause of hypotension. A GCS of 11/15 suggests a significant degree of deterioration; however, intubation is not necessary at this stage unless airway compromise is suspected. Fluid resuscitation is absolutely needed before, during and after surgery; however, a repeat CT scan of the abdomen is not only unnecessary in making the diagnosis but may in fact endanger the patient by delaying surgery.

32 e. In this case we are provided with three pieces of clinical information:

↓ chest expansion unilaterally

↓breath sounds on the affected side

↓ percussion note on the affected side

These features are all leaning towards a diagnosis of an extensive collapse or pneumonectomy. A lobectomy would be unlikely to provide such dramatic signs as the remainder of the lung normally expands to fill the void left by removal of a single lobe. Characteristic findings of a pleural effusion would be ↓ chest expansion on the affected side, stony dullness to percussion, with bronchial breathing above the effusion. Other scenarios are widely available in clinical textbooks although there is no substitute for clinical practice for compounding your knowledge.

33 b. The symptoms and biochemical markers of renal failure and lung involvement, i.e. haemoptysis, should raise the concern of hepatopulmonary diseases such as Goodpasture's syndrome. A proliferative glomerulonephritis associated with pulmonary infiltrates causing haemoptysis (sometimes massive in nature) is the pathological hallmark of this aggressive disease. Antibodies to basement membranes affecting both glomeruli and alveoli are the typical antibodies exhibited by patients with Goodpasture's syndrome.

ANCAs are more strongly associated with systemic vasculitides such as Wegener's granulomatosis (PR3-ANCA), microscopic polyangiitis and Churg–Strauss disease (MPO-ANCA). Anti-SCL 70 is classically associated with systemic sclerosis, antimitochondrial antibodies are often seen in cirrhosis of liver and biliary tree, and rheumatoid factor is associated with rheumatoid disease and associated syndromes, e.g. Felty's syndrome. It is worth noting, however, that no antibody is entirely specific or sensitive to a particular disease and there are many patients without any disease who will exhibit positive antibody titres.

34 b. This history is classical of bladder cancer. The one major clue is *painless* haematuria; this is a classical feature of bladder cancer and 95% of cases present in this way. Predisposing factors to bladder cancer include working in the rubber industry with exposure to carcinogens, smoking and schistosomiasis. Other risk factors include chronic bladder stones and a congenital abnormality of the urinary tract. Most bladder cancers are transitional cell histologically and spread by direct invasion initially but by lymphatic spread to the peri-aortic nodes and haematogenous spread to the liver and lungs eventually.

BPH presents with urgency and difficulty in initiating urination and terminal dribbling with an incomplete sense of emptying. Prostatism is an acutely painful condition.

35 c. Although radiologically the cervical spine X-rays are clear and clinically the patient complains of no tenderness, it is important that a CT scan of her neck is organized urgently and her neck is kept immobilized in the meantime. The key feature in this history is the fractured distal radius and iliac wing as well as the history of a fall from a height of approximately 4.5–6 m. Having sustained other serious injuries, this patient is not in a position to confirm or deny any cervical spine tenderness. In the presence of distracting injuries further imaging should be sought before removal of cervical spine protection. If you ever have any doubts, the case should always be discussed with a senior colleague as the consequences of any error is potentially life threatening.

36 a. Flow volume loops can be difficult to interpret for the inexperienced student. The x-axis represents time, while the y-axis is a measure of both inspiratory and expiratory flow (the negative deflection is the inspiratory component, while the positive is expiratory measured in litres per second). Flow volume loop **a** shows a typical loop of a person that does not suffer with respiratory disease. The expiratory curve shows maximal peak expiratory flow and the straight line joining up to the inspiratory curve suggests a non-collapsible airway. Curve **b** represents a patient suffering from emphysema. The expiratory curve shows early airway collapse and the inspiratory phase is reduced in volume compared with the normal patient. Curve **c** represents fixed upper airways obstruction, curve **d** represents variable upper airways obstruction while curve **e** shows a restrictive pattern.

37 e. Carpal tunnel syndrome is commonly associated with rheumatoid arthritis but lesser known but important other associations include dialysis, pregnancy, diabetes mellitus and hypothyroidism. Symptoms are always in the distribution of the median nerve and are characteristically described by patients as affecting them at night and are relieved by shaking the hands out. The symptoms can often be brought on in clinic by Tinel's test (tapping over the extended wrist) and, less reliably, by Phalen's test (forced flexion at the wrist). Treatment options in chronological order of trial should include:

- wrist splinting,
- local steroid injection (symptomatic relief only),
- consideration of surgical decompression of the carpal tunnel indicated in cases of either prolonged symptoms or neurological symptoms, e.g. thenar eminence wasting.

Plain radiographs of the wrist and hand are unlikely to be of any use in the management of carpal tunnel syndrome; however, they may provide useful baseline views for assessing radiographic progression of rheumatoid disease.

38 d. The cause of the obstruction is at the level of the ureteric orifices as suggested by the dilated ureters and kidney and small bladder volume. Insertion of a suprapubic catheter will be of no use in this situation, as there is no evidence of bladder outflow obstruction. IV antibiotics are useful for treating a suspected urinary tract infection, as evidenced from the urine dipstick, but are not the modality that will ultimately aid in recovery. IV fluids are useful in the management of urinary tract infection and sepsis; however, without surgical decompression of the renal tracts this is likely to overload the cardiovascular system. The indications for renal dialysis can be remembered by the mnemonic *AEIOU* in cases refractory to medical treatment and include: *a*cidosis; *e*lectrolyte derangement; *i*ngestion/intoxication – mainly useful for toxins that are renally cleared; *o*verload of fluid; and *u*raemia severe enough to cause complications such as pericarditis.

39 d. Loss of pulse is a very late sign; if compartment syndrome is not suspected before this sign is present the outcome is likely to be poor. Signs of compartment syndrome include the '5 Ps':

- *p*ain in the affected limb disproportionate to the injury,
- *p*allor,
- *p*aralysis (often difficult to asses due to presence of cast),
- *p*araesthesiae,
- *p*ulseless limb.

If there is any doubt about the integrity of a compartment, the intracompartmental pressure should be measured. As a guide, if it is >40 mmHg urgent treatment, for example fasciotomy, should be considered. Senior review should be sought if you suspect a diagnosis of compartment syndrome.

40 e. This patient is suffering from ischaemia of the bowel or mesenteric ischaemia. This condition is most commonly seen in elderly men, particularly in known arteriopaths. Commonly, the disease involves the superior mesenteric artery, which provides blood supply to both the small and large bowel. It is characteristically identified by severe abdominal pain after eating, which results in anorexia to avoid the pain and subsequent weight loss. Angiography would be useful to confirm this diagnosis.

A congenital cause of a bowel abnormality would more than likely have presented itself before the age of 67 years and a psychogenic cause can be ruled out due to physical signs being present. Imaging, including barium enema and colonoscopy, would identify the large majority of colonic neoplasms and therefore these can be ruled out, although they are important differentials in an elderly patient with weight loss.

41 e. The Chi-squared test is most often used in situations where raw data are being examined for effect and is similar to the paired *t*-test in generating *P* values; however, the paired *t*-test is used for comparison of the means of two populations. *P* value generation describes the number generated by calculation of the squared difference between the observed and expected values as a fraction of the expected values. This value is then converted to a *P* value relative to the degrees of freedom associated with the number of rows and columns involved.

P values are useful determinates of whether an observation (or set of observations) generated is likely to be due to chance. For example, setting a *P* value of <0.05 is often taken to herald significance (meaning that you are confident that there is only a 5% risk that the data are due to chance events rather than the ordered effect of a true measurable difference). Limits for significance cut-off can be set at higher or lower levels, for example in a small population it may only be appropriate to use a cut-off value of < 0.01 (i.e. 1%) to attain significance, although in practice this may be difficult to achieve.

Positive predictive value refers to the predictive power of a test and is defined as the number of true positives who tested positive for a disease. It is a useful method of assessing the accuracy of a test and, as it is linked to the prevalence of a disease in a population (number of active cases per population per unit time), it will become more reliable with higher prevalences due to reduction of the statistical error generated by small sample size.

Odds ratio is used to approximate the relative risk of an event occurring and is used most often in examining data from case-control studies.

The Mann–Whitney U test is a non-parametric test that compares two unpaired groups (they do not have to follow a normal distribution and the variance within the population from which the data are selected does not have to be equal). The test compares two medians to assess whether the samples are from the same population or not. For sake of simplicity, it is essentially a non-parametric, i.e. does not have the same constraints on population variance and distribution as the *t*-test but allows a comparison to be made between two data sets.

42 d. *Streptococcus pneumoniae* is the commonest cause of community-acquired pneumonia. Students are often under the misconception that the organism most likely to be responsible for community-acquired pneumonia is *Staphylococcus aureus*. *Haemophilus influenzae* is another common organism responsible for community-acquired pneumonia. Patients suffering from COPD are more likely than those without lung disease to get chest infections caused by *Moraxella catarrhalis*, due to their underlying lung condition.

43 c. The Glasgow criteria for predicting the severity of pancreatitis can be used for pancreatitis due to any cause, though the Ranson criteria are reserved for pancreatitis due to alcoholism. The mnemonic '*PANCREAS*' is useful for remembering the Glasgow criteria.

> $pO_2 < 8\,kPa$
> *A*ge > 55 years
> *N*eutrophils $> 15 \times 10^9/L$
> *C*alcium $< 2\,mmol/L$
> *R*aised enzymes – lactate dehydrogenase (LDH)/aspartate transaminase (AST)
> *E*levated urea $>16\,mmol/L$
> *A*lbumin $<32\,g/L$
> *S*ugar $>10\,mmol/L$

44 b. In this scenario we should consider the possibility of a posterior shoulder dislocation. On a single antero-posterior (AP) X-ray, it is not possible to exclude a posterior dislocation of the shoulder as on a single AP view this can look normal. This injury is usually caused by an epileptic fit, electric shock or fall from a motorbike. It is usually due to a forced internal rotation of the abducted arm or a direct blow to the front of the shoulder and can usually be reduced in the A&E department. Anterior dislocations of the shoulder are visible on AP views and are commonly caused by falls backwards on to an outstretched hand or by forced abduction and external rotation of the shoulder. This causes the head of the humerus to be driven forward, tearing the capsule or avulsing the glenoid labrum. Associated fractures are occasionally seen.

45 c. Antibiotic use in community-acquired pneumonia varies with both GP experience and preference. The recommended antibiotic for a simple case is amoxicillin (provided that the patient is not allergic to penicillins). Amoxicillin is derived from ampicillin and is better absorbed than ampicillin. It produces higher plasma and tissue concentrations and its absorption is not affected by the presence of food in the gut.

Augmentin (co-amoxiclav) is a compound preparation of amoxicillin and the beta-lactamase inhibitor, clavulanic acid. The clavulanic acid protects the amoxicillin from the penicillinases produced by virtually all staphylococci and therefore this should not be given as first-line therapy since staphylococcus is not one of the most common infective organisms. Metronidazole provides cover for anaerobes and works by breaking DNA strands. Erythromycin may be used in patients with allergies to penicillins.

46 a. Femoral hernias are more common in women. The small bowel herniates through the femoral canal underneath the inguinal ligament, medial to the femoral artery (remember from lateral to medial in the femoral canal – *n*erve, *a*rtery, *v*ein, *e*mpty space, *l*ymphatics '*NAVEL*'). The neck of femoral hernias is narrow and therefore strangulation ensues.

Indirect hernias pass through both the deep and superficial inguinal rings, ventral hernias also known as incisional hernias are most commonly seen in those patients with particular risk factors, including obesity, old age, wound infection postoperatively and violent coughing. Direct hernias do not protrude into the scrotal sac, although inguinal hernias cannot be classified adequately until surgery is performed.

47 c. This question is included to remind the clinician that the management of disease should always remain with the patient as a central focus. The indicators specified may all be associated with disease activity, although the role of early involvement of biological agents is currently being evaluated. However, subjectively from a patient's perspective, the useful function that is managed comfortably in rheumatoid arthritis is the best indicator of disease activity. Appearances are often deceiving, with 'normal' radiographs disguising disabling pain and loss of function while long-term deformities of the hands may mask surprising dexterity and adaptation.

48 a. While several other species of genus *Legionella* have been identified, *L. pneumophila* is the most frequent cause of human legionellosis and a relatively common cause of community-acquired and nosocomial pneumonia in adults. The organism can be found in natural aquatic habitats (freshwater streams and lakes, etc.) and artificial sources (cooling towers, potable water distribution systems). *Legionella* organisms are cleared from the upper respiratory tract by mucociliary action. Any process that compromises mucociliary clearance (e.g. smoking) increases risk of infection. *Legionella* organisms may infect other parts of the body, including the lymph nodes, brain, kidney, liver, spleen, bone marrow and myocardium.

Staphylococcus aureus is usually a hospital-acquired pneumonia and pneumococcal pneumonia usually presents as a lobar infiltration.

49 c. Fractures in children can be difficult to assess, particularly in areas such as the elbow where there are several growth plates involved. The history in this case is of a minor injury with very limited clinical findings, which suggests that the X-ray is unlikely to show anything significant. The mnemonic for remembering which of the growth plates fuse around the elbow is '*CRITOL*' and the ages at which they close is roughly ages 2, 4, 6, 8, 10 and 12 years.

C – capitulum
R – radial head
I – internal epicondyle
T – trochlear
O – olecranon
L – lateral epicondyle

Variations in these do occur among children and, if there is any doubt or difficulty in interpreting the X-rays, comparison views of the unaffected side should be taken and compared.

50 c. The history of colicky pain radiating from the loin to groin and occasionally down to the testis is classical of ureteric stones. He is within the right age group for this problem and microscopic haematuria is seen with calculi. Calculi may develop or be the cause of associated urinary tract infections, although most stones pass without any surgical intervention. Investigation should include a full set of bloods and a plain abdominal X-ray since 90% of urinary calculi are radio-opaque. Other useful investigations include urine culture and IVU, which can identify the level of the stone if indeed one is present.

51 **b.** This patient has acute infection of the parotid gland or acute parotitis. Patients with poor dental hygiene and those who have been intubated are most at risk. *Staphylococcus aureus* is the organism most commonly responsible. Most often treatment requires surgical drainage and antibiotics. Mumps, although now only seen in outbreaks usually among children and young adults that have failed to be immunized, is a common cause of parotitis. Haemorrhage into the gland is incredibly rare and trauma during this surgery is unlikely due to its position. Sialolithiasis, or stones in the salivary glands, could be the cause of this presentation, although there is no relationship between stone development and surgery.

52 **d.** Antiphospholipid syndrome is a spectrum of SLE, often associated with vascular thromboses. The vascular involvement may manifest most strikingly as stroke, MI and multi-infarct dementia in a younger population with no obvious identifiable risk factors, or more insidiously with migrainous symptoms and recurrent miscarriages. The presence of lupus anticoagulant and anticardiolipin antibodies with this clinical presentation strongly suggests antiphospholipid syndrome.

Reiter's syndrome typically presents with a triad of urethritis, conjunctivitis and arthritis in a young man associated with sexually transmitted or gastrointestinal infections. Systemic sclerosis is a disorder mainly affecting skin, gastrointestinal tract and respiratory system while dermatomyositis, as the name suggests, affects skin and muscles mainly. Marfan's syndrome typically affects the aorta and aortic valve, lens of the eye and skeletal system due to mutations in the fibrillin-1 gene.

53 **d.** This clinical picture points towards a lung abscess. Most frequently, a lung abscess arises as a complication of aspiration pneumonia caused by gastrointestinal anaerobes. Abscesses can be primary or secondary in origin. A primary abscess is infectious in origin, caused by aspiration or pneumonia in the healthy host, while a secondary abscess is caused by an underlying condition (e.g. obstruction), spread from a distal site, bronchiectasis, and/or an immunocompromised state. It is possible to classify abscesses by the infectious organism, e.g. *Staphylococcus* lung abscess and anaerobic or *Aspergillus* lung abscess.

In this case, the important factors to identify are the swinging fever and the recurrence of cough with foul-smelling sputum shortly after a chest infection. These are both factors that should raise suspicion of an abscess. In addition, the X-ray findings of a walled cavity should raise the possibility of the diagnosis. Empyema is defined as inflammatory fluid and debris within the pleural space and may result from an untreated pleural-space infection that subsequently progresses into a collection in the pleural space.

54 b. A ruptured spleen must be considered with blunt trauma to the chest or upper abdomen, particularly if rib fractures are involved. Splenic trauma can be diagnosed by peritoneal lavage, CT scan or radionucleotide scanning; however, in this situation surgery is necessary immediately due to the development of shock and to assess the level of damage to the spleen and potentially prevent its removal.

The location of the injury and the associated hypovolaemia argue against both transection of the abdominal aorta and injury to the liver capsule. Trauma to the lungs is unlikely to lead to normal breath sounds on examination.

55 e. Prednisolone is used as a treatment option in SLE and has not been widely reported to be associated with drug-induced lupus in the literature. A useful mnemonic for remembering four drugs commonly associated with drug-induced lupus is 'It's not HIPP to have lupus' (Hydralazine, Isoniazid, Procainamide, Phenytoin). The associated lung and skin manifestations usually resolve on cessation of drug therapy.

56 b. The main differential diagnosis here should be between lung cancer and bronchiectasis. Bronchiectasis is the abnormal and permanent distortion of one or more of the conducting bronchi or airways, most often secondary to an infectious process. It can be categorized as a COPD manifested by airways that are inflamed and easily collapsible, which in turn results in air flow obstruction and impaired clearance of secretions. It may be congenital or acquired, although the congenital form is normally diagnosed during childhood. The condition results in destruction of muscular and elastic components of the bronchial walls, which impairs mucociliary clearance and predisposes to recurrent infections.

Impaired clearance of secretions causes colonization and infection with pathogenic organisms, contributing to the common purulent expectoration noted in patients with bronchiectasis.

The result is further bronchial damage and a vicious cycle of bronchial damage, bronchial dilation, impaired clearance of secretions, recurrent infection and more bronchial damage.

Diagnosis is usually based on a compatible clinical history of chronic respiratory symptoms, such as a daily cough and viscid sputum production, as well as typical findings on CT scan.

57 b. The case in question is describing a Weber C fracture (a fracture arising above the syndesmosis). Ankle fractures were described by Weber and his simple classification is still used in orthopaedics today:

- Weber A – fibular fracture below the syndesmosis,
- Weber B – fibular fracture through the syndesmosis,
- Weber C – fibular fracture above the syndesmosis.

Management of these fractures depends on the classification. Weber A are always managed conservatively, Weber B fractures are sometimes managed surgically and sometimes managed conservatively, and Weber C fractures as a rule are always managed operatively. These rules apply for isolated fibular fractures; when other injuries coexist management may change.

58 d. There are many causes of round opacities on chest X-rays. Their location may provide a clue to the likely diagnosis but often it is necessary to revert back to the history and examination for clues. Tuberculosis tends to present in the apices due to the apparent improved oxygenation. Both lung cancer and carcinoid tumour can present anywhere in the lung fields as round lesions.

Sarcoidosis or sarcoid is a multisystem disorder, characterized by non-caseating epithelioid granulomas. Other commonly involved organ systems include the lymph nodes, skin, eyes, liver, heart and the nervous, musculoskeletal, renal and endocrine systems. Patients usually complain of non-specific symptoms, including weight loss and fatigue. Chest symptoms are fairly common among sufferers of the disease. Chest X-rays tend to show generalized signs, including upper zone fibrosis or bilateral hilar adenopathy rather than well-demarcated lesions.

59 a. Anticardiolipin and lupus anticoagulant antibodies are most strongly associated with antiphospholipid syndrome. Antireticulin antibodies are commonly found in coeliac disease and other enteropathies, antinuclear antibodies are raised in a variety of conditions such as SLE, Sjögren's syndrome, systemic sclerosis, chronic active hepatitis and rheumatoid arthritis. Anti-Ro antibodies are found in Sjögren's syndrome and SLE and ANCA are raised in systemic vasculitides such as Wegener's granulomatosis, microscopic polyangiitis and Churg–Strauss disease.

60 b. Paraphimosis is frequently seen as a result of urethral catheterization. This unfortunate complication can be avoided by careful attention to replacing the foreskin after catheterization and by regular inspection of the penis while a catheter is *in situ*. Phimosis is usually picked up in childhood by a concerned parent if a child has problems passing urine or if his foreskin balloons up on passing urine. The condition is due to a narrowing of the preputial orifice and will usually require correction by circumcision.

Epispadias is a defect in penile development where the urethra opens on the dorsal aspect of the penis. The 'opposite' defect, hypospadias, is more commonly found where the urethra opens on the ventral aspect of the penis in an abnormal position anywhere from base of the shaft to the glans penis. Peyronie's disease manifests as an angulation of the erect penis due to fibrosis. It is associated with Dupuytren's contracture and atheroma.

Extended Matching Questions

61 a. In the postoperative patient there are several potential causes of fever and shortness of breath. In this situation, the answer is atelectasis. This is most likely to be the cause of any shortness of breath or fever in the first 24 hours postoperatively. Pneumonia is more likely to be the cause 2–3 days postoperatively. In either case, it is important to confirm the diagnosis by sending off blood tests, blood cultures and requesting a chest X-ray in addition to a clinical assessment.

62 f. This man has suffered a massive pulmonary embolus which culminated in cardiac arrest. Given a history of being treated for an embolus and suspicion that this is the cause of his arrest, streptokinase may be used during the resuscitation process. As advised on the advanced life support course, during a cardiac arrest reversible causes should be sought including the 'four Hs and four Ts':

*H*ypokalaemia/hyperkalaemia	*T*ension pneumothorax
*H*ypothermia	*T*oxicity (drugs)
*H*ypoxia	*T*hromboembolism
*H*ypovolaemia	*T*amponade

By working through these potential causes of cardiac arrest, it is possible to treat these reversible causes effectively. During every cardiac arrest call that you attend, you should always be thinking about the cause in each particular case as quick thinking can be life saving.

63 **c.** This man has suffered an aspiration pneumonia secondary to a stroke. If patients are not carefully monitored by the ward staff they may continue to eat and drink, despite having altered neurological status. If a patient's ability to swallow is impaired then they can develop aspiration pneumonia. The commonest part of the lung to be affected by an aspiration pneumonia is the right lower lobe, due to the angulation of the right main bronchus which means that food or any aspirate will preferentially end up there. However, this can vary due to the position of the patient; for example, the upper lobes may be affected if the patient is lying supine after the aspiration event. Presentation of an aspiration pneumonia is identical to that of a normal pneumonia. Although the history may vary, the key difference is in the management. Aspiration pneumonia will require coverage for organisms normally found in the gastrointestinal tract and this will usually include cephalosporins and metronidazole.

64 **b.** Given the details in the history, it is sensible to be suspicious of a malignancy. Although this patient is young it is not uncommon for malignancies to present in this age group. Further delving into the history revealed a gradually worsening shortness of breath with a long history of cigarette smoking. The clinical findings of an effusion fit with the diagnosis of a lung cancer and analysis of the fluid would characteristically show an exudate with >30 g/L of protein and presence of malignant cells. While other causes of pleural effusions should be considered, the presence of malignant cells confirms the diagnosis and further imaging tests should be carried out to confirm the location and subgroup of the cancer.

65 **e.** This scenario is clearly describing an exacerbation of COPD. This is commonly caused by concurrent infection. In this case, it appears that omission of her inhalers has resulted in reduced lung function and an opportunist infection has exacerbated the problem. With this subgroup of patients, it is important to ensure that the infection is treated and that they are back on their usual bronchodilators and steroids before discharge in order to optimize their chances of coping once discharged. It is always important to make appropriate follow-up arrangements to prevent similar episodes occurring in the future.

66 b. Rheumatoid arthritis affects females three times more commonly than males. Its peak age of onset is between the ages of 30 and 50 years old. It can be described as a symmetrical polyarthropathy affecting both small and large joints. Common symptoms are swollen, painful, stiff hands and feet which are worse in the mornings and patients may describe a recent history of constitutional symptoms and fatigue. Patients with suspected rheumatoid arthritis should always be referred to a rheumatologist for commencement of disease-modifying drugs as soon as the diagnosis is confirmed in order to reduce the amount of joint damage sustained.

67 a. In acute gout there is often severe pain, redness and swelling in the affected joint. The metatarsophalangeal joint of the big toe is most commonly affected. Deposition of sodium monourate crystals in the joint space is responsible for the symptoms and attacks may be precipitated by trauma, surgery, starvation or commencement of diuretics. Risk factors include a high-protein diet, alcohol and obesity. Aspirin is known to increase serum urate. Allopurinol can be used to reduce the level of urate in the circulation but it must not be commenced within 3 weeks of an acute attack, as it can precipitate another incident.

68 h. This patient is suffering from arthritis mutilans – telescoping of the joints in her ring finger on her right hand. This arthritis is a form of psoriatic arthropathy, associated with the skin condition psoriasis. There are several similarities in this skin condition to rheumatoid arthritis; therefore it is important to consider psoriasis in any new patient presenting with rheumatoid features as the joint conditions may present before the skin lesions.

69 f. At the age of 16 years, ankylosing spondylitis is six times more common in males than females. By the age of 30 years it is twice as common in males. Typical presenting symptoms are morning back stiffness and progressive loss of spinal movement. Other features include hip and knee involvement and plantar fasciitis, as eluded to in this case study. Diagnosis is clinical but strongly supported by radiology, for example squaring of the vertebrae, formation of a 'bamboo spine' and obliteration of the sacroiliac joints. This is a rare example of a rheumatological condition being more common in males than females.

70 c. Osteoarthritis is the commonest joint condition. It is usually primary but may be secondary to any joint disease or joint injury. Its mean age of onset is 50–60 years old. Pain is defined as being worse after periods of activity and towards the end of the day, with some eventual joint deformity and reduction of movements. Radiologically, there are four main features: loss of joint space, subchondral sclerosis, cyst formation and marginal osteophytes. Treatment is mainly by NSAIDs for pain relief, and reduction of risk and exacerbating factors.

71 **d.** This scenario is describing a dislocation of the hip. This is commonly caused by trauma to the leg, including a dashboard injury during a road traffic accident or injury involving a motorbike. From the examination, the important features to remember are the positioning of the leg. Although shortening is seen in both fractures and dislocations, internal rotation is characteristic of posterior dislocations of the hip. In cases of fractures or dislocations, patients may well experience difficulty in weight bearing after the injury and therefore this does not distinguish one from the other. The other possible diagnosis in this case is a peri-prosthetic fracture; this will usually be clearly visible on X-ray if it is present.

72 **a.** This child is suffering from an irritable hip. Many hip conditions in children have a similar presentation during their early stages and thus are difficult to distinguish. The commonest cause of this condition is a transient synovitis, which usually resolves within a couple of weeks. In a child of this age it is important to consider other paediatric conditions, including Perthes' disease and slipped upper femoral epiphyses, although both of these would have some positive findings on X-ray. Although his hip joint neither feels hot nor looks erythematous, the possibility of a septic arthritis needs to be investigated by a battery of blood tests, including inflammatory markers and aspiration of the joint. In children, and particularly in the case of a hip joint, this aspiration is best done under general anaesthetic in the operating theatre. The fluid obtained should be urgently sent to microbiology for microscopy, Gram staining and culture.

73 **b.** This patient has suffered a fractured neck of femur. This diagnosis should always be considered in elderly patients with a history of falls, particularly in those patients who are unable to weight bear due to pain. There are different types of neck of femur fractures and their management varies in accordance with the type of fracture sustained. Fractures may be either intracapsular or extracapsular:
- *Intracapsular fractures* are classified by the level of the fracture line in the neck into subcapital, transcervical and basal

fractures. In this group, the proximal fragment often loses part of its blood supply and hence the union of this fracture is difficult. This is a serious injury in the elderly patient. In the very old and debilitated, it can precipitate a crisis in the precarious metabolic balance. It can become a terminal illness due to uraemia, pneumonia, bed sores, etc.

- *Extracapsular fractures* are all grouped as trochanteric fractures of various types.

Patients with intracapsular fractures are managed by hemiarthroplasty, while extracapsular fractures are managed with a dynamic hip screw.

74 **e.** This woman has suffered a periprosthetic fracture. This is a potential risk in patients undergoing any kind of procedure involving insertion of prostheses. It is believed that some of these fractures are caused at the time of insertion although they are too small to be picked up at the time and it is only when they become symptomatic that they are discovered. It is a particular complication with a resurfacing prosthesis and should this happen the management involves removing the prosthesis and inserting a more traditional hip replacement. For patients complaining of such symptoms so soon after surgery, periprosthetic fractures should be considered as a potential differential diagnosis.

75 **h.** In this scenario the diagnosis is septic arthritis until proven otherwise. He has a fever and severely limited range of movement in the affected joint, which are characteristic findings of a septic joint. Normally, the joint is hot and swollen though, in the case of the hip joint, it is not possible to assess this due to the depth of the joint. The raised white cell count and inflammatory markers make the diagnosis more likely and confirmation is achieved by aspirating a sample from the joint. In the case of the hip, this is often done under general anaesthesia. In this particular case, if the metalwork has become infected it is more than likely that it will need to be removed and occasionally replaced.

76 **a.** Viral hepatitis presents with a patient who is unwell with lethargy and malaise and who may present with jaundice and abdominal pain. There is often hepatomegaly, which is smooth and tender (unlike the non-tender craggy hepatomegaly of carcinoma or metastasis) and the patient may feel nauseated, anorexic and have experienced some weight loss. Intrahepatic cholestasis causes a deepening jaundice and derangement of liver enzymes, notably the aminotransferases, indicating hepatic

inflammation. Groups at risk from hepatitis infection include haemophiliacs prior to the 1980s (when routine screening for blood-borne viruses was not undertaken in donated blood products), IV drug users, those engaging in risky sexual practice, healthcare workers and those at risk from vertical transmission.

77 d. Lower lobe pneumonia may present with abdominal signs and indeed may occasionally be investigated from the general surgical standpoint. In a confused patient from a nursing home, infection should always be at the top of the differential and a septic screen should be performed. This involves a urine dipstick, chest radiography, blood cultures, urine, sputum and faeces culture, as well as routine blood tests. If this does not reveal any source of infection then other causes of confusion must be rule out and CT scan of the head, thyroid function tests (TFTs), syphilis serology and haematinics may be clinically indicated. In this particular case, there is strong suspicion that the patient may have aspirated, as she is PEG fed and was observed to have regurgitated her feed. Starting antibiotics such as cefuroxime and metronidazole for an aspiration pneumonia would be appropriate if clinical and/or radiographic findings confirmed the diagnosis.

78 f. Diabetic ketoacidosis is almost exclusively seen in type I diabetics requiring insulin injection. Diabetic ketoacidosis can be precipitated by acute disease such as surgery, infection and even an MI. Insulin requirements increase in time of homeostatic stress and a failure to increase or even take insulin during a period of illness may cause blood glucose levels to become very high. This causes a lack of glucose metabolism and an increase in ketone formation due to the increased availability of circulating free fatty acids. Ketone bodies are acidic in nature and cause a metabolic acidosis, which is compensated for by an increase in ventilation rate to blow off carbon dioxide. The treatment of diabetic ketoacidosis hinges around adequate fluid rehydration (up to 5 L in an 18-hour period) and reduction of blood glucose with suppression of ketogenesis. The latter two are achieved by insulin infusion at a rate of 3–6 units of short-acting insulin an hour. In addition, potassium replacement is almost always required as insulin will drive potassium intracellularly and an apparently 'normal' level may quickly become low once therapy is instituted.

79 b. Cholecystitis is often depicted as a disease affecting a population described as 'Fat, Female, Forty and Fertile'. While slightly outdated in approach, this *aide memoire* provides some useful guidelines when considering those at risk for gallstone disease. Only 10% of gallstones contain calcium and thus are radio-opaque on plain abdominal radiographs (in stark contrast to over 90% of renal stones) and thus the first line investigation for suspected cholecystitis is ultrasound. This patient additionally exhibits a sonographic-positive Murphy's sign – the patient will typically 'catch their breath' on inspiration with the ultrasound probe placed at the right upper quadrant as the inflamed gallbladder descends on inspiration and impinges on the probe. The presence of pericholecystic fluid and a thickened gallbladder wall as well as the presence of gallstones aids in the diagnosis of cholecystitis. Intrahepatic duct dilatation suggests common bile duct obstruction and many centres suggest further imaging of the biliary tree with magnetic resonance cholangiopancreatography.

80 **h.** Subphrenic collection is a recognized complication of liver and biliary tree surgery. The patient typically presents with a fever, pain in the right (or left) upper quadrant and raised inflammatory markers. Septic screen results may return normal and the surgical aphorism, '*pus somewhere, pus nowhere, pus under the diaphragm*' reminds the clinician to consider subphrenic abscess as the cause of a patient's pyrexia. Small abscesses may respond to a conservative approach with antibiotic therapy and may resolve. Larger abscesses merit drainage and infrequently surgical evacuation. More importantly, however, is the source of the collection and if a biliary leak is suspected upon evaluation of the evacuated fluid, a determination of the anatomical site should be undertaken. An endoscopic retrograde cholangiopancreatogram (ERCP) has both diagnostic and therapeutic (endoscopic sphincterotomy with stent placement) benefit in these cases.

81 **a.** Reiter's syndrome presents classically with a triad of urethritis, conjunctivitis and arthritis. It is sometimes subclassified as part of reactive arthritis, which presents similarly after a gastrointestinal infection. Reiter's syndrome typically affects young males with a sexually transmitted infection, such as non-specific urethritis. Joint involvement is usually limited to a few large joints.

82 **g.** Psoriatic arthropathy may present with a range of arthritis patterns, the most common of which is arthritis affecting the distal interphalangeal joints. Evidence of nail changes is very

strongly suggestive and manifest as nail pitting, nail dystrophy and onycholysis (lifting of the nail from the nail bed). For reasons still not entirely clear, between 5 and 8% of individuals with psoriasis develop a seronegative arthritis. Radiologically, the erosions of psoriatic arthropathy are central in the joint and present with thinning of the distal end of a phalanx (pencil) in a relatively spared proximal end of the adjacent phalanx (cup) giving a pencil-in-cup appearance.

83 **h.** Enthesopathy is an inflammation at the junction of ligament or tendon and bone and occurs more frequently with seronegative arthritides than other arthritides, for example rheumatoid arthritis. Typically presenting as plantar fasciitis or Achilles tendonitis, patients usually complain of pain and stiffness at the affected site. The pathogenetic basis of enthesopathy is still not known; however, molecular mimicry and cross-reaction between infective organisms and joint components are thought to play a role.

84 **d.** Ankylosing spondylitis is more common in males than females and presents with back pain, morning stiffness, decreased thoracic excursion and chest pain, as well as extra-articular features such as uveitis, enthesopathy and, rarely, aortitis. A reduction in back flexion to <5 cm as assessed by Schober's test in a young male with sacroiliac pain is almost diagnostic of ankylosing spondylitis. Radiological changes are marked with local erosion of bone at the junction of spinal ligament and bone with bone healing at these sights (syndesmophyte formation) causing ankylosis (fusion) of the vertebrae. Ankylosing spondylitis and other spondyloarthritides are all associated with the HLA-B27 subtype.

85 **b.** Enteropathic arthropathy can be seen in between 10 and 15% of sufferers of ulcerative colitis and Crohn's disease. As with many of the seronegative arthritides, the joints are affected in an asymmetrical pattern with the large lower limb joints preferentially affected. Interestingly, the arthritis symptoms may occur some time before the gastrointestinal disturbance. Gastrointestinal bypass surgery has also been linked to the development of an arthritis picture similar to that associated with inflammatory bowel disease. This is thought to be due to the introduction of antigens, normally protected from the immune system, by changes in the normal mucosal uptake of the gastrointestinal tract as a consequence of surgery.

86 g. The most useful test in this case is a PEFR. It will give instant results and allow the status of her asthma to be quickly and quantifiably assessed. By using results charts based on sex, height and weight, we can tell whether her PEFR values are optimal and this helps in deciding on her management. Although this girl claims to be using her inhalers regularly, in a person of her age, non-compliance is a big problem with chronic disease management and must be considered as an important cause for deterioration in her normally well-controlled asthma.

87 c. In any patient with reducing saturations it is very important to get an ABG. Although saturation monitors on the ward give fairly accurate readings, in those patients where the readings are very important it can be useful to get an arterial sample, which gives more accurate readings. In patients whose clinical condition is deteriorating, it will give an idea of respiratory function and any associated metabolic function and is a quick and easy test to both perform and interpret.

88 b. This patient has suffered a pneumothorax. The most appropriate investigation is a chest X-ray to confirm the diagnosis. Pneumothoraces are common in tall people, those with pre-existing lung disorders and those with connective tissue diseases. Treatment depends on the size of the pneumothorax. If it is small, it can be left to be reabsorbed; larger ones require insertion of a chest drain.

89 f. This woman requires a CT-PA scan to investigate for a pulmonary embolus. She has clinical symptoms consistent with a diagnosis of a pulmonary embolus and associated risk factors. Since her chest X-ray is clear, a V/Q scan is an option but a CT-PA is considered to be the gold standard.

90 d. This patient requires a high-resolution CT of his chest. The diagnosis under consideration is of pulmonary fibrosis and this may be confirmed on CT. The characteristic appearance on chest X-ray is a ground glass appearance while on CT scan it is linear opacities and honeycombing. Although ABG studies will show a change from the norm, these will not be diagnostic and neither will lung function tests.

PAPER 4

Answers

Single Best Answer Questions

1 b. This man provides a history that raises suspicion of subarachnoid haemorrhage. He requires an urgent CT scan of his brain to rule this out and to assess for raised intracranial pressure. A CT scan is usually indicated in order to proceed with a lumbar puncture to assess for xanthochromia, as up to 10% of subarachnoid haemorrhages can be missed on CT scan alone. An MRI scan of this man's brain would provide a detailed view of his cerebral parenchyma, although this is not the first-line investigation in this case. The history given gives no mention of fever and therefore looking for a systemic infective cause with blood cultures is unnecessary, while neurological observations and regular analgesia, although important, are unlikely to aid with the diagnosis and, therefore, not first line.

2 d. There is no association between iron-deficiency anaemia and peripheral neuropathy. This finding is associated with a vitamin B12 deficiency. There are approximately 500 million cases of iron deficiency anaemia worldwide. It most commonly affects premenopausal women. The small bowel is responsible for absorption of iron and it is stored in the body in the form of ferritin. Signs of iron deficiency include koilonychia (spoon shaped nails – both fingers and toes), angular stomatitis and glossitis. Other general signs of anaemia include fatigue and pallor.

3 e. Haematuria is seen in nephritic conditions such as glomerulonephritis and is not associated with nephrotic syndrome by definition. Components of the nephrotic syndrome are proteinuria, defined as protein loss in the urine at a rate of >3 g in a 24-hour period, hypoalbuminaemia, defined as an albumin level <30 g/L and oedema. Fourth and fifth elements are sometimes

---

EMQs and SBAs for Medical Finals, Second Edition. Jonathan Bath,
Rebecca Morgan and Mehool Patel.
© 2011 John Wiley & Sons, Ltd. Published 2011 by John Wiley & Sons, Ltd.

described as part of the syndrome and are hypercholestero-laemia and normal renal function, respectively. Nephrotic syndrome can occur as a primary event or a secondary phenomenon but this definition is not clinically of great benefit in the management of cases of nephrotic syndrome as treatment is supportive in the first instance while the underlying cause is sought. Management focuses on the use of diuretics to reduce oedema, along with fluid and salt restriction, adequate nutrition to replace protein loss (approximately 1–2 g/kg/day) and venous thromboembolism prophylaxis, unless contraindicated. This is due to the loss of clotting factors with heavy proteinuria and predisposes those with the nephrotic syndrome to thromboembolism. Hypercholesterolaemia usually requires no active treatment and will resolve alongside the nephrotic syndrome; however, if persistent, a role for statins may be indicated.

4 d. Sickle cell disease is most commonly seen in patients of African, Arabian or southern European descent. Carriers have one normal and one sickle gene and usually remain asymptomatic. Those individuals homozygous for the sickle chain suffer with sickle cell disease. The red blood cells are of an abnormal sickle shape and therefore 'clog' smaller blood vessels, resulting in ischaemia of distal tissues and associated pain.

Clinical features include pallor as a result of the anaemia. Splenomegaly is seen in early disease but, as it progresses the spleen shrinks as due to the lack of blood supply. Bone crises are often predisposed by infection, cold or hypoxia; the initial management of a sickle crisis is to apply oxygen and provide some symptomatic relief. Pigment gallstones are seen in the condition due to the haemolysis of red blood cells. Vesicular rash is not seen in this condition.

5 c. Lesions of the cerebellum provide characteristic signs that can be remembered by the mnemonic '*DANISH P*': *d*ysdiadocho-kinesia, *a*taxia, *n*ystagmus, *i*ntention tremor, *s*lurred speech, *h*ypotonia, *p*ast pointing.

This woman's lesion is in the cerebellar vermis, as she has bilateral signs of cerebellar disease. Lesions of the bilateral basal ganglia would be incredibly unusual and provide Parkinson's-like features, including a rest tremor. A lesion of the left temporo-parietal lobe would provide a dysphasia (assuming this is her dominant hemisphere) and some visual field defects, in addition to hemisensory neglect. Lesions of the frontal lobe would result in personality changes and dysphasia, thus not in keeping with the clinical details in this case.

6 c. Cystic fibrosis is characterized by a defect in a chloride-channel transporter and is usually due to a single amino acid substitution at position 508. Children usually suffer from multiple recurrent chest infections, usually due to *Pseudomonas*, failure to thrive and malabsorption. Cystic fibrosis should be at the forefront of a differential diagnosis of any chest problems and failure to thrive in any infant.

PAS-positive macrophages refer to a finding in Whipple's disease caused by the Gram-positive rod *Tropheryma whippelii*. Whipple's disease usually causes malabsorption in men over 50 years. Cobblestone appearance is a typical finding on barium enema in Crohn's disease, which is a disease affecting any part of the gastrointestinal system, unlike ulcerative colitis. A double bubble on abdominal X-ray is occasionally seen associated with Down syndrome due to duodenal atresia. Abnormal bone marrow cytology refers to the possibility of a haematological malignancy, such as AML and unlikely to present in this manner.

7 c. Treatment of acute severe hyperkalaemia (potassium level >6.5 mmol/L or ECG changes) is managed first by IV injection of 10 ml of 10% calcium gluconate as cardioprotection. Second, infusion of 10 units of short-acting insulin with 50 ml of 50% dextrose over 30 minutes will shift potassium intracellularly. Correcting the underlying cause, for example hypovolaemia, may stabilize the potassium level. However, depletion of total body stores of potassium may be indicated and can be achieved by using calcium resonium (although this may take up to 6 hours or more to take effect).

Other modalities used are beta-agonists such as salbutamol but this is less commonly employed. Haemodialysis is indicated in conditions of uraemic complications, for example pericarditis, metabolic acidosis or hyperkalaemia refractory to drug treatment, and fluid overload refractory to drug treatment. Patients may exhibit few signs or symptoms but may complain of fatigue, weakness and paraesthesia. ECG changes seen in hyperkalaemia depend on the level and duration of hyperkalaemia and in summary can be broken down into peaked T waves, shortened QT interval and ST depression initially progressing to bundle branch blocks with associated widening of the QRS complex with PR shortening and P wave flattening. Eventually irreversible changes occur, leading to sinusoidal character of the ECG and eventual ventricular fibrillation and asystole.

8 c. Of the listed investigations, CT scan is the most important to obtain. This man is displaying signs of a vascular event;

distinguishing between an infarct or haemorrhage is vital and this can be done by CT scan. Although an INR level will give us vital information about his anticoagulation state, in the short term this is not imperative. A carotid duplex scan could be a helpful adjunct to a cardiovascular examination in identifying a cause of an ischaemic episode if that transpires to be the case. ECG and echocardiogram would again identify a cardiac cause of any emboli if the CT scan showed an infarct; however, these are not first-line investigations to make a diagnosis but may well help in classifying the aetiology.

9 d. This girl is, in the eyes of the law, a legal minor and under common law is the responsibility of her parents. However, a landmark legal case in 1985 (Gillick vs West Norfolk and Wisbech Area Health Authority), brought to court by the parents of a teenage girl who was prescribed contraception without the knowledge of her parents, clarified the legal standpoint on medical treatment for those under the age of 16 years. This standpoint is often referred to as Gillick competence (or the Fraser guidelines after the representative of the House of Lords who conceived the guidelines) in reference to this test case and reasons that young people in England and Wales (and Northern Ireland) under the age of 16 years can consent to medical treatment if they have sufficient maturity and judgement to enable them fully to understand what is proposed. A similar law, The Age of Legal Capacity (Scotland) Act 1991, exists in Scotland.

However, the Fraser guidelines are open to interpretation by the agent assessing whether a minor is Gillick competent and thus it is the duty of the doctor or healthcare provider responsible for medical care and treatment of that minor to assess whether the ability to understand, retain and act upon information in an informed manner is present in those under the age of 16 years. If deemed the case, then the minor assumes the same rights as any competent adult seeking medical treatment.

In this case, referral to a family planning clinic is appropriate as it is the girl's wish and will also serve to provide support, education and contraceptive advice if sexual activity continues. Counselling about sexual intercourse and contraceptive options is of vital importance in increasing the awareness of the merits and disadvantages of teenage pregnancy and the risk of sexually transmitted infection and blood-borne virus exposure.

Offering a sexually transmitted infection screen should occur in conjunction with counselling, as she has been engaging in unprotected intercourse. Most importantly, she should also be encouraged to discuss the pregnancy and her feelings regarding sex with her parents. However, it must be stressed that any information shared with a healthcare professional can only be passed on to her parents with her express consent (if she is deemed Gillick competent).

10 b. This patient has Wilson's disease. It is an autosomal recessive disorder affecting the lenticular nuclei (globus pallidus and putamen) and the liver, hence the description of hepatolenticular degeneration. Copper deposits can also be seen in the cornea–scleral junction. Copper and caeruloplasmin screening should reveal the diagnosis, which can be confirmed with a positive family history. Wilson's disease should be considered in patients with acute mental state changes or impaired mental development for their age.

Porphyria is most likely to present with colicky abdominal pain, vomiting and fever. It is a low-penetrant autosomal dominant condition. Glycogen storage disorders, for example Hunter's syndrome, usually present as gargoylism in children. Presentation of Parkinsonism at this age, unless drug related, is rare and the symptoms and signs are not identified in this case.

11 b. This clinical picture represents ALL. The bone marrow is taken over by immature, abnormal lymphocytes which spill over into the bloodstream. The majority of cases occur in children, although it remains an uncommon condition (approx 450 children are affected in the UK each year). The child is in the right age category, i.e. approximately 4–8 years of age. Symptoms of this condition may be split into bone marrow failure, systemic symptoms and local symptoms. Systemic symptoms include malaise and weight loss with sweats or anorexia being the most common. AML commonly presents in the elderly, i.e. around 70 years. A chest X-ray may be helpful in the diagnosis and a mediastinal mass is occasionally seen. For confirmation of the diagnosis, a trephine bone marrow biopsy is required.

12 a. The patient's history is of a young man with recurrent aerodigestive tract bleeding and haemoptysis and non-specific symptoms that would be consistent with renal failure. A clinical impression (confirmed with biochemical tests of renal function) would be of a process affecting both kidneys and lungs. Pulmonary–renal syndromes must be excluded as a matter of some urgency, as therapy is dependent upon early diagnosis and treatment. This clinical scenario lies at the more extreme end of the presentation spectrum. An autoantibody screen, comprising antineutrophil cytoplasmic antibodies (ANCAs), antiglomerular basement membranes (anti-GBM), complement, lupus antico-agulant, cardiolipin antibodies and double-stranded DNA (ds-DNA) antibodies, is an easily performed screening tool for vasculitic and autoimmune processes. Goodpasture's syndrome (to which the clinical vignette alludes) comprises the triad of glomerulonephritis/renal impairment, pulmonary haemorrhage and anti-GBM antibodies.

Renal biopsy will definitively provide histological confirma-tion of the disease, with immunofluorescent staining demon-strating linear deposition of antibody (usually immunoglob-ulin G [IgG]) along the GBM. However, this should not be undertaken until after simple screening blood tests. CT chest aids definition of the extent of pulmonary involvement, but again can be pursued at a later date. High-dose immunosuppression plus plasmapheresis forms the mainstay of medical treatment for Goodpasture's syndrome.

13 d. This is in line with the current UK immunization guidelines. BCG immunization is given in certain high-risk areas at birth or 6 weeks of age. The first meningitis C vaccination is given at 3 months of age. MMR vaccination is not administered until 13 months.

14 a. Superficial temporal arteritis is 'never' seen in patients of this age. It is a disease of over 55-year-olds and is more prevalent in women than men. There is a 25% association with polymyalgia rheumatica, which manifest with symptoms of scalp and tempo-ral artery tenderness while brushing hair, pain while eating and, most drastically, sudden blindness in one eye. Thus, any suspi-cion of superficial temporal arteritis should prompt immediate twice-daily 40–60 mg prednisolone until the diagnosis has been disproven. All the other causes of headache are commonly ex-perienced in the general practice setting and could reliably cause the pattern of symptoms exhibited by this patient.

15 c. Urine analysis is a cheap, simple and non-invasive screen-ing tool for a variety of conditions and should be performed as standard in the investigation of suspected renal or urinary tract disease. Red-cell casts are simply impressions of the renal tubules that have been formed by compaction of red cells. These are almost always pathological and are associated with glomeru-lonephritis and vasculitic processes and occasionally seen in ma-lignant hypertension with renal involvement.

Glucose can be detected on urine dipstick analysis once the renal threshold for glucose reabsorption has been surpassed, for example in conditions such as pregnancy, renal tubular damage, diabetes and with altered reabsorption of solutes, such as in chronic renal failure. Bilirubin can be seen in the urine with obstructive jaundice (posthepatic jaundice), as water-soluble bilirubin, conjugated in the liver, overflows into the systemic circulation and is excreted by the kidneys. Nitrites are commonly seen in urinalysis with conditions such as urinary tract infection and high-protein meals (as nitrites are breakdown products of protein metabolism). Cystine crystals are diagnostic of the rare condition, cystinuria.

16 c. It is CML that involves the translocation of the so-called Philadelphia chromosome. All the other options are correct.

17 d. Papilloedema is congestion of the optic disc, invariably associated with raised intracranial pressure. It is most often bilateral. General features reflect the underlying disease process but a choked disc is characteristic, although differentiation from papillitis may be difficult.

In the acute setting, vision is rarely affected but peripheral vision may be lost in chronic cases where it is frequently accompanied by transient visual obscurations. Papilloedema results from raised intracranial pressure where the subarachnoid space surrounding the optic nerve is patent, thus papilloedema is not necessarily a consequence of raised intracranial pressure.

The most common causes include:
- intracranial space-occupying lesions, e.g. tumours, especially of the posterior fossa due to restricted space; cerebral abscesses; subdural haematoma,
- any condition that results in hydrocephalus in an adult, e.g. subarachnoid haemorrhage, meningitis, head injury,
- venous sinus thrombosis due to congestion,
- benign intracranial hypertension – most likely in patients with visual complaints but otherwise normal,
- malignant hypertension – bilateral with other signs of hypertensive neuropathy,
- central retinal venous occlusion, ischaemic optic neuropathy, optic neuritis – unilateral with sudden loss of vision,
- chronic carbon dioxide retention.

Other rare causes include:
- metabolic:
  - hypoparathyroidism,
  - diabetic ketoacidosis,
  - chronic carbon dioxide retention,
  - obesity,

- haematological – anaemia, leukaemia,
- toxic – tetracycline, lead, oral progestational agents, corticosteroid withdrawal,
- spinal cord tumours.

18 c. Chronic renal failure is associated with small, shrunken kidneys and ultrasound is in fact a useful guide in determining whether renal impairment found clinically or on blood tests is an acute phenomenon or whether it has been persistent for some time.

Amyloidosis is an unusual and rare disease of extracellular deposition of an abnormal protein that is particularly resistant to breakdown (amyloid). Classified as primary or secondary (reactive), or localized versus systemic, there are various inherited forms of amyloid that are associated with organ failure with renal, cardiac and liver being the most commonly affected. Deposition in the kidneys causes bilateral enlargement of the kidneys, detectable ultrasonographically, and leads to renal failure by a mechanism that is thought to be mechanical disruption of tissue architecture in the main. Compensatory hypertrophy of a single kidney allows maintenance of normal renal function and manifests as a larger and thicker remaining kidney.

Polycystic kidney disease results in an irregularly enlarged kidney filled with cysts, easily detectable and reliably diagnosed on ultrasound scan. Renal cell carcinoma is the most common primary tumour of the kidney, representing over 90% of all renal cancers. Presentation is frequently as an abdominal mass, palpable on clinical examination, associated with loin pain and haematuria.

19 a. The diagnosis in this case is Hodgkin's disease. Approximately 50% of patients with this condition test positive for Epstein–Barr virus. The condition occurs in young, fit people and the elderly. There is an increased risk in family members of the affected patient or in those who have suffered from infectious mononucleosis. Symptoms are divided into categories A and B, with B including constitutional symptoms such as weight loss and night sweats. The diagnosis is confirmed by lymph node biopsy. Histology characteristically shows Reed–Sternberg cells (multinucleated giant cells). Treatment depends on the staging and location of the lymphoma.

20 c. In early disease there are no clinical findings. With disease progression, myoclonus and gait disorder may be seen but these are very unlikely to be present at the onset of the condition. A

CT scan of the brain may show diffuse cortical atrophy in late disease but again in early disease there are often no radiological signs. Two of the commonest features to develop are memory impairment and language dysfunction and dominant inheritance is seen in some families with an approximate age of onset of 50–60 years. While insight remains, depression is a common feature. As the disease progresses and insight is lost, depression understandably becomes a less common feature.

21 e. Scaphoid fracture is one of the most commonly injured bones of the carpal row, thought to be due to the higher stresses imposed on the scaphoid due to its unique position spanning both proximal and distal rows of the carpal bones. Falling on an outstretched hand is the mechanism of injury usually encountered in this type of injury, occasionally complicated by neurovascular compromise as with any fracture. Tenderness in the anatomical snuffbox forms a useful clinical reckoner if scaphoid fracture is suspected.

22 b. The most common cause of acute renal failure post-surgery is dehydration and hypovolaemia. In this particular case, acute renal failure can be deduced by the normal renal function preoperatively and acute onset of biochemical derangement postoperatively. Remaining nil by mouth prior to surgery with inadequate fluid maintenance on top of any pre-existing dehydration, in addition to increased losses such as vomiting in this case, all contribute to dehydration and reduction of blood flow to the kidneys if volume loss is significant. Acute rather than chronic renal failure can also be reasoned if there is a disproportionate rise in urea relative to creatinine.

Analgesic nephropathy typically causes an interstitial nephritis but would be unlikely to manifest with therapeutic doses of analgesia used over a short period of time. Renal metastases would be unlikely to present acutely post-surgery with no stigmata preoperatively and is an uncommon site for metastases from an isolated colonic carcinoma. Postsurgical rhabdomyolysis is not the cause of renal failure in this case; muscle injury is usually significant in cases of rhabdomyolysis and is usually associated with crush injuries, acute drug reactions or elderly patients immobile on a hard surface for a period of time. If rhabdomyolysis is suspected as a cause of renal failure, CK levels and urinary myoglobin assay will usually aid diagnostic uncertainty. Urinary retention post-surgery is very common in the elderly population, especially males with pre-existing prostatic hypertrophy; however, it is a less likely cause in this case. Urinary catheterization with replacement fluids if a palpable bladder or a significant bladder residual volume is usually all that is required.

23 b. Placenta praevia occurs when the placenta abnormally implants in the lower segment of the uterus. Bleeding is usually painless unlike the other common cause of antepartum haemorrhage, abruptio placentae (placental abruption). Physical signs are usually few; breech or oblique presentation is occasionally seen due to the mechanical obstruction to birth canal outflow. Routine ultrasound scans may overestimate the prevalence of this condition as the lower segment grows cephalically late in the last trimester and it is estimated that up to 10% of placentae are low lying before 37 weeks.

Cervical cancer would be a diagnosis not to be dismissed; however, as cervical smears are usually recommended as part of antenatal care, this makes this option unlikely. Placenta accreta is usually encountered at Caesarean section, often with catastrophic effect and does not usually present with antepartum haemorrhage.

24 c. In a case such as this one, a diagnosis of a subarachnoid haemorrhage needs to be excluded. From the history it sounds as though the patient is quite well but she is describing the characteristic history of the worst pain ever experienced with no exacerbating or relieving factors. Subarachnoid haemorrhage can be fatal if it is not diagnosed and discussed with the neurosurgical team promptly. In many cases it can lead to fluctuations in the GCS, requiring intensive monitoring and nursing.

While meningitis is important to rule out, the history is not classical for this. Subdural haemorrhages are most commonly seen in the elderly or in patients who abuse alcohol. Benign intracranial pressure is most commonly seen in younger patients (20–40 years), usually females, particularly those with a raised body mass index (BMI).

25 d. *Gardnerella vaginalis* produces an offensive brown discharge; it causes an inflammation of the vagina in women or the glans of the penis in men. It often results in dysuria. Both chlamydia and gonorrhoea result in urethritis. While most infections can be distinguished by colour or quality of discharge, the most reliable method is by taking appropriate swabs.

26 c. In older males, a dilated abdominal aorta is a common finding. Other risk factors include those patients with a family history. In approximately 10% of cases, an associated popliteal artery aneurysm will be found. Smaller aneurysms (below 4 cm) are considered to be benign and grow at a rate of 1–2 mm per year. The most feared complication of AAA is rupture. *Approximately 5% of aneurysms over 6 cm rupture spontaneously.* Resection is usually advised in those aneurysms 5–6 cm in diameter. Complications of this surgery include renal failure since the renal artery ostia are often compressed during the procedure when the aorta is cross-clamped. Other complications include myocardial infarction (MI) as coronary artery disease is usually present in those people with aortic compromise. As a result of cross-clamping of the aorta the back pressure on the heart increases, which increases the workload of the heart. This, coupled with the metabolic stress that occurs when the legs are reperfused, may precipitate an MI.

27 **e.** Reversal of renal failure once the end-stage has been reached is extremely unlikely and usually represents a misdiagnosis of the initial cause or an acute event that requires supportive therapy until intrinsic renal function is restored. Dialysis has been implicated in the development of cardiovascular disease and incidence of such disease related to the process of dialysis itself has been shown to be higher in dialysed patients. Complications associated with β_2-microglobulin amyloidosis, associated with dialysis for periods >5 years, have been well described and include bony fractures due to bone weakening by formation of amyloid-related bony cysts, carpal tunnel syndrome due to accumulation of amyloid in tendon sheaths and arthralgia.

Aluminium toxicity, with the associated risk of dementia and cognitive impairment, is a phenomenon seen less frequently with current dialysis methods but has been described in patients dialysed using non-aluminium-depleted dialysate. Bleeding tendency may occur with long-term dialysis and is due to platelet dysfunction that may be exacerbated by anticoagulants used to prevent clotting while on the dialysis machine.

28 **c.** This woman has suffered a deep vein thrombosis. Risk factors for deep vein thrombosis include: past history, pregnancy, malignancy, antiphospholipid syndrome, oral contraceptive pill use, nephrotic syndrome, recent surgery, pelvic mass, recent childbirth and obesity.

While she has no past history, she is pregnant and therefore has a pelvic mass. In pregnancy, patients may be reluctant to take anticoagulants. Once the diagnosis is considered, treatment with a low molecular weight heparin should be commenced as venous thromboembolism is a major cause of maternal morbidity and mortality. If investigations are negative, treatment can be stopped.

29 e. Medullary infarction results in damage to the nucleus of cranial nerve VII, which provides upper motor neurone signs.

Head injuries may result in basal fractures to the petrous temporal bone which can result in damage to cranial nerve VII. Although uncommon, cranial sarcoid may be bilateral and can affect cranial nerves III, V, VI and VII. Lyme disease is caused by infection by *Borrelia burgdorferi* via tics. The commonest neuropathy associated with this condition is of the facial nerve and can once again be bilateral. Guillain–Barre syndrome is usually symmetrical and ascending in its symptoms. In severe cases, cranial nerves may be involved although in less severe cases its pathology remains in the limbs and trunk.

30 e. This woman is suffering from toxic shock syndrome. It was first described in 1978 and is caused by the exotoxin *Staphylococcus aureus*. In extreme cases the condition may progress on to staphylococcal multiorgan failure. Other clinical symptoms include a fluctuation in the level of consciousness and a widespread erythematous macular rash. The biggest clue to the diagnosis comes from the history of recent menstruation and useful investigations include vaginal examination, blood tests such as urea and electrolytes, LFTs, clotting screen, full blood count and arterial blood gas (ABG). Other useful tests include an ECG and a chest X-ray to exclude other causes of these symptoms.

31 a. Staging CT scan of the chest, abdomen and pelvis will be of most help in assessing the extent of any presumed metastatic spread and may provide information regarding a primary focus if malignancy is strongly suspected. However, computed tomography is of most diagnostic use when contrast medium is used and this is contraindicated in renal failure, as a potential side-effect of contrast use is contrast-induced nephropathy. Around 5% of the population will experience this side-effect, with those already exhibiting renal failure at a 5–10 times increased risk above this baseline.

Ultrasonography of the liver is a useful, non-invasive and safe tool if liver enzymes are elevated and should be considered in patients in whom metastatic cancer (especially breast and colon) is suspected. Thoracic radiography requires no contrast and may demonstrate bony metastases in this woman who is experiencing mid-back pain. Breast examination should be carried out possibly with mammography or breast ultrasound, depending on age and breast characteristics, if clinically indicated. Bony metastases are an extremely common presentation of cancer and may manifest as bone pain, pathological fractures, hypercalcaemia and a raised alkaline phosphatase. Thyroid, breast, lung, kidney, colon and prostate are the most common sites of primary neoplasm metastasizing to bone.

32 a. This history is representative of Crohn's disease. It is a chronic inflammatory condition of the gastrointestinal tract, characterized by transmural granulomatous inflammation. Crohn's disease may affect any part of the gut from the mouth to the anus but favours the terminal ileum and proximal colon. Unlike ulcerative colitis, there are parts of the bowel that are unaffected in between lesions. A total of 15% of patients with Crohn's disease have a positive family history and there is a 3–4 times increased risk in smokers. Extraintestinal signs include erythema nodosum, clubbing, conjunctivitis, episcleritis and arthritis. Investigations include blood tests, sigmoidoscopy and biopsies, and small bowel enema. Exacerbations are managed with IV steroids and rehydration with topical treatment if necessary.

33 d. Holmes–Adie pupil is usually large but can be small after prolonged light exposure. In acute retrobulbar neuritis pupils are of normal size; often an afferent defect may be seen on the affected eye. Amitriptyline overdose gives large pupils due to the anticholinergic effect. Unequal pupil size, or anisocoria, is seen in syphilis. Pontine haemorrhage gives a bilateral sympathetic lesion, probably associated with parasympathetic overactivity, which results in constricted pupils.

34 a. This woman has myeloma. The mean age of presentation of myeloma is 65–70 years of age. This disease is caused by the monoclonal proliferation of B-lymphocyte plasma cells infiltrating the bone marrow and causing it to produce a paraprotein M. This prevents the bone marrow from functioning normally and leads to anaemia. The production of normal immunoglobulin is suppressed, which results in an increased risk of developing infection. Bone marrow normally produces equal amounts of light and heavy chains, which make up the immunoglobulin ratio; in myeloma more light chains are produced (Bence–Jones proteins). The median survival is approximately 3 years and disease control is achieved in over half of patients with chemotherapy. Allogenic bone marrow transplant has been used in small number of young patients with a moderate success rate. Myeloma has a characteristic blood picture including: ↑ calcium, ↑ or normal phosphate and normal alkaline phosphatase.

35 c. This girl is suffering from pelvic inflammatory disease. This disease ascends from the cervix to the uterus and the fallopian tubes. On examination, it is common to find a low-grade pyrexia with lower central abdominal pain. There may be associated nausea and vomiting with tenderness on vaginal examination and cervical excitation commonly exhibited. Ninety per cent of these infections are sexually transmitted and the commonest age group to be involved is between 15 and 20 years of age. The commonest causative organism is *Chlamydia trachomatis* but *Neisseria gonorrhoea* is often implicated. Following pelvic inflammatory disease, there is a five times increased risk of developing an ectopic pregnancy and infertility.

36 b. Metformin is primarily excreted by the kidneys and dosing is dependent on the intrinsic renal function. Although the biguanides are not directly nephrotoxic when used at therapeutic doses, in the face of renal failure and oliguria or anuria, metformin levels may build up to toxic levels in peripheral tissues. This in turn may rarely lead to an increase in lactate production and lactic acidosis. Metformin therefore should not be continued in cases where contrast injection (such as CT scanning) is necessary. It should be withheld on the day of the planned study (occasionally on the day before, if renal failure is significant) and for at least 48 hours post-contrast with documentation of the renal function on a daily basis. Once normal renal function has been demonstrated, metformin can be instituted with adequate hydration. This is especially important in the elderly and those not able to take in adequate oral hydration, for example surgical patients and these patients should be well hydrated prior to undergoing any contrast procedures with diligent monitoring of renal function. Shortness of breath in this case is related to a degree of acidosis caused by both renal failure and the build-up of lactic acid due to metformin use and thus respiratory compensation in the form of hyperventilation. An ABG, possibly with a plasma lactate, will help to confirm the diagnosis and assess the extent of the acidosis.

37 a. He is suffering from rheumatic fever. This infection remains common in developing countries, although it is a dreaded complication of a streptococcal sore throat in developed countries. Diagnosis is made on a group of criteria.

Major criteria are the following:

- carditis – tachycardia or new murmurs,
- arthritis – usually a migratory arthritis,
- subcutaneous nodules,
- erythema marginatum – rash with raised red edges and a clear centre,
- Sydenham's chorea.

Minor criteria are the following:

- fever,
- raised erythrocyte sedimentation rate (ESR) or C-reactive protein,
- arthralgia,
- prolonged P-R interval,
- previous rheumatic fever.

Using the revised Jones' criteria, there must be evidence of a recent *Streptococcus* infection and two major criteria *or* one major and two minor criteria.

38 e. Myelodysplasia is a clonal disorder of the bone marrow in which morphologically and structurally abnormal blood cells are produced. Patients tend to have a macrocytic anaemia, leucopenia and thrombocytopenia. In most cases, no cause is identified but occasionally radiotherapy or cytotoxic drugs are found to be the cause. Clinical features include recurrent infections, pallor and easy bruising and bleeding. Management involves symptomatic relief, i.e. treating infections, blood transfusions as well as platelet transfusions to help in haemorrhage resulting from thrombocytopenia. Allogenic bone marrow transplants are an option in younger patients if donors can be found. After 2–3 years this condition may progress to AML, which is refractory to treatment.

39 c. A spastic paraparesis is usually seen in upper motor neurone lesions. It is a fairly common feature of multiple sclerosis, often due to plaques affecting the cervical and thoracic cord. Other causes of a spastic paraparesis include vitamin B12 deficiency and Friedrich's ataxia.

In the case of syringomyelia, the syrinx acts as a mass effect often affecting the cervical cord resulting in upper motor neurone signs, most commonly in the legs, with a wasting and weakness affecting the trunk and arms in a cape-like distribution. In the case of a meningioma, the symptoms are caused by a mass effect. Since the spinal cord terminates at the level of L1–2, any pathology affecting the lumbo-sacral spine will result in lower motor neurone signs and therefore weakness would be seen most commonly.

40 d. Renal vein thrombosis typically presents in association with nephrotic syndrome or sometimes in cases of thrombophilic states such as malignancy. Loss of clotting factors as part of the nephrotic syndrome causes an increase in venous thrombosis, particularly seen in association with membranous glomerulonephritis causing the nephrotic syndrome. Pain over the affected kidney with haematuria, in addition to the stigmata of nephrotic syndrome, coupled with occasionally palpable renal enlargement and progressive renal failure, provides a clue to the diagnosis.

Pyelonephritis is a reasonable differential for the clinical presentation but the absence of temperature, lack of sensitive indicators in the urine dipstick (leucocytes and nitrites) and markedly raised D-dimer make this less likely. Diagnosis is by renal vein Doppler ultrasound, CT scan or rarely with renal angiography. Treatment is similar to that for pulmonary embolus, with oral anticoagulation for up to 6 months.

Pancreatitis does present with abdominal pain and can cause deterioration in renal function when severe; however, the clinical picture is one of renal pathology.

Addisonian crisis can occur when patients are taken off long-term steroids abruptly due to suppression of the normal hypothalamo–pituitary–adrenal axis and manifests clinically with hypotension, lethargy, hyperkalacmia, hyponatraemia and hypoglycaemia.

Pulmonary embolus may indeed mimic abdominal pain if thrombosis involves the lower lobe blood supply; however, usually signs of hypoxia, tachypnoea and tachycardia prevail. D-dimer findings are raised in any venous thrombosis but may be raised in a variety of disorders and this is only of clinical value in ruling out venous thrombosis. ABGs aid the diagnosis and should be considered in any patient with signs of respiratory compromise.

41 a. Ninety per cent of cervical cancers are squamous. Of the remaining 10%, the majority are adenocarcinoma. It is a disease that is heavily screened for but symptoms are all too often ignored by those affected. There is a national screening programme in which all women aged 25 years and over (or younger in socially deprived areas) are invited to attend a 3-yearly screening program. There is a vaccine programme in the UK for girls for some strains (type 16 and18) of human papilloma virus (HPV). A common presentation is intermenstrual bleeding or postcoital bleeding, which should always prompt an internal examination using a speculum. Any patient that has an abnormal-looking cervix should be referred to a gynaecologist for further review and testing.

42 **e.** Hypercalcaemia may result in vague limb pains but not muscle cramps. Low calcium may account for twitching or tetany, as will hyponatraemia or hypokalaemia. Cramps have been reported in cases of hyponatraemia. Central pontine myelinolysis usually results from a rapid correction of hyponatraemia, the neurological symptoms that develop are believed to be secondary to oedema of the cells in the pons. Hyperthyroidism is known to result in proximal limb myopathies, tremor, hyperreflexia and occasionally seizures, as can hyponatraemia. A rare complication of hypoglycaemia is hemiparesis. It is occasionally seen in infants and children but is easily treatable with IV glucose, which normally results in a complete recovery.

43 **b.** This vignette represents a clinical picture of coarctation of the aorta. In this picture, there is narrowing of the aortic lumen just distal to the subclavian artery. This results in left ventricular hypertrophy as a result of increased afterload and hypertension secondary to reduced renal perfusion. The reduced blood flow results in the mottled appearances of the lower limbs. Cyanosis does not usually occur in this condition unless the patient is severely anaemic.

44 **d.** Non-steroidal anti-inflammatory drugs (NSAIDs) act on cyclo-oxygenase to reduce formation of prostaglandins, thereby dampening the inflammatory response as well as reducing pain sensation. Prostaglandins play an important role in vasodilatation of renal vasculature. Inhibiting the production of prostaglandins adversely affects the flow of blood to the kidney. This can cause huge changes in glomerular filtration rate (and hence renal function and urine output) in patients with already compromised renal function and thus should be avoided in cases of moderate to severe renal impairment. Simply stopping the offending medication and rehydrating the patient should bring the renal function back to the pre-existing baseline.

Analgesia is often difficult in patients with severe renal failure as doses, for example of morphine, may need to be reduced to prevent the build-up of drug and toxic metabolites; however the reduced dose may not always provide effective pain relief. Amoxicillin should be given at a reduced dose; although it is not strongly associated with intrinsic renal damage it has a tendency to cause crystalluria and rashes in severe renal failure. Clarithromycin should be used at half the normal dose if the glomerular filtration rate is <30 mL/minute. Paracetamol and sodium docusate are safe to use at normal doses in renal failure.

45 e. Polycythaemia is an increase in haemoglobin by >2 g/dL. Increased haemoglobin occurs in myeloproliferative diseases. Most commonly, polycythaemia is secondary to chronic hypoxaemia from chronic lung disease and heavy cigarette smoking with systemic hypertension (Gaisbock's syndrome). Other causes include cyanotic heart disease and dehydration. Rarer causes include kidney tumours that secrete excess erythropoietin. Polycythaemia may be asymptomatic or produce a hyperviscosity syndrome. Most polycythaemia is secondary to other causes and therefore investigations should include ABGs and LFTs. Venesection is occasionally used to provide symptomatic relief.

46 b. Signs of an ischaemic limb include the '6 Ps': *p*allor, *p*ulseless, *p*araesthesiae, *p*ainful, *p*aralysis and *p*erishingly cold. From the history, we know that this woman is suffering from pallor and pulselessness. She has a present femoral pulse but no pulse below that level, which suggests an embolus at the mid-femoral level. Potential sources of emboli in this case include from the left atrium, heart valves and the aorta. This woman went on to have an embolectomy and postoperative management with unfractionated heparin.

The symptoms are not indicative of arterial insufficiency and there has been no mention of an abdominal mass to suggest an abdominal arterial aneurysm. In cases of venous ulceration you would expect to see changes in the skin including, breakdown of the epidermal level which is not described here.

47 c. The nerve supply to the thenar muscles of the hand is the median nerve, while the nerve supply to the intrinsic small muscles of the hand is supplied by the ulnar nerve. A lesion of the ulnar nerve at the elbow would result in damage to the hypothenar and small muscles of the hand but would have no effect on the thenar eminence.

Syringomyelia provides weakness and muscle wasting in a cape-like distribution and wasting in the arms is a fairly common peripheral symptom of amyotrophic lateral sclerosis. While osteoarthritis of the lower cervical and upper thoracic spine is uncommon, it does occur and would result in similar problems to those defined in this case.

48 a. Severe psychiatric illness is an absolute contraindication to renal transplantation, except in very exceptional cases where a patient has been assessed by a psychiatrist and deemed fit to comply under very rigorous criteria. An ability to attend regularly for follow-up appointments, total compliance with post-transplantation medical care and a high level of motivation and understanding of the drastic lifestyle implementation required with a transplanted kidney are crucial factors in selecting candidates for receipt of organs. Relative contraindications, which may be considered on an individual basis, include cardiac disease assessed by a cardiologist to be compatible with the demands of immunosuppression and transplantation, chronic non-active hepatitis, minor treatable infections (excluding active tuberculosis and HIV) and quiescent or well-treated cancer. Renal transplantation is the modality of choice for diabetic nephropathy and paediatric patients with end-stage renal failure but due to a worldwide shortage of suitable donors the average wait for an available organ may be in excess of 2 years. The life expectancy at 3 years for a first renal transplant is approximately 90%, with between 2 and 6% of those on the waiting list for a transplant dying before transplantation.

49 d. During pregnancy the pressure at the lower oesophageal sphincter is reduced, which results in the patient developing symptoms of heartburn. Other common findings include reduced gut motility, which can lead to constipation and raised platelets, ESR, cholesterol and fibrinogen. With the physiological changes taking place in the vascular compartment, a systolic flow murmur is common while water retention occurs, leading to ankle oedema and carpal tunnel syndrome.

50 d. Tetralogy of Fallot is the most common congenital cyanotic heart abnormality. The abnormality is characterized by variable obstruction to the right ventricular outflow due to pulmonary stenosis, dextroposition of the aorta, overriding of the ventricular septum, ventricular septal defect and right ventricular hypertrophy. Due to the ventricular septal defect, there is a shunt of blood from the left to the right side of the heart. Children have learned that squatting decreases the cyanosis and the hypoxaemia. This increases the left ventricular afterload and decreases the left to right shunt. Other mechanisms listed in the question do not have any effect on the left to right shunting of the blood flow in the heart.

51 b. The history of a crush injury with radiographic confirmation of extensive soft tissue swelling with deranged renal function makes the diagnosis of rhabdomyolysis the most likely explanation. When interpreting renal biochemical tests, it is important to have an idea about a patient's baseline creatinine as the investigation and treatment strategy of acute renal failure is very different to that of chronic renal failure. Muscle injury from trauma, ischaemia, cold or toxins releases myoglobin and protein fragments that are nephrotoxic and cause tubular damage. Urine myoglobin levels (where available) or CK levels are useful tests to aid the diagnosis.

Renal contusions may present with varying degrees of haematuria but usually there is a history of damage to the renal angle and for acute renal impairment to occur usually bilateral involvement (or, rarely, a lone damaged kidney) is required.

Cholesterol embolus should be suspected if a net-like rash (livedo reticularis) is associated with renal failure in association with invasive procedures such as cardiac catheterization or multiple trauma but usually occurs with a background of atherosclerosis.

Acute interstitial nephritis is well associated with certain medications, most notably the penicillins and NSAIDs, but a typical history usually includes haematuria, proteinuria, eosinophiluria and raised eosinophil count due to the type IV hypersensitivity reaction.

Urethral rupture should be considered in any case of trauma with pelvic injury and a failure to pass urine and digital rectal examination may reveal a free-floating prostate. Urinary catheterization should not be attempted until this diagnosis has been excluded due to the risks of creating a false passage or in fact exacerbating any pre-existing anatomical disruption.

52 a. CK and myoglobin urinalysis are two useful screens for assessing the likelihood of rhabdomyolysis causing renal failure. Often the diagnosis is self-evident from the history; however, in the elderly and unconscious there may be a lack of clinical information regarding possible muscular damage. A typical scenario for rhabdomyolysis outside of the sphere of trauma is an elderly patient who is brought to hospital with a fall who has been lying on a cold hard floor for hours to days.

A renal ultrasound scan is a useful and non-invasive investigation of renal failure without a readily identifiable cause and may show obstruction, renal masses and kidney size that may guide further investigation.

A 24-hour urine protein collection is a useful test for quantifying proteinuria, which in the nephrotic syndrome is found in the urine at a rate of 3 g/24 hours. Normal range of proteinuria is up to 150 mg/24 hours but can be elevated above this level (but <3 g/24 hours) in times of stress, heavy exercise, infection and in children.

Bence–Jones protein is an assay for the light-chain breakdown products of monoclonal immunoglobulins that are excreted by the kidney in excess in myeloma. It is commonly encountered in elderly patients who may present with bone pain, signs of hypercalcaemia and even pathological fractures associated with signs of renal failure.

Renal artery Doppler scans would be a useful investigation of suspected renal artery stenosis and allows waveform morphology and flow velocity in the renal and peri-renal aorta to be assessed. A reduction in flow below a threshold velocity indicates a significant degree of stenosis. Bilateral renal artery stenosis is a contra-indication to using angiotensin-converting enzyme (ACE) inhibitors and renal function must be watched when starting ACE inhibitors in case this condition is present.

53 e. Risk factors for developing an ectopic pregnancy include:
- pelvic inflammatory disease,
- pelvic surgery/adhesions,
- previous ectopic pregnancy,
- endometriosis,
- assisted fertilization,
- IUCD,
- progesterone-only pill,
- congenital anatomical variants,
- ovarian/uterine cysts and tumours.

Although previous Caesarean section may result in development of adhesions, it is not in itself responsible for future progression to an ectopic pregnancy.

54 a. Creutzfeldt–Jakob disease is caused by a mutation in a naturally occurring prion protein. A typical presentation is by a progressive dementia with psychiatric symptoms. The new form of the disease is thought to be much slower in onset, developing over the course of a few years rather than a few months. Although a link to infected meat is a suspected cause, this has not been confirmed. However, there is evidence to suggest that infection may be transmitted by surgical procedures and corneal transplants. While imaging may provide diagnostic information, tonsillar biopsy provides a tissue diagnosis.

55 d. Thalassaemia is a spectrum of genetic conditions affecting the blood. Their severity ranges from asymptomatic to life-threatening, for example thalassaemia major. Thalassaemia is most common in people whose family origins are Mediterranean or Asian. Most well-treated thalassaemic patients survive into their 30s and 40s. Thalassaemia is associated with a microcytic anaemia. The other associations are correct.

56 d. The case describes a history of a transient ischaemic attack; there is no residual neurological deficit 24 hours after onset of symptoms. Risk factors for transient ischaemic attacks include: male sex, age, smoking, diabetes, hypercholesterolaemia, hypertension and past history of cardiovascular disease.

This man went on to have his carotid vessels scanned and this showed an 80% stenosis, which means that he is at a high risk of developing a further transient ischaemic attack or cardiovascular accident in the following months. With such findings on carotid scanning, the patient should be referred to a vascular surgeon with a view of carrying out a carotid endarterectomy to reduce the chances of an embolus being dislodged.

57 c. The median nerve innervates most of the flexor compartment of the forearm. It does not pass around the lateral epicondyle – in fact this is the course of the ulnar nerve, which is often damaged following injuries to the elbow or distal humerus fractures. The median nerve does provide sensation to the lateral $3\frac{1}{2}$ digits of the hand on the palmar aspect of the hand and may become trapped in the carpal tunnel as it passes deep to the flexor retinaculum at the wrist which may result in pain, paraesthesia and weakness in the distribution of the nerve.

58 a. Primary postpartum haemorrhage is defined as vaginal blood loss in the first 24 hours after delivery of the baby. The bleeding is often related to retained products and blood loss.

59 c. The most likely diagnosis given the history and clinical findings is of pyloric stenosis. This condition is usually seen in newborn males and results in forceful vomiting immediately after meals. The condition is most likely to occur in first-born males. The most cost-effective and useful investigation to make this diagnosis is an abdominal ultrasound, which will reveal hypertrophy of the pylorus. Management of this condition is surgery to make an incision in the hypertrophied muscle to relieve the pressure.

60 e. Acute pyelonephritis itself usually does not cause hypertension and blood pressure is usually within the normal range. However, hypotension may in fact be seen due to systemic sepsis and the systemic inflammatory response syndrome causing systemic release of inflammatory mediators, which in turn causes peripheral vasodilatation and a drop in blood pressure.

Recurrent urinary tract infections, especially in childhood when associated with abnormalities of the urinary tract (most commonly vesicoureteric reflux), can lead to renal scarring seen on renal ultrasonography. This in turn predisposes to hypertension by a mechanism thought to be due to the abnormal blood flow through scarred regions. Interestingly, only reflux of infected urine has been linked to renal scarring; sterile refluxing urine requires only low-dose prophylactic antibiotic to prevent infection that will lead to scarring.

Renal artery stenosis is often diagnosed after an ACE inhibitor has been started, with a sharp rise in urea and creatinine shortly after commencement. This is due to glomerular efferent arteriole tone being lost when levels of angiotensin II (the end-product of ACE) fall secondary to use of ACE inhibitor. As those with renal artery stenosis have a reduced flow through the glomerular afferent arteriole, they require an intrinsically high tone at the efferent arteriole to maintain an adequate glomerular filtration pressure. Once the efferent tone is reduced then the glomerular filtration rate tails off rapidly and renal failure ensues. The intrinsic reduction in blood flow to the kidney in renal artery stenosis is detected by the juxtaglomerular apparatus, which is responsible for upregulating renin–angiotensin levels to increase blood pressure to maintain adequate perfusion and thus these patients often present with hypertension.

61 f. Although there are several conditions that could mimic this history, the most serious is Wilms' tumour. They arise from the kidneys and may present with haematuria. Owing to the nature of their presentation, these tumours can often become large before producing any symptoms or signs. Any patient with a suspected malignancy or suggestion of a mass should be sent for appropriate imaging, either CT scanning or ultrasound and an appropriate surgical referral should be made in anticipation of the result.

62 a. This vignette is describing a case of intussusception. It affects children between the ages of 6 months and 4 years old and results in abdominal pain. Since the affected children are young they often appear to be unwell, occasionally vomit and characteristically pass redcurrant jelly-like stools. Other clinical features include a fever and a palpable abdominal mass. Abdominal X-rays may appear to be entirely normal or may show an absent caecal shadow. Diagnosis may be confirmed or indeed managed by air or barium enema; it characteristically reveals a coiled spring or sudden termination of barium. These patients should be urgently referred to the surgical team.

63 d. The case in question is describing midgut volvulus. This occurs when a segment of bowel rotates on its mesentery, resulting in bowel obstruction, vascular compromise and abdominal distension with associated pain. It is most frequently seen with congenital malrotation but it can occur in other scenarios, including adhesions from previous surgery or Meckel's diverticulum. The best management involves a high index of suspicion with urgent gastrointestinal contrast evaluation and surgical referral in order to preserve viable bowel.

64 b. This is a case of pyloric stenosis. It is most common in firstborn males and most frequently occurs between the ages of 2 and 10 weeks. Vomiting is characteristically projectile in nature, with progressive dehydration and constipation. The vomiting is unaltered food and in severe cases a hypochloraemic acidosis may be seen. On examination, a palpable mass in the epigastrium may represent the thickening of the pylorus and is most easily felt during a feed. The diagnosis can be confirmed on ultrasound scan and surgical management is necessary to relieve the obstruction.

65 e. Acute appendicitis should always be considered in a child presenting with acute abdominal pain with fever. However, in this case it is important to be cautious that her symptoms do not relate to her reproductive tract. Further probing in the history revealed commencement of the pain in the centre of the abdomen some 24 hours earlier, with radiation of the pain down to the right iliac fossa. Gynaecological causes of pain tend to originate in the appropriate iliac fossa. To confirm the diagnosis, an ultrasound scan should be obtained as this can be useful in excluding diagnoses such as ovarian cysts in addition to confirming appendicitis.

66 c. Multi-infarct dementia (vascular dementia) usually presents in patients who have suffered multiple cerebrovascular events, such as transient ischaemic attacks or strokes. Typically there is a step-wise deterioration of cerebral function with each event and relatives will often remark that the patient never recovered to the level he or she was before the stroke. Multi-infarct dementia accounts for about 25% of all strokes and should be considered in those with a history of cerebrovascular disease with global impairment of cognition.

67 g. Lewy-body dementia, as the name suggests, is characterized by the presence of Lewy bodies in the brainstem and cortex, with a myriad of features of dementia and parkinsonism. The difficulty in treating patients with this dementia is that using traditional antiparkinsonian drugs may lead to delusions, which themselves are a common finding in dementia, and using neuroleptic drugs to counter delusions will worsen features of parkinsonism.

68 a. Alzheimer's dementia should be suspected in adults who demonstrate long-lasting problems with spatial navigation and visual awareness; this usually manifest as wandering or becoming lost. The mini-mental state examination is a relatively sensitive tool for screening for dementia but an ideal diagnosis requires exclusion of other reversible causes of dementia along with neuro-imaging and histology. Found more commonly with increasing age, there is evidence that 20% of those over 80 years old have dementia. Many people with Down syndrome manifest signs of dementia earlier than 40 years of age.

69 h. Pseudo-dementia is a psychiatric illness that can mimic the apparent cognitive decline of true dementia. It is linked to depression and will characteristically ameliorate once the depression has been treated. The mini-mental state examination is not as sensitive a test for dementia in these cases, as motivation plays a large part in determining a representative score. Clues to the diagnosis tend to come from the patient's affect and mood; however, as with any apparent dementia, it is important never to ascribe a reduction in cognition to pseudo-dementia without ruling out any organic cause. Coexisting depression in patients with a diagnosis of dementia has been described.

70 e. This patient is too young to fit into the typical patterns of dementia and thus it is important that all organic causes for his behaviour be explored. The patient's nationality has an important bearing on narrowing down possible diagnoses and in a patient from sub-Saharan Africa it is important to consider whether the patient's HIV status is a factor. In these cases, appropriate treatment of the HIV virus can reveal fairly rapid improvements in the cognitive state.

71 a. Combined oral contraceptives should be started with caution in patients. Questions should be asked about past or family history of venous thrombosis. Other factors that should be discussed include obesity, immobility and varicose veins; two or more of these risk factors should urge you to think again about contraceptive solutions. In this case, she is a young healthy girl who wants to control excessive bleeding and the combined oral contraceptive should help reduce the proliferation of the uterine endometrium and in turn the associated pain and bleeding.

72 d. This woman has too many risk factors or contraindications for the standard option of the combined oral contraceptive pill. The remaining options for regular contraceptives include progesterone-only solutions including a pill, intrauterine system or an IM injection. Since she is known to be forgetful, the option of a daily progesterone-only pill is less than ideal. Standard progesterone-only pills require to be taken at the same time every day and the window is shorter than for the average combined oral contraceptive. The IUCD should be ruled out since she cannot have adequate cervical smears taken and visualization of the cervix is required for insertion of the coil. The other option is the progesterone-only injection; it is a 3-monthly preparation that is injected intramuscularly, which avoids the need to remember a daily pill.

73 g. This woman has sought advice at the correct time. When a patient commences on any contraceptive solution, they should be advised that in the presence of any intercurrent illness either abstinence or a barrier method of contraception should be sought. In this case, this girl has essentially had unprotected sexual intercourse and therefore the most appropriate contraception is the emergency contraception (or 'morning after pill'), which can be used up to 72 hours after the event.

74 b. Any oral contraceptives require regular checks on simple observations, including blood pressure. For those patients whose blood pressure is found to be outside of the upper range of normal on a combined oral contraceptive, there are a few options. A progesterone-only option should be considered, in addition to a low-oestrogen combined pill or a period without hormonal treatment. In this case, since the patient is a medical student with a regular schedule, it is assumed that she could be trusted to take the pills at the same time each day. This is a good alternative for those patients with blood pressure problems.

75 c. This woman is a good candidate for an IUCD. There are two options: a hormone-based device or a copper device. These are rarely used in nulliparous women. The hormonal device is impregnated with progesterone and works in a similar way to the progesterone-only pills. The copper device is well known to have the side-effect of heavy bleeding but can be used as emergency contraception up to 5 days after unprotected sexual intercourse or up to 5 days prior to the next predicted ovulation.

76 a. Benign prostatic hyperplasia (BPH) and prostate cancer can cause haematuria, although this is a rarer clinical finding in BPH due to prostatic vein congestion. BPH most commonly presents with lower urinary tract symptoms, which can be neatly summed up by the mnemonic '*WISE FUN*': *w*aiting to pass urine, *i*ntermittency, *s*training to pass urine, *e*ffortless passing (incontinence), *f*requency, *u*rgency and *n*octuria. Conversely, prostatic hyperplasia tends not to cause these symptoms until it is very advanced due to neoplastic growth of the peripheral rim of prostatic tissue rather than the central enlargement of the prostatic core seen in BPH. A digital rectal examination is vital in the assessment of prostatic enlargement due to hyperplasia or neoplasm and prostatic-specific antigen (PSA) levels may help monitor treatment for confirmed malignancy. Typically, the enlargement of the prostate gland felt in BPH is smooth, while that of prostatic carcinoma is craggy and nodular. Surgical therapy to ameliorate BPH is usually performed via the urethra (transurethral resection of the prostate [TURP]) and consists of coring out the enlarged peri-urethral prostate to relieve the symptoms of bladder outflow obstruction.

77 d. Bladder carcinomas in Western populations are overwhelmingly transitional cell carcinoma, with a very small number showing histology of other cell types such as squamous cell or adenocarcinoma. Although transitional cell carcinoma of the bladder is often of unknown aetiology, associations between chemical exposure (in particular aniline dyes, hair dye and smoking – nitrosamines are present in carcinogenic quantities in cigarette smoke) have been described. Chronic infection with organisms such as schistosomiasis and bladder stone disease have been linked to an increased incidence of squamous cell carcinoma. Embryological abnormalities, such as a persistent urachal remnant communicating between umbilicus and bladder, have also been shown to predispose to bladder carcinoma. Seen more commonly in men than women, and in the latter during the later decades of life, bladder carcinomas are the second most common urological cancer after cancer of the prostate and the most frequent malignant tumour of the urinary tract. Painless haematuria is the most common presenting complaint but may be complicated by clot retention, i.e. where the build-up of clotted blood inside the bladder obstructs the bladder outflow tract causing urinary retention. Treatment of clot retention is by insertion of a three-way urinary catheter into the bladder and constant irrigation until the urine runs clear.

78 c. Schistosomiasis affects over 200 million people in the tropics and is found commonly in those from the Middle East and Africa. Three main strains of *Schistosoma* cause disease in humans: *Schistosoma mansoni*, *S. japonicum* and *S. haematobium*, of which *S. japonicum* is most commonly linked to severe disease. The life cycle of *Schistosoma* first involves an intermediate host, the water snail, before being released into water where they attempt to penetrate the mucous membrane and skin of the human host.

Each strain of *Schistosoma* presents slightly differently and *S. mansoni* primarily affects the large bowel with migration to the liver resulting in diarrhoea, hepatitis and portal hypertension. *S. japonicum* affects both the large and small bowel as well as the liver but may also cause neurological and respiratory symptoms if migration to the brain and lung occur. *S. haematobium* (bilharzia), as the name suggests, usually affects the bladder and causes painless haematuria with progressive obstructive symptoms such as bladder inflammation which increases in severity, and hydronephrosis, renal failure and loin pain may develop. The treatment for trematode disease is praziquantel tablets at a dose of 40 mg/kg taken with food. The aim of treatment is not necessarily to eradicate the disease but to reduce the effect of chronic infection, of which a serious complication is squamous cell carcinoma of the bladder.

79 f. Urinary tract infection is a common cause of transient haematuria, which is often only discovered on urine dipstick as microscopic haematuria. It is one of the commonest causes of confusion in the elderly. Any patient who presents with confusion should have a urine dipstick and sample sent for microscopy, culture and sensitivity, as this is an easily treatable and thus reversible cause of confusion and should never be missed. The signs of pyrexia accompanying suprapubic tenderness point strongly to a diagnosis of urinary tract infection and the clinician must be quick to treat empirically on the basis of clinical suspicion while sensitivities and organisms are awaited, to prevent development of the more serious pyelonephritis, which in compromised patients may be life threatening.

A cephalosporin such as cefuroxime or, alternatively trimethoprim if a 'simple' urinary tract infection is suspected, for a period of 3–7 days depending on severity is usually enough to resolve the infection. A single urinary tract infection in a young male prompts investigation of at least blood glucose (for diabetes) and occasionally a renal tract ultrasound to assess for renal tract abnormalities, as this type of infection is uncommon in this population and may point to an underlying, hitherto undiscovered, cause.

80 h. Renal trauma can be divided into categories based upon type of injury to the kidney, i.e. laceration, vascular disruption or contusion (bruising) and the mode of injury causing the damage, i.e. blunt or penetrating injury. When assessing a patient with suspected renal trauma, it is of paramount importance that a systematic method is adopted, such as the ABCDE (*a*irways, *b*reathing, *c*irculation, *d*isability, *e*xposure) approach to trauma. Assessing the airways and cervical spine should be the first priority with any immediate intervention, for example airway adjuncts, performed before moving to assess other systems. A quick assessment of breathing, starting with the presence or absence of breath sounds, symmetry of lung expansion and any abnormal findings should be treated with appropriate interventions as necessary. Circulation should then be assessed, starting with examination of pulses and vital signs (blood pressure, capillary refill, etc.). Disability refers to any deficit in function that may have occurred as a result of trauma, for example neurological upset and musculoskeletal problems such as fractures and dislocations.

A more complete examination may be performed once the clinician is satisfied that the airway, breathing and circulation are stable. Abdominopelvic examination should always be considered as exsanguination (catastrophic and fatal blood loss) can quickly and insidiously occur with abdominal and pelvic visceral or bony injury. *Exposure* forms the last part of the primary survey, with assessment of areas previously not examined, such as the spine (normally accessed by log-rolling patients until the cervical spine has been radiologically and clinically cleared of injury) and the level of exposure to the environment, for example temperature, soft tissue injury and wound assessment.

81 g. It is important to remember that children are not simply small adults. There are a range of conditions that are specific to children and as a result their baseline observations vary.

Age (years)	Respiratory rate (breaths/minute)	Heart rate (bpm)	Systolic blood pressure (mmHg)
<1	30–40	110–160	70–90
1–2	25–35	100–150	80–95
2–5	25–30	95–140	80–100
5–12	20–25	80–120	90–110
>12	15–20	60–100	100–120

82 c. By the age of 9 months it is expected that a child will be able to sit up unaided. In all of these cases, gestational age needs to be taken into account and any pre-term births need to have allowances made when assessing for normal development. Between the ages of 13 and 18 months it is expected that a child will be able to walk unaided.

83 a. The vaccination schedule in the UK starts at the age of 2 months. At 2, 3 and 4 months, infants are immunized against diphtheria, tetanus, pertussis, polio, *Haemophilus influenza B* and meningitis C. At the age of 12–15 months, children are immunized against MMR. Between the ages of 3 and 5 years, booster doses of diphtheria, tetanus, pertussis, polio and MMR are administered. The next step in the schedule is BCG at 10–14 years which provides approximately 75% protection against tuberculosis. The final step is a booster dose of diphtheria, tetanus and polio at approximately 18 years old.

84 a. This is a presentation of acute bronchiolitis. It is most commonly seen in those children under the age of 6 weeks or in those with chronic respiratory cardiac or neurological deficits. The commonest causative organism is the respiratory syncytial virus, which accounts for 75% of cases. Those infants in respiratory distress may require non-invasive ventilation in the acute phase in addition to inhaled bronchodilators and there is some evidence for the use of ribavirin, a nucleoside analogue. Long-term consequences may include obstructive bronchiolitis.

85 **a.** By 6–8 weeks it is believed that babies are able to follow movements with their eyes. At this age experts believe that their eyesight is developing and their vision extends up to a distance of approximately 30 cm. This is one of the reasons that babies are believed to form a strong bond with their mother, as they can focus their gaze on them while feeding.

86 **e.** This history is of cavernous sinus thrombosis. Although the symptoms seem vague, a high index of suspicion is required to make the diagnosis. Clinical features include:
- fevers and rigors,
- pain in the eye and forehead – ophthalmic division of the trigeminal nerve,
- exophthalmos and, occasionally, papilloedema,
- cranial nerve palsies – III, IV, VI,
- oedema of the periorbital structures and forehead due to blockage of venous drainage,
- symptoms are most usually unilateral, but can extend via the circular sinus to become bilateral.

87 **c.** The history describes a subdural haemorrhage. It is most commonly seen in people with pre-existing cerebral disease, in the elderly due to atrophy of the brain or in alcoholics. Subdural haemorrhages result from rupture of cortical bridging veins. These connect the venous system of the brain to the large intradural venous sinuses and lie relatively unprotected in the subdural space. Acute subdural haemorrhage is usually associated with severe brain injury following trauma. It can occur at any age.

88 **a.** This is a case of a tension headache. It is believed that four out of every five people suffer with these over the course of their lifetime and approximately 40% of the population will suffer with them each year. Characteristically, they are bilateral and the pain is band-like and exerts a pressure over the head. There is no neurological deficit associated with these episodes and patients should be reassured and given adequate analgesia.

89 **b.** This case is describing a subarachnoid haemorrhage. The headache is sudden in its onset and described by patients as feeling like being kicked in the head. The severity of the symptoms will depend on the extent of the bleed. It is bleeding from the

intracranial vessels that is accrued in the subarachnoid space. Its incidence is approximately 1 in 10 000:

- 80% are due to 'congenital'/berry aneurysms that rupture, resulting in a bleed,
- 10–15% are due to other aneurysms:
  - arteriosclerotic/fusiform,
  - inflammatory/mycotic,
  - traumatic,
- 5% are due to arteriovenous malformations – commoner in younger patients,
- less than 5% are due to:
  - bleeding diathesis anticoagulants, e.g. warfarin,
  - tumours.

90 g. This patient is suffering from sinusitis. This can often cause the symptom of headache and often follows close after an upper respiratory tract infection. On further questioning, patients may occasionally complain of feeling congested with increased amounts of nasal secretions. Sinusitis is the inflammation of the mucous membranes of the paranasal sinuses. It usually results from inadequate drainage of the sinuses secondary to physical obstruction, infection or allergy.

PAPER 5

Answers

Single Best Answer Questions

1 d. The transverse colon is spared many of the complications that are commonly seen in the sigmoid colon, the site of most pathology in the gastrointestinal tract. A host of conditions, including diverticulitis, volvulus, colorectal carcinoma and angiodysplasia, to mention but a few, afflict this area. Ruptured aortic aneurysms are most often seen in older men; however, the clinical picture of upper abdominal pain, raised inflammatory markers and a high amylase level in a clinically unstable patient should prompt investigation to rule out this fatal condition. Pancreatitis is one of the most likely causes of the above clinical picture and an amylase level less than the often-quoted limit of four times normal (360 IU/L) does not exclude this common condition.

2 e. Syndrome of inappropriate antidiuretic hormone (SIADH) secretion is associated with small cell lung cancer. Release of antidiuretic hormone (ADH) results in the dilution of the serum, which in turn gives a relative hyponatraemia.

Depending on the location of the lung cancer, local spread can apply pressure on to the superior vena cava, resulting in reduced blood return to the heart from the upper half of the body. The superior vena cava is the major drainage vessel for venous blood from the head, neck, upper extremities and upper thorax. It is located in the middle mediastinum and is surrounded by relatively rigid structures, such as the sternum, trachea, right main bronchus, aorta, pulmonary artery, and the perihilar and paratracheal lymph nodes. It is a thin-walled, low-pressure, vascular structure. This wall is easily compressed as it traverses the right side of the mediastinum. Clinical features include venous distension of the neck and chest wall, facial oedema,

EMQs and SBAs for Medical Finals, Second Edition. Jonathan Bath,
Rebecca Morgan and Mehool Patel.
© 2011 John Wiley & Sons, Ltd. Published 2011 by John Wiley & Sons, Ltd.

upper extremity oedema, mental changes, lassitude, cyanosis, and even coma.

Pressure on the recurrent laryngeal nerve can result in a palsy of the vocal cords and a hoarse voice, while growth into the sympathetic system can lead to Horner's syndrome: ptosis, meiosis and anhydrosis on the ipsilateral side.

Pulmonary oedema is not a complication of lung cancer.

3 e. Chronic alcohol abuse lowers the seizure threshold and can put drinkers at risk of withdrawal fits. Hypoglycaemia is the most common metabolic cause of seizures and may be seen in poorly controlled diabetics or alcoholics who are prone to dropping their blood sugars. Any form of cerebral mass can result in seizures; depending on its location the mass itself may be responsible as can the surrounding oedema and raised intracranial pressure. Overdosing of antidepressants is known to result in seizures. While epileptics are more prone to subdural haemorrhages than non-epileptics, subdural haemorrhages do not result in generalized tonic–clonic seizures.

4 c. Rigler's sign is a radiographic finding of bowel perforation. It manifests as a dual-enhanced image of the bowel, owing to the presence of air in the peritoneum and in the lumen of the bowel. Murphy's sign is positive when pain is elicited over the right upper quadrant when two fingers are placed here and the patient is asked to breathe in. An inflamed gallbladder will cause the patient to catch his or her breath. Rovsing's sign relates to pain felt in the right iliac fossa when pressure is applied to the left iliac fossa and is associated with appendicitis. Kerr's sign is pain felt in the shoulder tips associated most classically with ruptured ectopic pregnancy. The pain is referred pain from blood irritating the diaphragm and emphasizes the common embryological relationship between the motor innervation of the diaphragm (C3, C4 and C5) and the sensory dermatome supplying the shoulder tips (C4). Trousseau's sign in the context of abdominal disease relates to crops of tender nodules affecting blood vessels (thrombophlebitis migrans) often associated with pancreatic malignancy.

5 e. The condition described is typical of retroperitoneal fibrosis (peri-aortitis). It is an autoimmune condition where there is progressive fibrosis surrounding the aorta, into which the ureters become embedded, causing renal obstruction, failure and retention. Methysergide has a particular association and may still be seen in use for resistant migraine. Paracetamol can lead to acute tubular necrosis as an adverse side-effect and acyclovir may cause crystal deposition in cases of dehydration. Gold injections should also be monitored regularly for renal side-effects by follow-up urinalysis for proteinuria. Rosiglitazone must be used with caution in patients with pre-existing renal impairment but has few renal side-effects in normal kidneys.

6 **e.** Respiratory failure is a syndrome in which the respiratory system fails in one or both of its gas exchange functions: oxygenation and carbon dioxide elimination. Respiratory failure may be classified as hypoxaemic or hypercapnic and may be either acute or chronic.

Type I ($\downarrow$ PaO$_2$; normal or $\downarrow$ PaCO$_2$) – acute diseases of the lung:
- pulmonary oedema,
- pneumonia,
- acute pulmonary embolus,
- acute exacerbation of asthma.

Type I, hypoxaemic respiratory failure, is characterized by a low PaO$_2$ with a normal or low PaCO$_2$. This is the most common form of respiratory failure and it can be associated with virtually all acute diseases of the lung that generally involve fluid filling or collapse of alveolar units.

Type II ($\downarrow$PaO$_2$; $\uparrow$PaCO$_2$) – chronic conditions of the lung:
- neuromuscular disease,
- chest wall abnormalities,
- drug overdose,
- severe airways disorders (e.g. asthma, COPD, chronic pulmonary emboli).

Type II, hypercapnic respiratory failure, is characterized by a low PaO$_2$ and a high PaCO$_2$ The pH depends on the level of bicarbonate, which, in turn, is dependent on the duration of hypercapnia.

7 **e.** In approximately 50% of cases no cause is found; however, many people can improve the severity and number of attacks that they experience by avoiding certain risk factors. Risk factors can be remembered by the mnemonic '*CHOCOLATE*': *ch*eese, *o*ral contraceptive, *c*affeine (or its withdrawal), alcoh*o*l, *a*nxiety, *t*ravel, *e*xercise. Depression is not a risk factor, although there is documented evidence that migraines can lead to depression.

8 **d.** Bile leak is a recognized complication of hepatobiliary surgery and presents within days postoperatively. Bile is a potent irritant to the peritoneum, causing a chemical biliary peritonitis

associated with rising biliary enzymes and bilirubin. Conservative management will often suffice for minor leaks; however, surgical intervention is the definitive treatment in severe cases. Accidental ligation of the common bile duct is a rare but catastrophic complication of cholecystectomy; however, this is not routinely seen in cyst fenestration.

Cholecystitis presents with a similar clinical picture but does not usually present with such marked derangement of liver enzymes without the coexistent bile duct involvement seen in biliary colic. Propofol is an agent commonly used as an anaesthetic-induction agent and although associated with hepatotoxicity in large doses would not normally cause significant hepatic injury. Biliary sepsis is always a high risk with hepatobiliary surgery but presents characteristically with relatively normal liver enzymes and signs of clinical sepsis.

9 c. Major risk factors for pulmonary emboli include:
- immobility,
- abdominal/pelvic surgery,
- malignancy (abdominal/pelvic/advanced metastatic),
- lower limb fracture,
- pregnancy,
- hip/knee replacement,
- previous venous thromboembolism.

Minor risk factors include the oral contraceptive pill, hormone replacement therapy and long distance travel.

10 d. Tuberculosis should always be in the forefront of the differential diagnosis of a patient who has recently come from a developing country and who exhibits weight loss and fever. This presentation is not classic for tuberculosis; however, the presence of a constitutional upset with a sterile pyuria is good enough cause to investigate for the disease. Treating for a urinary tract infection with antibiotics or antifungals is not correct without first excluding growth of alcohol and acid fast bacilli in culture specimens. An IVU may be necessary down the line to investigate any specific blockage to the urinary tract but a chest X-ray is mandatory for any suspicion of tuberculosis so that prompt treatment and barrier nursing precautions can take place if necessary. Cystoscopy is unlikely to be helpful as there has been no mention of any haematuria and may be considered at a later stage if indirect imaging is inconclusive.

11 a. Respiratory distress is a complication of upper torso burns that must be closely monitored. Surgical escharotomy may be required to release the mechanical restriction to breathing caused by circumferential burns to the chest wall. Infection may result in the intervening period as wound breakdown occurs but does not present such an emergency. Loss of peripheral pulses is again treated with surgical release of constricting tissue, most often associated with circumferential burns of the limbs, and may influence the decision to transfer an otherwise stable patient to a specialist Burns Unit rather than at a general treatment centre. Acute stress ulceration (Curling's ulcer) is managed with proton pump inhibition and has been robustly shown to be effective in treating this complication. Severe dehydration is a close second for the most important complication to be vigilant for in severe burns; however, younger patients can tolerate a larger degree of fluid loss than the elderly. Although not clinically validated, a rough indication to prognosis following burns can be estimated using the formula below:

Patient's age + % burn > 100 = poor chance of survival

(e.g. 48 year old + 35% burn = 83, i.e. moderate chance
of survival).

12 **e.** In cases such as this one, investigations are not always necessary. After appropriate examinations have been carried out, if you are happy that it is purely a syncopal attack then no further tests need to be done. In this case, there is a clear and obvious role for an ECG and blood tests are self-explanatory, i.e. looking for any undiagnosed hypoglycaemia or anaemia. An echocardiogram may have a role if a murmur is heard on auscultation or if there is any concern on cardiovascular examination. A CT scan of the head is unlikely to yield any information in this case and should be reserved for cases when no cause can be found on other simple tests.

13 **b.** Acute pulmonary emboli normally present with type I respiratory failure, i.e. low PaO_2 and normal or low $PaCO_2$. This option represents type II respiratory failure, which is seen in the context of chronic pulmonary emboli. The diagnosis of a pulmonary embolus should be considered in patients with hypoxia and tachypnoea in the absence of any clinical signs such as pneumonia. Occasionally, on chest X-ray a pulmonary embolus can cause a wedge-shaped infarct (due to loss of blood supply to an area of lung) but more commonly the chest X-ray is clear. In cases of large pulmonary embolus, rarely a characteristic $S_IQ_{III}T_{III}$ pattern may be seen on ECG, more commonly a tachycardia and right axis deviation is seen. Calf swelling unilaterally

virtually confirms the diagnosis in a patient who has become acutely short of breath; in fact, guidelines state that in patients with a confirmed deep vein thrombosis with acute-onset shortness of breath the diagnosis of a pulmonary embolism should be assumed and treatment continued for the appropriate length of time, usually 6 months.

14 d. Causes of proximal myopathy are varied. Patients will notice that they have difficulty in climbing up stairs or difficulty in standing from a low chair. Causes include: metabolic problems, including hyper- or hypocalcaemia; alcoholism; steroid use; thyroid disease; inflammatory myositis; and myasthenia gravis. Syphilis infection is known to cause a sensory deficit resulting in a high-stepping gait but not a proximal weakness and waddling gait.

15 a. Pulmonary embolus is an often overlooked risk of laparoscopic procedures. During surgery, the peritoneum is insufflated with carbon dioxide to a pressure of around 15 mmHg. Occlusion of the venous system draining through the abdomen including the great vessels has been reported to increase the incidence of postoperative venous thromboembolism. Thromboembolic deterrent stockings are recommended for 4 weeks, with daily injection of subcutaneous low molecular weight heparin for any patient who has recently undergone laparoscopic procedures. Pulmonary embolus is associated with pleuritic chest pain, tachycardia, and the often-quoted but rarely seen deep S-wave in lead I, deep Q-wave in lead III and inverted T-wave in lead III (S_1,Q_3,T_3), with haemoptysis or silently. Beware the elderly patient on beta-blocking medication who does not mount a tachycardia, a useful warning sign of pulmonary embolus.

16 a. This patient is likely hypovolaemic from inadequate fluid resuscitation that probably started in the operating room. The commonest cause of a rise in creatinine, mild hypotension, mild tachycardia and low urine output following a standard abdominal procedure is hypovolaemia. Supplying the patient with a 1-L bolus of fluid after a clinical assessment of fluid status is the first step in reversing intravascular volume depletion and low urine output postoperatively.

Foley catheterization is a reasonable course of action if the bolus does not appear to have improved the patient's fluid status; however, it is preferably performed after documentation of a bladder with a significant volume of urine in place. This can be elicited either by clinical examination or bedside ultrasound (bladder scan) that can be performed by any provider after some simple instruction. A residual volume of >300 ml urine is evidence enough that a patient may benefit from urethral catheterization until the bladder is able to empty normally again.

A renal ultrasound often forms part of the work-up of a rise in creatinine in the setting of new-onset oliguria to assess for a mechanical obstruction as manifest by a dilated urinary system. It also can assess the renal vasculature in more complex cases such as renal transplantation where a number of causes may inhibit the renal inflow leading to a reduction in urine output that must be dealt with expeditiously.

Urine electrolytes also form part of the work-up of new-onset renal failure with a fractional excretion of sodium (FENa) defined as (urine Na × plasma Cr) / (plasma Na × urine Cr) × 100. Values <1% suggest prerenal causes such as dehydration or acute glomerulonephritis while values >3% suggest cases of acute tubular necrosis or severe bilateral obstruction of the kidneys. This would be a secondary measure if the above patient were in renal failure.

Finally, 20 mg furosemide is never indicated in this setting for two main reasons: (i) if a patient is thought to be dehydrated then diuresis will exacerbate matters; and (ii) a healthy 55-year-old man after a colectomy should be able to offset fluid overload by manifesting an increase in urine output spontaneously. Diuretics should not be needed to start the process of fluid offloading in a healthy patient in the setting of oliguria. There are other aetiologies at work here and these should be investigated.

If a patient is suspected to be fluid overloaded in the setting of acute renal failure and the reason for use of furosemide is to test the ability of the kidney to regulate fluid balance to avoid the need for dialysis, then a small dose such as 20 mg furosemide will inevitably fail. A higher dose will be required with an increased creatinine level. Some nephrologists use doses of up to 200 mg furosemide to see if the kidney can be encouraged to make urine. If this dose does not allow adequate urine output, then dialysis is almost always required.

17 d. Patients with underlying lung conditions are more likely to develop pneumothoraces than those without. Young, tall men are at risk of developing pneumothoraces spontaneously, simply due to their body shape. This diagnosis should always be considered in a young patient with acute-onset shortness of breath (with or without pain). Although most small pneumothoraces will be re-absorbed, larger ones will require treatment with a chest drain and underwater seal while tension pneumothoraces require emergency treatment.

Pulmonary emboli do not predispose to pneumothoraces, as they are not predominately a condition of the lung parenchyma but of the associated vasculature.

18 **b.** D-dimer is a test useful only in the process of ruling out a pulmonary embolus. A negative result predicts a high likelihood of absence of pulmonary embolus; a positive result is almost meaningless diagnostically. D-dimers are expected to rise postoperatively and thus should not form the first line of investigation for a suspected pulmonary embolus.

ABGs and electrocardiography are invaluable for the investigation of dyspnoea, for both quantifying the respiratory compromise and in stratifying the differential to either cardiac or respiratory causes. Chest radiographs may demonstrate pneumonic processes or pneumothoraces and form part of the standard investigation of breathlessness. CT-PA forms the most definitive imaging in cases of suspected pulmonary embolus but may return equivocal results in the presence of pre-existing lung pathology.

19 **e.** This case describes a right-sided homonymous hemianopia (homonymous = same side; hemianopia = loss of half a field of vision) with macular sparing. The macular sparing suggests that the lesion is not in the occipital cortex. The bilateral symptoms suggest that the lesion is at a place in the pathway where fibres for both eyes will be affected (posterior to the optic chiasm). Causes for this man's symptoms may be an infarct, a haemorrhage or a tumour producing a mass effect. Isolated lesions of the upper or lower optic radiation provide a quadrantanopia and lesions of the optic nerve alone will affect only one eye.

20 **b.** The ideal anticoagulation regime for management of a pulmonary embolus is commencement of warfarin (with a loading dose) and in addition administration of low molecular weight heparin until the dose of warfarin becomes therapeutic. One of the benefits of using low molecular weight heparin rather then unfractionated heparin is that its effect does not need to be monitored.

Low molecular weight heparin exerts its effect on factor Xa in the clotting cascade, thus requires no monitoring. Once administered, it becomes effective immediately and its effects last for approximately 24 hours. Warfarin is a vitamin K antagonist and its effects need to be monitored. When commencing a patient on warfarin, it is important to remember that it is procoagulant for the first 24 hours and it takes up to 3 days for its effect to be exerted. For patients being treated for a pulmonary embolus, the target international normalizing ratio (INR) range is 2–3, which means that their blood will be two to three times thinner than a patient who is not being anticoagulated. To maintain this, regular blood tests are required as over-anticoagulation can be dangerous and under-anticoagulation may result in development of further clots.

Both aspirin and clopidogrel have antiplatelet action and therefore are not useful in the management of pulmonary emboli. While unfractionated heparin is an adequate choice, its effects require monitoring up to 4-hourly. This requires the patient to be hooked up to an infusion pump and therefore this option is less desirable than low molecular weight heparin. However, a benefit of unfractionated heparin is that once stopped its effects will be reversed after 4–6 hours, whereas with low molecular weight heparin it takes 24 hours after administration for the effects to normalize and with warfarin it takes about 3 days for the effects to be reversed.

21 c. Inguinal hernias present the greatest diagnostic challenge when defining the subtype of hernia; indirect hernias were often said to be controlled by pressure over the internal (deep) inguinal ring at a point 1–2 cm above the femoral pulse once reduced. However, this clinical distinction is frequently inaccurate in even the most experienced hands. A more useful definition is that direct hernias pass medially to the inferior epigastric artery with indirect hernias passing laterally. This can be neatly summed up as 'MDs don't Lie' (Medial Direct, Lateral Indirect). Confusion between inguinal and femoral hernias can be avoided by remembering that inguinal hernias present above and medial to the pubic tubercle with femoral hernias presenting below and lateral. Spigelian hernias are located at the lateral border of the posterior rectus sheath, passing through the arcuate line to present as a mass in the lower abdominal wall. Ventral hernias are often seen in the elderly and are associated with a widening of the recti muscles (divarication of the recti).

22 d. Multiple sclerosis is one of the most common of a group of inflammatory conditions affecting the central nervous system. The disease has a relapsing and remitting course but ultimately most patients develop progressive permanent neurological symptoms. It is a fairly common disease and normally presents in younger patients. Its effects are wide reaching and in addition to the physical disability that develops, there are often accompanying psychological problems. At present there is no proven treatment, β-interferon has been shown to reduce the relapse rate of exacerbations but not alter the disease progression. Patients are plagued with a combination of eye problems, motor weakness, sensory loss, cerebellar and brainstem lesions, in addition to spinal cord damage. Its investigation remains challenging due to the intermittent course that the disease initially undertakes.

23 c. Ibuprofen and other NSAIDs should be avoided if possible in anything other than mild renal failure (arbitrarily defined as a glomerular filtration rate of between 20 and 50 mL/minute). The mechanism of action of the NSAIDs is to inhibit cyclo-oxygenase enzymes thus decreasing the amount of prostaglandin production (PGE_2 and PGI_2 especially). Prostaglandins are involved in the inflammatory cascade but additionally have effect on the maintenance of renal blood flow, especially at the site of the glomerular afferent arterioles. Thus the decrease in production of prostaglandins in patients who are susceptible to changes in renal homeostasis (such as those with renal impairment) can cause decompensation of function. Alternative analgesic modalities that can safely be used in patients with suboptimal renal function should be sought.

24 b. There are two significant congenital diaphragmatic abnormalities that usually require intervention: large central tendon defects; and herniation through the foramen of Bochdalek. Congenital herniation of abdominal contents through the foramen of Morgagni are usually small and insignificant and usually require no further treatment. Trauma to the diaphragm can occur with both blunt or penetrating injury to the abdomen and usually affects the relatively unprotected left hemidiaphragm. The liver usually takes the brunt of right-sided injury, resulting in relative right hemidiaphragm sparing. Congenital diaphragmatic hernias usually require surgical intervention; however, respiratory distress is usually present at birth and is best stabilized prior to repair. Embryologically, the diaphragm is made up of the *s*eptum transversum, *p*leuroperitoneal membrane, *m*esentery of the *d*orsal oesophagus and the *d*orsal body wall, neatly summed up by the mnemonic '*Several Parts Make Diaphragm*'.

25 d. The analysis of the pleural fluid shows that the effusion is an exudate (protein content <30 g/L = transudate, >30 g/L = exudate). Causes of transudates can be grouped as failures (e.g.

heart failure, renal failure, liver failure, etc.). The following conditions cause transudates:

- congestive heart failure,
- cirrhosis,
- atelectasis (which may be due to malignancy or pulmonary embolism),
- nephrotic syndrome,
- myxoedema,
- constrictive pericarditis.

In contrast, exudates are produced by a variety of inflammatory conditions and often require more extensive evaluation and treatment. The more common causes of exudates include:

- parapneumonic,
- malignancy (carcinoma, lymphoma, mesothelioma),
- pulmonary embolism,
- tuberculosis,
- asbestos-related,
- pancreatitis,
- trauma,
- drug-induced,
- sarcoidosis.

26 b. Post-streptococcal glomerulonephritis is associated with streptococcal upper respiratory tract infections and usually presents anywhere between 1 and 3 weeks post-infection. Haematuria, often described as dark or smoky rather than frank blood, is frequently encountered. Oedema, especially of the peri-orbital region, is a common presentation in children with post-streptococcal glomerulonephritis and accompanies proteinuria, hypertension and oliguria. Treatment is usually supportive with spontaneous resolution being the rule.

Minimal change glomerulonephritis is the most common cause of the nephritic syndrome in children. Symptoms are similar with oedema, hypertension and association with upper respiratory tract infection; however, thromboembolic events due to loss of anticlotting products in the urine make the diagnosis more likely. Corticosteroids form the mainstay of treatment.

Henoch–Schönlein purpura is a vasculitis of small vessels that affects young males twice as frequently as females and manifests as punctate bleeding points associated with abdominal pain and gastrointestinal bleeding. Characteristic 'bruising' occurs over the buttocks and lower limbs and may sometimes be mistaken for non-accidental injury in a child.

Berger's disease is the commonest primary glomerulonephritis worldwide. Immune complex deposition is thought to be part of the pathophysiology of Berger's disease with ensuing glomerular damage and renal failure. Treatment may be supportive only if the degree of renal failure is mild.

Rapidly progressive glomeruloncphritis describes a pathological reduction in glomerular filtration rate over a short space of time and may be associated with anti-glomerular basement membrane (anti-GBM) antibodies, immune complex deposition or vasculitis-associated disease. Immunosuppression is the treatment modality of choice.

27 a. In a patient with a confirmed diagnosis of bacterial meningitis we would expect to see a raised opening CSF pressure. Normal pressure is seen in cases of viral infection and sometimes encephalitis but not in bacterial meningitis. Protein levels are elevate and glucose is low due to the active bacteria affecting the fluid and >50 polymorphs should be seen. Confirmed cases are public health issues and the appropriate departments should be contacted.

28 a. Being of female sex affords a certain amount of resistance to the development of duodenal ulceration and this is markedly seen during pregnancy. Steroid use has been shown to predispose to the formation of ulcers by mechanisms that involve both a disturbance in acid regulation and secretion, and interference with the normal protective mucosal layer of the stomach. Cushing's ulcer is the eponymous name given to the development of acute peptic ulceration secondary to head injury, major surgery or acutely stressful conditions and a strong association between ulcer formation and severe burns has also been described (Curling's ulcer). These findings form the basis for the routine use of proton pump inhibitors such as omeprazole as part of the gastrointestinal prophylaxis of the critical care bundle in situations of acute stress.

29 c. The results of the ABG can be broken down into components:
- pH 7.4 – this is within the normal range (7.35–7.45)
- pO_2 7.3 kPA – this is clearly suboptimal. Even in patients suffering from COPD the pO_2 should be >8.0 kPA.
- pCO_2 4.8 kPA – this is also within the normal range. Some patients with COPD retain CO_2, which can suppress their respiratory drive.

On balance, this patient is hypoxic with a normal pCO_2, therefore the main problem is hypoxia, which can be improved by administering oxygen. If too much supplementary oxygen is administered it could raise her CO_2 level, thus its best to adopt a stepwise approach and start with 1 L. In these patients it is always important to be on the look out for the signs of CO_2 narcosis, particularly when increasing concentrations of oxygen.

30 d. Hyperkalaemia is associated with chronic renal failure and is most important in the setting of acute on chronic renal failure when levels can be rapidly elevated due to a sharp fall in glomerular filtration rate. Treatment of acute severe hyperkalaemia (potassium level >6.5 mmol/L or ECG changes) is managed first by IV injection of 10 mL of 10% calcium gluconate as cardioprotection. Second, infusion of 10 units of short-acting insulin with 50 mL of 50% dextrose over 30 minutes will shift potassium intracellularly. Correcting the underlying cause, for example hypovolaemia, may stabilize the potassium level; however, depletion of total body stores of potassium may be indicated and can be achieved by using calcium resonium.

Other electrolyte abnormalities may be a dilutional hyponatraemia secondary to fluid retention, hyperphosphataemia and associated hypocalcaemia due to reduced renal hydroxylation of vitamin D, with uraemia and metabolic acidosis due to impaired hydrogen ion excretion. Neurological manifestations of chronic renal failure include restless legs syndrome, peripheral neuropathy and non-specific signs such as dizziness and headache associated with dialysis.

31 b. The condition that this case alludes to is an acute cord compression (cauda equina). Any history of niggling pain is a red herring. While that may be significant, in the acute setting the worry is that he is unable to pass urine and is complaining of saddle anaesthesia. While in a scenario such as this one spinal X-rays may provide some information and clues, the diagnosis will be made on MRI scan. Any evidence of acute cord compression, regardless of cause, should be discussed with a neurosurgical centre for potential surgery to decompress the lesion. There is no evidence that these symptoms are caused by a cerebral lesion and blood tests are unlikely to be of diagnostic value alone.

32 a. Sarcoidosis is a multisystem inflammatory disease of unknown aetiology that mainly affects the lungs and intrathoracic lymph nodes. Sarcoidosis is manifested by the presence of non-caseating granulomas in affected organ tissues. It is more common in men than women (2:1) and peak incidence occurs from ages 25 to 35 years, with a second peak in women aged 45 to 65 years. Characteristic appearance on chest X-ray is bilateral hilar lymphadenopathy, although there are many other presentations.

Pulmonary fibrosis presents with a ground glass appearance on chest X-ray and rarely has symptoms manifest outside of the chest. In a person of this age, it is unlikely that this would be malignancy. In lung cancer, unilateral hilar lymphadenopathy is seen but rarely is this bilateral.

33 e. Postoperative ileus is a common recognized sequel of abdominal surgery where handling of the bowel leads to a period of inactivity. It is commonly seen in open, as opposed to laparoscopic, procedures due to the greater manipulation of the bowel required in this type of approach. The initiation of oral intake is often subjective and will depend on factors such as the length of operation and the difficulty of the procedure; for example, a case of ruptured appendix will normally result in a greater period of bowel inactivity than an intact but inflamed appendix.

Anastomotic leak is a serious complication more often seen during large bowel procedures due to the relatively poor blood supply to this part of the gastrointestinal tract. It is usually heralded by a tense, rigid abdomen, absence of bowel sounds and a patient who is unwell. Adverse reactions to anaesthetic agents are relatively common; however, they usually present soon postoperatively or soon after induction of anaesthesia. Small bowel obstruction can be a long-term complication of any abdominal surgery; however, is almost never the cause of such a clinical picture so soon after appendectomy.

34 d. The prescription of antiemetic medication should always be with caution. The cause for vomiting should be assessed and a diagnosis made before starting antiemetics. Serious causes of vomiting, for example gastrointestinal obstruction, must be excluded. Erect chest radiographs are useful if perforation is suspected; however, in this case the clinical index of suspicion is low and would not be a useful investigation. Abdominal radiographs are useful only in cases of suspected gastrointestinal obstruction, as a crude assessment of renal tract stones (a kidneys, ureter and bladder radiograph is far superior) and often as a useful method of confirming constipation in elderly patients who complain of abdominal pain and difficulty in passing stool. Nasogastric tube passage would be an option if vomiting were severe or unlikely to settle with antiemesis; however, it would not be necessary to feed a patient like this via nasogastric tube in the short term and thus would be an unnecessary hindrance to recovery of normal oral intake. Proton pump inhibitors such as omeprazole are not required in a young patient without documented peptic ulcer disease and in this example would not afford any significant benefit in the immediate management of vomiting caused by postoperative ileus.

35 d. Cystic fibrosis occurs in one in approximately 3000 births. It is a multisystem disorder, affecting the respiratory tract, pancreas, gastrointestinal tract (including hepatobiliary) and reproductive systems. The majority of cases are diagnosed before their first birthday. On examination of the chest in a patient suffering from cystic fibrosis, you would expect to hear coarse inspiratory crackles due to the production of thick secretions and difficulty of the mucociliary system in clearing these. The result is coarse crepitations heard on auscultation.

36 c. Frusemide is an example of a loop diuretic and has action at the loop of Henlé. Other loop diuretics include ethacrynic acid and bumetanide. The mechanism of action is one of inhibition of the sodium/potassium/chloride cotransporter in the thick ascending limb of the loop of Henlé and inhibition of reabsorption of the above electrolytes at this site. Renal losses of sodium of up to 15–20% are seen, causing a loss of concentrating power at the loop and thus loss of free water.

Acetazolamide is a carbonic anhydrase inhibitor acting at the proximal convoluted tubule, causing increased excretion of sodium bicarbonate with resultant loss of sodium, potassium and free water. The effect is self-limiting as levels of bicarbonate fall producing a temporary diuresis.

Osmotic agents are not commonly used in the treatment of fluid overload and are more useful in the management of raised intracranial pressure; however, mannitol is an example of an osmotic agent that acts on parts of the nephron freely permeable to water (proximal convoluted tubule, descending limb of the loop of Henlé and collecting tubule). Water is drawn into the tubular lumen by osmosis with relatively marginal effect on sodium loss from the kidney.

Thiazide drugs such as bendroflumethiazide and newer agents such as indapamide act at the distal convoluted tubule to reduce sodium and chloride reabsorption. Potassium loss is significant with the thiazide diuretics and is due to a relative increase in the electrolyte gradient in the collecting duct, essentially flushing away potassium. Spironolactone, amiloride and triamterene are examples of potassium-sparing diuretics. Spironolactone is especially useful in conditions of hyperaldosteronism, such as Conn's disease (primary aldosteronism) and hepatic cirrhosis.

37 d. Tight control of blood sugars in diabetic patients is essential to reduce the risk of developing later complications. Bilateral pupillary abnormalities are caused by an autonomic neuropathy. The pupils have a poor reaction to light but react better to accommodation. The third nerve palsy results from a microvascular lesion to the nerve trunk, often the pupil is spared in this condition. Hemiparesis may occur transiently due to hypoglycaemia or due to a transient ischaemic attack. There is no evidence that headaches are associated with diabetes.

38 b. Oliguria is not an indication for dialysis itself and the cause, for example hypovolaemia, should be investigated and treated. However, manifestations of oliguria, such as fluid overload refractory to treatment or build-up of toxins such as urea and nitrogenous compounds, may influence the decision to dialyse. A useful mnemonic for remembering the indications for dialysis is *AEIOU* standing for *a*cidosis, *e*lectrolyte abnormalities, *i*ngestions, *o*verload and *u*raemic symptoms. Severe or worsening metabolic acidosis with a pH <7.2 and persistent hyperkalaemia >7 mmol/L are good markers of the need for dialysis. Fluid overload, manifest as pulmonary oedema, that is likely to cause respiratory embarrassment and/or cardiovascular instability may be adequately managed with dialysis when medical therapy has failed. In the setting of acute overdose, especially with metabolic derangement as may be seen with aspirin overdose, dialysis can be a useful means of stabilizing a patient until adequate acid–base homeostasis is achieved.

39 e. Causes of fibrosing alveolitis are vast and varied. When all causes have been excluded and the diagnosis is certain, it can be said that the patient is suffering with cryptogenic fibrosing alveolitis of unknown cause. Rheumatoid arthritis, Sjögren's disease and ulcerative colitis are all systemic conditions that are known to cause fibrosing alveolitis. Aspergillus is associated with extrinsic allergic alveolitis as it causes an immune response by which it mediates its effect.

40 a. This case describes trigeminal neuralgia. It commonly affects the maxillary and mandibular divisions of the trigeminal nerve and occasionally affects the ophthalmic division. It can be an intensely painful condition and result in the face completely screwing up. The symptoms may be precipitated by washing, brushing or simply touching the overlying skin. It has a number of causes including idiopathic, a cerebellopontine angle tumour, multiple sclerosis or a vascular malformation. Although the condition may resolve spontaneously, drugs such as carbamazepine and phenytoin directed at the nerve ganglion may provide relief.

41 a. Alport's syndrome is an inherited disease of the kidney affecting young boys between 5 and 20 years of age. Inheritance is in three forms: X-lined dominant, autosomal dominant or autosomal recessive. The clinical presentation is one of asymptomatic haematuria with progressive sensorineural deafness and eye disorders (lenticonus). Treatment is to support the progressive renal failure. Renal transplantation may be considered; however, there is a risk of anti-GBM nephritis even after transplantation.

Anderson–Fabry disease is an X-linked recessive disorder of trihexoside deposition. Clinical features include a burning sensation in distal limbs associated with a characteristic blue-hued rash (angiokeratoma corporis diffusum).

Goodpasture's syndrome is a pulmonary–renal syndrome manifest as pulmonary haemorrhage and massive haemoptysis associated with proliferative glomerulonephritis. Linear anti-GBM deposits are seen on immunofluorescent staining of biopsy specimens. Treatment involves aggressive immunosuppression with or without plasmapheresis.

Wegener's granulomatosis is a necrotizing granulomatous vasculitis affecting the respiratory tract and kidney. Typically, sinusitis with epistaxis, haemoptysis and renal failure all coexist. Autoantibody assay returns a positive ANCA, which responds to corticosteroid and cyclophosphamide. Von Hippel–Lindau syndrome is an oncologic vascular disorder manifest in many different organs with renal cysts and tumours, phaeochromocytoma, retinal angiomas and haemangioblastomas of brain and spinal cord being most frequently seen. Clinical clues to the diagnosis are posterior fossa symptoms of dizziness, ataxia and headache in young adults, often with retinal detachment detectable on fundoscopy.

42 a. The diagnosis is strongly suggested by two salient features in the history: the presence of high blood glucose in an elderly man with no previous history of diabetes mellitus, and jaundice. Compression of the distal end of the common bile duct by the head of the pancreas causes back pressure leading to jaundice. The presence of new-onset diabetes mellitus in the elderly should always be treated with suspicion and a diagnosis of diabetes mellitus should never be made until an attempt to rule out malignancy has been undertaken.

Cholangiocarcinoma presents with weight loss, jaundice and deranged liver enzymes; however, the presence of raised blood glucose is more suggestive of pancreatic cancer. Choledocholithiasis (literally = stone in biliary tree) can cause an intermittent jaundice and right upper quadrant pain; however, weight loss and new-onset elevated blood glucose suggest a more sinister cause. Hepatitis is usually associated with tender hepatomegaly and does not usually accompany raised blood glucose.

43 e. Males are usually more affected than females as malignant mesothelioma is associated with a history of asbestos exposure. In most cases, the exposure is approximately 40 years prior to onset of the symptoms and discovery of the cancer. It is believed that some women suffer from mesothelioma after exposure via their husband's work overalls; others have become exposed by living down-wind from an asbestos factory. Men usually have a good history of occupational exposure to asbestos. Pleural mesothelioma is 1.6 times more common on the right side than on the left. Prognosis of the condition from diagnosis is poor.

44 d. Myeloma should always be kept in mind when considering the differential diagnosis of an elderly patient with back pain and renal failure. The simple and non-invasive urine test for Bence–Jones protein, the light-chain fragment of the B-cells overexpressed in myeloma, makes this investigation one that should not be overlooked in the diagnostic work-up of patients with renal failure. The mechanism of renal failure in myeloma is thought to be a directly toxic effect of light chains on the nephrons and leads to the characteristic 'flea-bitten' appearance of the myeloma kidney.

Paget's disease is a disorder primarily of bone remodelling leading to alternating osteoclastic bone resorption followed by abnormal osteoblastic woven bone formation. Symptoms usually include bone pain, excessive warmth over the affected bony sites due to hypervascularity, bony deformity and neuropathy due to nerve compression (especially the vestibulocochlear nerve).

Sarcoidosis is characterized by the presence of non-caseating granulomata and is most classically a disease of the respiratory system; however, renal involvement is seen in rare cases.

Hyperparathyroidism can lead to a raised calcium and is usually seen as the by-product of failing kidneys. However, chronic hyperparathyroidism itself may manifest as renal stones, uraemia and eventual renal failure. Bony involvement is common and may be seen as an erosive arthropathy, subperiosteal bone resorption at the phalangeal tufts or a 'rickets-type' picture.

Osteosarcoma presents typically with pain and soft tissue swelling and classically Codman's triangle is seen on radiographs, indicative of periosteal tenting from underlying bone. Radiographic appearances are usually a mixed lytic/sclerotic picture but purely lytic or sclerotic lesions can be seen.

45 d. Patients suffering from Parkinson's disease develop a typical gait. It is normally a shuffling gait with difficulty both initiating and stopping movements. As the condition progresses, the posture becomes increasingly flexed. Other characteristic gait findings include:

- spastic – circumduction of legs,
- frontal – difficulty getting feet off floor,
- cerebellar – wide-based gait,
- myopathic – waddling and difficulty climbing stairs.

46 c. Caeruloplasmin and serum copper are useful tests in the investigation of liver disease of unknown aetiology and are sensitive indicators of the presence of Wilson's disease (hepatolenticular degeneration). A renal ultrasound scan is useful to identify any obstruction, scarring from previous infection or altered renal size indicative of long-term renal damage or chronically reduced renal blood flow. Safe and non-invasive to perform, this should always be considered in the investigation of renal disease.

Complement levels (C3 and C4) as well as double-stranded DNA (ds-DNA) and erythrocyte sedimentation rate (ESR) should be used as a screen for SLE (lupus) nephritis. Generally, an elevated ESR and anti-ds-DNA and low C3 and C4 levels are associated with active nephritis. ANCA are useful in the detection of vasculitic diseases affecting the kidney, such as Wegener's granulomatosis and Churg–Strauss disease. Bence–Jones protein (light-chain fragment) is a simple and effective screening tool for suspected myeloma with associated light-chain nephropathy and should never be omitted from the diagnostic work-up of renal failure.

47 b. Chest radiography is the investigation most likely to aid with diagnosis of the cause of breathlessness. The history is consistent with an element of heart failure with peripheral as well as pulmonary oedema; however, a large unilateral pleural effusion should raise suspicion of a localized respiratory lesion, for example infection or malignancy.

An echocardiogram will not be useful diagnostically as the clinical signs point to a degree of heart failure and an ECG, although a useful screening tool for suspected pulmonary embolus and signs of cardiac disease, can be performed later once localized disease has been ruled out. Pleural tap and drainage are the most useful diagnostically and therapeutically; however, in the non-acute situation radiographic confirmation of the diagnosis and extent of pleural effusion is useful. Finally, there is a tendency to start antibiotics empirically in elderly patients without accurate history or diagnosis. The minimal history and examination are not strongly suggestive of pneumonia and it is sensible to await chest imaging before considering antibiotics.

48 a. Sleep apnoea is mainly a problem of overweight middle-aged men. It is believed that the weight of the additional fat surrounding their necks places pressure on their trachea during sleep and subsequently they have apnoeic episodes. Owing to this interruption to their sleep, daytime somnolence is a common feature as is morning headache. Reduced libido and cognitive function are associated with sleep apnoea although rarely considered to be part of the same condition, as sleep apnoea is commonly overlooked. Cough is not a feature of this condition.

49 b. This is a classical history of an extradural haemorrhage. They commonly follow head injuries, particularly those causing fractures of the temporal or parietal bones resulting in damage to the middle meningeal artery and vein. Damage to the dural venous sinus will also result in an extradural haemorrhage. Important signs to look out for include deterioration in the level of consciousness and a lucid interval that may be mistaken for an uncomplicated recovery. This lucid interval may last for anything from hours to days as the blood accumulates between the bone and dura. The bleed finally declares itself with a reducing level of consciousness, rising intracranial pressure and increasingly severe headaches. Vomiting and confusion may also be features and hemiparesis and upgoing plantars may be seen as the deterioration progresses. Management of this bleed is by the neurosurgeons releasing the pressure through burr holes in the skull.

Subdural haemorrhages are most common in the elderly or among alcoholics. A subarachnoid haemorrhage is often described as being kicked in the back of the head while a cerebrovascular accident would provide neurological evidence at presentation.

50 a. Renal ultrasonography should be the first-line investigation. Other useful investigations to be considered initially are a urine dipstick, urine pregnancy test and a bedside blood glucose level. Blood pressure is markedly elevated in this otherwise well middle-aged woman and the deterioration in renal function is significant. The additional clue from the history that two relatives suffered strokes at a 'young age' should prompt strong consideration of a diagnosis of autosomal dominant polycystic kidney disease, which is associated with cerebral (berry) aneurysms, cysts in other organs such as liver, pancreas and spleen, and cardiac valvular defects. Renal failure is progressive and may lead to end-stage renal disease. Renal ultrasound scan is a very sensitive and specific tool in detecting cystic abnormalities of the kidneys and may well confirm the suspected diagnosis.

CT scan of the head should not be rushed into on the basis of a lack of neurological signs until other simple investigations have been performed and would only be indicated if blood pressure control did not ameliorate symptoms. Renal biopsy is not without serious risks and should never be undertaken unless knowing histology will influence management. A 24-hour urine collection for metanephrines is indicated in cases of suspected phaeochromocytoma and, along with adrenal CT scanning, aids diagnosis of this rare cause of hypertensive crisis. Carotid and vertebral Doppler scans are sometimes indicated in cases of stroke secondary to suspected arterial stenosis such as atherosclerotic disease. A history of multiple transient ischaemic attacks or strokes in the absence of a good cause, such as atrial fibrillation, may prompt examination of carotid arterial flow waveform. A similar process may occur in the vertebrobasilar system (so-called posterior circulation stroke) and manifests as symptoms of dizziness, vertigo, nausea and lower cranial nerve abnormalities.

51 b. This woman is most likely to be suffering from delirium, otherwise known as an acute confusional state. It is a fairly common condition in hospitalized patients and occurs in approximately 5–15% of inpatients on general medical or surgical wards. Symptoms and signs include:
- Impaired consciousness with acute onset over hours to days. It will fluctuate throughout the day often being worse in the late afternoon to evening.

- Disorientation in time, place and person.
- Altered behaviour, including quietness and reduced speech to agitation and aggression.
- Thinking may be slow and muddled and occasionally paranoid.
- Mood is likely to be labile and depressed.
- Memory is often impaired.

All presentations similar to this should have a full screen of tests carried out to discover the underlying cause. Dementia is much slower in its onset and more chronic in its course. While it is easy to assume that this presentation could be due to a psychiatric illness, other organic causes should first be excluded.

52 e. Acute asthma does not cause cor pulmonale. It is caused by chronic conditions that result in high pressures in the lungs leading to high back pressure being transmitted to the heart, which ultimately has a re-modelling effect on the right sided heart chambers. Chronic asthma has been associated with the development of cor pulmonale but acute lung diseases do not cause this problem. The main symptom is shortness of breath and occasionally chest pain. If the condition is prolonged both sides of the heart become involved and symptoms such as bipedal oedema will develop.

53 d. Liver failure presents with a plethora of physical signs: jaundice, fluid shift leading to pulmonary oedema and effusion, ascites and peripheral oedema, and biochemical derangement of liver function, for example increased clotting time, decreased protein/immunoglobulin synthesis, etc. Fluid collections associated with liver failure tend to be transudates rather than exudates (transudates <30 g/dL protein; exudates >30 g/dL). *Ex*udates *ex*ceed 30 g/dL protein is one way of remembering this association. Transudates are mainly associated with failures (e.g. heart failure, liver failure, thyroid failures, kidney failure (nephrotic syndrome). On the contrary, exudates are mainly associated with infection (e.g. pneumonia, tuberculosis), inflammation (c.g. rheumatoid arthritis, SLE) and malignancy (e.g. bronchial carcinoma, lymphoma and mesothelioma).

The most likely diagnosis from the pleural tap would be malignancy in this case and must be excluded

54 c. The most useful diagnostic investigation is bilateral renal biopsies. CT scanning of the abdomen has a role in the diagnosis of a suspected Wilms' tumour; however, staging CT of the chest, abdomen and pelvis must be performed to assess for metastatic spread of tumour. Chest radiography is a useful baseline investigation to assess for pulmonary metastases but again if Wilms' tumour is identified then staging CT is performed. Albumin/creatinine ratio is a very useful investigation in the work-up of renal disease of various origins and can detect microalbuminuria (defined as the presence of albumin in the urine of 30–300 mg/day), which is one of the pathological hallmarks of early renal disease. Especially useful in the investigation of patients with diabetes and cardiovascular disease it should be performed on a regular basis to guide secondary prevention strategies, for example tight blood pressure or glucose control and as a prognostic indicator of the level of renal deterioration.

55 c. Drug-induced interstitial nephritis presents acutely typically following commencement of penicillins although it has been described in association with diuretics such as frusemide, NSAIDs and sometimes with infections. Acute renal failure associated with fever, arthralgia, rash and eosinophils in both blood and urine helps to make the diagnosis.

Haemolytic uraemic syndrome is a vascular disorder with the formation of platelet aggregates. A triad of symptoms is usually seen: microangiopathic haemolytic anaemia, thrombocytopenia and acute renal failure. It is the commonest cause of acute renal failure in children and usually occurs following a diarrhoeal disorder, although many infections may cause haemolytic uraemic syndrome.

Cholesterol embolus is rarely seen but can be catastrophic when it occurs. Clinically, it manifests with disturbance of renal biochemistry associated with eosinophilia and purpura of limb, usually in those with arterial disease. A net-like rash (livedo reticularis) is sometimes described similar to that seen in SLE and this may aid diagnosis.

Acute tubular necrosis is a common and spontaneously resolving cause of acute renal failure and is associated with hypovolaemia, drugs that are nephrotoxic, and rhabdomyolysis by a direct insult to the renal tubules from excess myoglobin in the glomerular filtrate. The typical clinical picture is of acute renal failure refractory to rehydration that eventually responds within days to weeks. Treatment is to ensure adequate hydration until tubule function is restored.

56 e. The causes of peripheral neuropathy may be remembered by the mnemonic '*DANG THERAPIST*':
- *d*iabetes,
- *a*myloid,

- *n*utritional (e.g. vitamin B1, B6, or B12 deficiency),
- *G*uillain–Barre syndrome,
- *t*oxic (e.g. amiodarone, arsenic),
- *h*ereditary,
- *e*ndocrine,
- *r*ecurring (10% of Guillain–Barre syndrome),
- *a*lcohol,
- *P*b (lead) or *p*orphyria,
- *i*diopathic,
- *s*arcoid,
- *t*umours.

57 d. Mid-line shift is a warning sign of impending raised intracranial pressure and eventual herniation of brainstem through the foramen magnum. Colloquially known as cerebral compartment syndrome, any space-occupying lesion such as tumour, infection, bleeding, etc. may cause a rise in the pressure inside the closed space with catastrophic effect. Extradural haematoma evacuation is a priority in cases of proven mid-line shift and/or localizing signs, for example pupillary inequality. Neuroradiological clipping or coiling of intracerebral aneurysm is not indicated here as the source of bleeding is external to the brain itself.

Modalities used for treating non-surgically amenable causes of raised intracranial pressure include:
- raising the head of the bed to 30 degrees,
- osmotic diuresis with mannitol,
- thiopentone infusion,
- hyperventilation (rarely performed).

58 c. The history is describing a tension pneumothorax, which is a respiratory emergency. With every additional breath that the patient takes, his pleural cavity is filling up with air and his lung is being pushed over to the opposite side of the chest. Not only is the pleural pressure causing the lung to deflate but it is also reducing venous return to the heart. In this situation urgent action is required.

Clinical symptoms include:
- tracheal deviation away from the affected side,
- increased resonance to percussion on the affected side,
- reduced breath sounds on the affected side,
- reduced chest expansion on the affected side.

In this clinical picture insertion of a large-bore cannula into the second intercostal space as soon as possible is lifesaving (always remember to remove the needle once inserted). A hissing sound should be heard if your diagnosis is correct and gradually the patient should find it easier to breathe as the lung re-inflates. You should always seek senior support in this scenario.

59 d. This man has developed a rare complication of renal cell carcinoma – a left sided varicocoele manifest due to venous congestion of the left testicle. In 1% of cases of renal cell carcinoma (also called Grawitz tumour) advancement of the tumour along the left renal vein can cause occlusion at the inlet of the left testicular vein. This complication is not seen on the right hand side due to the differential anatomy of the venous drainage on the right hand side. To respect laterality, the left testicular vein drains into the left renal vein, which then crosses the mid-line to drain into the inferior vena cava. On the right hand side, the right testicular vein drains directly into the inferior vena cava thus a right-sided varicocoele is 'never' seen in right renal vein tumours.

60 a. Causes of pin-point pupils include both an opioid overdose and a pontine event, including a haemorrhage.

Extended Matching Questions

61 a. Appendicitis is both one of the easiest surgical conditions to diagnose and simultaneously one of the most difficult. The classical presentation of a young male or female with central colicky abdominal pain associated with nausea and vomiting, which subsequently localizes to the right iliac fossa (with local peritoneal involvement) causing rebound tenderness and guarding, leaves little else on the list of differentials. However, the variable position of the appendix and often relatively uncharacteristic presentation can often cause diagnostic conundrums. It must be heeded that torsion of the testis may present with the same clinical findings as appendicitis and there are cases of missed necrotic testes that were only discovered on the table when preparing the patient for appendectomy. The abdominal exam must always include examination of the external genitalia, hernial orifices and consideration of digital rectal examination.

62 c. Diverticulitis is often colloquially referred to as the 'left-sided appendicitis'. It presents with many of the features of appendicitis: nausea, vomiting, rebound tenderness and guarding, and localized pain in the left iliac fossa. The sigmoid colon is the unhappy recipient of the brunt of gastrointestinal disease for reasons still unknown and diverticulitis is most commonly found here. Terminology in diverticular disease is precise and should be used correctly:

- *diverticulosis* – diverticula that are present and asymptomatic,
- *diverticular disease* – refers to symptomatic diverticula,
- *diverticulitis* – active inflammation of diverticula,
- *complicated diverticulitis* – the presence of complications of diverticulitis, e.g. fistula, abscess or perforation.

The Hinchey classification grades perforated diverticulitis from stage 1 to 4, depending on the extent of peritoneal contamination, and forms a useful guide to the severity of diverticulitis complication.

63 i. Rectosigmoid carcinoma may present with local, general or metastatic features. A change in bowel habit, large bowel obstruction, perforation, stricture or fistula associated with fresh rectal bleeding may all occur. General features associated with cancer are malaise, weight loss and a pyrexia of unknown origin caused by activation of inflammatory cytokines and anaemia. As a rough guide, right-sided tumours are more inclined to cause large bowel obstruction while those presenting on the left-side, for example caecal carcinoma, may present purely with an anaemia. Any unexplained anaemia or episode of rectal bleeding in older patients merits outpatient investigation such as colonoscopy if there is any suspicion of malignancy. More recently, a national screening programme for colon cancer has been introduced in the form of faecal occult blood testing.

64 f. Epigastric pain, vomiting and features of peritonism should alert the clinician to the possibility of a perforated peptic ulcer. Risk factors for ulceration include drug therapy, especially NSAIDs and steroids, smoking, excess alcohol intake, presence of *Helicobacter pylori*, severe burns (Curling's ulcer), acute stress reaction (Cushing's ulcer) and Zollinger–Ellison syndrome. Perforation is investigated by both clinical examination and erect chest radiograph. Air under the diaphragm can help to confirm clinical suspicion and is present in more than 70% of cases of perforation.

65 b. Pancreatitis can be a complication of a myriad of causes. These are best summarized by the mnemonic '*GET SMASHED*': *g*allstones, *e*thanol, *t*rauma, *s*teroids, *m*umps, *a*utoimmune disease, *s*corpion venom, *h*yperlipidaemia (also *h*ypertension, *h*ypercalcaemia, *h*ypothermia), *e*ndoscopic retrograde cholangiopancreatogram (ERCP) and *d*rugs, rarely but significantly

HMG-CoA reductase inhibitors (statins) and antiepileptic medication. Surgical signs associated with pancreatitis are the oft-quoted but rarely seen Grey Turner's sign (bruising discoloration in the flanks) and Cullen's sign (bruising discoloration around the umbilicus). Reactive pleural effusions can occur secondary to systemic inflammatory response evoked by severe pancreatitis and can be significant enough to affect the respiratory system.

66 **h.** Henoch–Schönlein purpura is usually seen between the ages of 2 and 11 years but approximately a quarter of cases may present in adulthood. It commonly presents with a diffuse purpuric rash over the lower limbs and buttocks that can often be mistaken for non-accidental injury in a young child (hence the incorrect and improper involvement of social services on admission to hospital) and is associated with abdominal pain, vomiting and oedema. Joint pain is also a common presenting feature and bloody stools indicate gastrointestinal involvement. The pathology is one of a small-vessel vasculitis with immune complex deposition in the vessels, thus predictably leading to glomerular inflammation and signs of glomerulonephritis. About half of those presenting with Henoch–Schönlein purpura describe a preceding upper respiratory infection, although many other putative triggers have been postulated. Treatment is supportive and usually requires admission to hospital for monitoring of renal and gastrointestinal complications. Resolution is the rule but corticosteroids have been trialled to ameliorate symptoms.

67 **b.** IgA nephropathy (Berger's disease) is the commonest cause of glomerulonephritis worldwide and is more prevalent in Asian populations. Berger's disease typically affects males more commonly than females and those in their 20s and 30s. The usual clinical presentation is with haematuria, which may be recurrent, usually following an upper respiratory tract infection. Less than 1 in 20 cases will present with acute renal failure and the nephrotic syndrome but spontaneous resolution does occur. An association with conditions such as gluten enteropathy and respiratory tract infections has led to the hypothesis that mucosal dysfunction is likely to play an important part in the development of the disease. Renal biopsy is the only modality to reliably diagnose IgA nephropathy and mesangial deposition of IgA and C3 seen on immunofluorescence is pathognomonic of the condition. Prognostically, between 20 and 40% of all patients will eventually progress to end-stage renal failure, requiring renal replacement therapy or transplantation.

68 a. Minimal change disease is the commonest cause of glomerulonephritis in children and can be difficult to distinguish from post-streptococcal glomerulonephritis as both can be brought on by preceding upper respiratory tract infections. An association in adults is with Hodgkin's lymphoma and this should be considered in adult patients presenting with signs of hypertension, proteinuria and oedema in whom a diagnosis of minimal change disease is considered. Renal biopsy should only be considered in children when tissue diagnosis is likely to alter management strategies and most renal physicians favour a therapeutic trial with corticosteroids with renal biopsy in more resistant cases. Histology by definition under light microscopy demonstrates little or no change, thus electron microscopy is relied upon to look for subtle changes in foot process (podocyte) anatomy with podocyte fusion and retraction being the most common pathology.

69 i. SLE is a systemic autoimmune condition with multiorgan involvement. Vasculitis is the underlying component that ties many of the organ dysfunction together, with renal involvement predicting a poorer prognosis. Characteristically exhibiting the malar rash (butterfly rash, so-called because of the double-winged appearance on either side of the nose, with a spectrum of symptoms ranging from neuropsychiatric to pulmonary, SLE can be difficult to diagnose unless it is borne in mind. Immune complex deposition of immunoglobulins directed against nuclear elements causes a glomerulonephritis often referred to as lupus nephritis with features on light microscopy graded by the World Health Organization from I to VI. Wire-loop lesions are seen in grade IV microscopic appearances and are due to hyaline deposits. Treatment is directed at medically stabilizing the patient until such time that they may require more definitive treatment of renal compromise, such as replacement therapy or transplantation. Corticosteroids are the first-line therapy for all but severe renal disease, at which point immunosuppressive agents such as azathioprine and cyclophosphamide improve renal function more significantly.

70 e. Rapidly progressive glomerulonephritis can manifest with a variety of conditions such as the systemic vasculitides, other systemic autoimmune conditions such as SLE, Goodpasture's disease, rheumatoid arthritis and glomerulonephritides of unknown or infectious aetiology. Malignancy and drug therapy, such as penicillamine and antituberculous drugs, can also cause a florid glomerulonephritis. As the name suggests, the decline in renal function to a level where intervention is required can be very rapid, occurring anywhere from days/weeks at its most aggressive to a few months. Early medical therapy is therefore key in trying to influence the course of disease. Pathological correlates on renal histology are primarily of fibrinoid necrosis, with crescent formation seen in over half the specimens biopsied.

71 j. Oesophageal carcinoma usually presents with progressive dysphagia, initially for solids then progressing to liquids. There is usually an associated marked weight loss due to both the anorexic effects of cancer and the inability to tolerate food. In the main, oesophageal carcinoma is squamous in histology but may be adenocarcinoma in the distal oesophagus. Risk factors include Barrett's oesophagus, Plummer–Vinson (Patterson–Kelly) syndrome, achalasia of the cardia, caustic stricture, excessive alcohol intake, coeliac disease, smoking and tylosis.

72 a. Mallory–Weiss tear is characteristically described following a large meal and alcohol ingestion, with subsequent severe retching and vomiting causing a tear in the oesophageal mucosa leading to fresh haematemesis that usually resolves spontaneously. This is a relatively benign type of oesophageal tear when compared with the catastrophic transaction of the oesophagus that is seen in Boerhaave's syndrome. This can also occur precipitated by vomiting after a large meal and causes severe chest pain with a collapsed patient. Chest radiography aids in the diagnosis; air seen in the mediastinum usually leads to acute mediastinitis and the clinical sign of surgical emphysema in the neck.

73 h. Aorto-enteric fistula is a rare but devastating complication of previous aortic surgery. Adhesion and erosion of the repair line into the adjacent small bowel can cause massive gastrointestinal haemorrhage, which may be fatal if not diagnosed and treated early. Patients have been described as experiencing a 'warning' bleed preceding massive and life-threatening haematemesis. The presentation of the patient described is one of florid hypovolaemic shock. Tachypnoea, signs of sympathetic activation and a markedly reduced GCS are important signs of shock as blood pressure may be maintained until approximately 30% of the blood volume has been lost.

74 e. Gastric ulceration can occur for a variety of reasons; postoperatively it is usually a combination of poor oral intake, acute stress reaction and the addition of NSAIDs as pain-relief. It is more likely to occur in patients with a history of dyspepsia and presents acutely with coffee ground vomiting due to altered blood by stomach contents, with occasional melaena (black tarry stools again due to altered blood) if the bleeding is significant. Treatment in the first instance is by stopping any gastric-irritant drugs, starting either high-dose proton-pump inhibitor, for example omeprazole, or a 72-hour infusion at a rate of 8 mg/hour depending on the severity of haematemesis/melaena. Fluid and/or blood resuscitation may be required if the patient is in hypovolaemic shock and uncontrolled bleeding may require urgent endoscopic therapy or emergency laparotomy.

75 g. Gastric carcinoma carries a very poor prognosis, mainly due to the relatively late presentation of disease in which the carcinoma is already established and may well have invaded local organs or metastasized to liver, lungs and bone. A feature of gastric carcinoma that is not seen in many other tumours is transcoelomic spread of tumour to peritoneal structures such as the ovaries, causing bilateral Krukenberg tumours. Tumours near the pylorus (as in this example) can cause pyloric obstruction leading to projectile vomiting following meals and may require endoscopic dilatation or surgical palliation. Risk factors for the development of gastric cancer include pernicious anaemia, partial gastrectomy, *Helicobacter pylori* infection (tentatively thought to be the cause behind the high rates of gastric cancer in the Japanese population), chronic peptic ulceration, blood group A and genetic predisposition, such as hereditary nonpolyposis colon cancer syndrome.

76 a. Pneumococcal pneumonia is the commonest bacterial pneumonia affecting all ages but is especially common in the elderly. Other groups commonly affected are alcoholics, patients after splenectomy, immunosuppressed patients and patients with chronic heart failure or those with pre-existing lung disease. Patients usually complain of fever and pleurisy. A classical chest X-ray appearance is one of a lobar pneumonia.

77 d. *Pseudomonas* is a common pathogen in those patients suffering with cystic fibrosis and bronchiectasis. It is often associated with an increasing mortality and a general deterioration in their clinical condition. The treatment is usually with antipseudomonal penicillins, for example piperacillin.

78 e. Mycoplasma pneumonia affects young, well people. It presents with general features that often precede the chest signs and symptoms by 4–5 days. Often physical signs in the chest are scanty and do not fit the clinical picture. The chest X-ray does not frequently correlate with the clinical state of the patient. Following diagnosis, treatment is usually with erythromycin. Occasionally, extrapulmonary features take over the clinical picture.

79 b. Staphylococcal pneumonia usually follows a viral illness and is especially seen in IV drug abusers or in those patients with indwelling central venous catheters. Chest X-ray appearances are normally of patchy consolidation, which can break down to form abscesses that form a cystic appearance on chest X-ray. Other complications include pneumothoraces, effusions and empyemas. The mortality with this form of pneumonia is approximately 25% and treatment with IV antibiotics (flucloxacillin) is usually advised.

80 f. This is most likely to be due to infection with *Legionella pneumophila* which infects water supplies to hospitals, hotels and workplaces. It characteristically follows a prodrome of a viral illness and symptoms include a high temperature and associated extrapulmonary features including diarrhoea, hyponatraemia and confusion. Once diagnosed either by sputum, bronchial washings or urine analysis, treatment is simple with clarithromycin, ciprofloxacin or rifampicin for 2–3 weeks.

81 b. SLE fits with the clinical scenario of multiorgan involvement that appears clinically fairly mild from the history and a simple autoantibody screen will aid the diagnosis in the first instance. Haematuria with slightly elevated urea and creatinine levels, along with positive urinalysis, are signs that there may be an element of renal glomerulonephritis but the rise in renal markers may be due to dehydration and thus renal biopsy may be indicated at some point in the future to indicate prognosis if the renal function has not ameliorated with steroids and rehydration. Daily urea and creatinine testing should be considered for this patient as it is important to see the trend in renal function; however, the diagnosis needs to be established first to allow future management and follow-up to be planned.

82 c. A renal tract ultrasound should be considered a first-line imaging investigation in renal disease as much reliable information can be gained easily and quickly. The history is consistent with that of autosomal dominant polycystic kidney disease, suggested by the previous stroke and renal failure in such a young woman. Renal ultrasonography has a high sensitivity and specificity for diagnosing polycystic kidney disease, in addition to picking up other renal masses, size of kidneys, obstruction to outflow, collections and bladder volumes. Other rare causes of 'enlarged' kidney include renal tumours, benign cysts, single kidney hypertrophy, amyloidosis and renal contusion and trauma. The association of polycystic kidney disease with subarachnoid haemorrhage due to rupture of a berry aneurysm should be noted as well as the association with cardiac valvular lesions (especially mitral valve prolapse) and diverticulitis.

83 **f.** Bence–Jones protein is an easily performed assay for multiple myeloma and should be considered in a patient who presents in the above fashion with new-onset renal failure. Myeloma causes a monoclonal gammopathy of mainly immunoglobulin G (IgG) (60%) and sometimes IgA (25%) and is the most common primary malignancy of the skeletal system. Light-chain fragments are found in abundance due to overexpression of a plasma cell clone and are nephrotoxic causing renal failure. Lytic lesions are sometimes seen on radiography and are associated with the development of hypercalcaemia causing abdominal pain, psychiatric disturbance, renal stones and bony pain – famously described as *'stones, bones, groans and psychic moans'*. Interestingly, although one immunoglobulin line is overexpressed, patients are susceptible to infection, especially from encapsulated organisms, and this is due to the resultant suppression of the other immunoglobulin lines. A pancytopenia may be present due to the suppression of other blood cell lines.

84 **a.** Although daily urea and creatinine levels are important to monitor in a young man with rapidly deteriorating renal function, it is vital that a renal biopsy is considered to make the diagnosis. In this case, the diagnosis appears to be one of rapidly progressive glomerulonephritis and diagnosis of any remediable cause is key to prognosis and survival. Autoantibodies are a useful screen to perform; however, for extent and tissue diagnosis a biopsy is key. A 24-hour urine protein collection would quantify the amount of proteinuria associated with glomerulonephritis and the nephrotic syndrome and could be performed as an inpatient; however, it is unlikely to alter the management.

85 **h.** Renal artery stenosis is often diagnosed on commencement of an ACE inhibitor and can lead to flash pulmonary oedema, a sharp rise in urea and creatinine levels associated with a sharp decline in renal function. Reduced renal perfusion with bilateral renal artery stenosis leads to a reliance on the intrinsic tone of

the glomerular efferent arteriole to maintain glomerular filtration pressure. Reducing this efferent tone markedly drops the filtration pressure and thus an acute deterioration in renal function can occur. The investigation of choice is renal artery ultrasonography and this has replaced the invasive renal arteriography as the first line in diagnosis. Doppler flow studies are very sensitive for stenosis and are able to quantify the degree of stenotic lesion. A form of renal artery stenosis may be seen in young women (fibromuscular dysplasia) and may present in a similar fashion. Radiographically definable via renal artery angiography, this manifests as a string-of-beads appearance.

86 a. This man has injured his common peroneal nerve. It is a branch of the sciatic nerve and may be damaged following trauma, application of a plaster cast or by repeated kneeling. It provides the motor supply to the muscles of the anterior and lateral compartments of the leg. It is the most commonly damaged nerve in the lower limb and is relatively unprotected as it traverses the lateral aspect of the head of the fibula. Clinical features include:
- foot drop,
- weakness of dorsiflexion and eversion of the foot,
- weakness of the extensor hallucis longus,
- loss of sensation over the lower lateral part of the leg and dorsum of the foot.

87 h. The axillary nerve winds around the head of the humerus. It is this tortuous course that puts it at risk from damage from trauma, for example from cast application or during rotator cuff surgery. It supplies the deltoid muscle and teres minor and therefore results in problems with shoulder elevation and abduction. It also provides sensation to the skin on the lateral aspect of the arm over the body of deltoid muscle.

88 b. This woman is describing symptoms of median nerve palsy. In addition to these symptoms, she may note a weakness in the muscles of her thenar eminence with associated wasting. This is likely to be caused by carpal tunnel syndrome which results in compression being applied to the median nerve as it passes under the flexor retinaculum on the palmar aspect of the wrist. If this is the cause, it can be treated with a carpal tunnel decompression, although since she is complaining of bilateral symptoms the cause may result in a lesion of the cervical vertebrae.

89 g. This woman has damaged her ulnar nerve. It runs in the cubital tunnel and may be damaged following injuries to the bones in that area. The symptoms resulting are those mentioned in the case as the ulnar nerve supplies sensation to the medial half of the ring finger and the little finger. It provides motor supply to the intrinsic muscles of the hand and therefore weakness and reduced function may ensue.

90 f. This patient is complaining of pain and burning sensation over the distribution of the lateral cutaneous nerve of the thigh. It passes from the lateral border of psoas major across the iliac fossa to pierce the inguinal ligament. It travels in a fibrous tunnel medial to the anterior superior iliac spine and enters the thigh deep to the fascia lata before continuing distally into the subcutaneous tissues. The nerve can become compressed as it passes under the inguinal ligament resulting in meralgia paraesthetica, provided there are no associated motor signs the treatment of this is conservative.

Topic Index

EMQs and SBAs for Medical Finals, Second Edition. Jonathan Bath, Rebecca Morgan and Mehool Patel.
© 2011 John Wiley & Sons, Ltd. Published 2011 by John Wiley & Sons, Ltd.

Oncology

Paper 1
Questions 1, 3, 16, 21, 42, 47, 50, 55.
Paper 2
Questions 17, 21, 32, 48, 52, 67, 78.
Paper 3
Questions 6, 15, 23, 30, 34, 64.
Paper 4
Questions 11, 16, 19, 31, 34, 41, 61, 77.
Paper 5
Question 2, 42–44, 59, 63, 71, 75, 83.

Ophthalmology

Paper 2
Questions 7, 10, 19, 25, 31, 40, 49, 58, 86.
Paper 3
Question 81.
Paper 4
Question 17.
Paper 5
Question 19.

Orthopaedics

Paper 1
Question 70.
Paper 2
Question 69.
Paper 3
Questions 3, 12, 18, 25, 35, 44, 49, 57, 73–75.
Paper 4
Question 21.
Paper 5
Question 89.

Paediatrics

Paper 1
Questions 18, 36.
Paper 2
Question 49.

Paper 3
Questions 2, 4, 49, 72.
Paper 4
Questions 6, 11, 13, 32, 37, 43, 50, 59, 61–65, 81–85.
Paper 5
Questions 24, 26, 33, 34, 37, 41, 49, 54, 61, 66, 68.

Psychiatry

Paper 2
Questions 8, 16, 18, 27, 38, 39, 41, 51, 56, 71–75, 82, 83, 90.
Paper 4
Questions 20, 54, 66–70.
Paper 5
Question 51

Public Health

Paper 1
Questions 61–65.
Paper 3
Questions 5, 19, 41.
Paper 4
Question 70, 78.
Paper 5
Question 10, 27.

Renal

Paper 1
Question 86.
Paper 3
Questions 8, 13, 16, 23, 33, 38.
Paper 4
Questions 3, 12, 15, 18, 22, 27, 40, 44, 48, 51, 52, 60, 61, 80.
Paper 5
Questions 5, 23, 26, 30, 36, 38, 41, 44, 46, 50, 54, 55, 59, 66–70, 81–85.

Respiratory

Paper 1
Questions 8, 65, 66, 67, 70, 77.

Keep up with critical fields

Would you like to receive up-to-date information on our books, journals and databases in the areas that interest you, direct to your mailbox?

Join the **Wiley e-mail service** - a convenient way to receive updates and exclusive discount offers on products from us.

> Simply visit **www.wiley.com/email** and register online

We won't bombard you with emails and we'll only email you with information that's relevant to you. We will ALWAYS respect your e-mail privacy and NEVER sell, rent, or exchange your e-mail address to any outside company. Full details on our privacy policy can be found online.

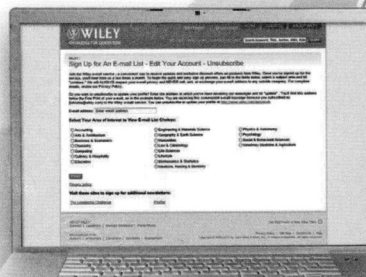

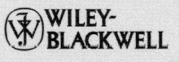
WILEY-BLACKWELL

www.wiley.com/email

17841